# Isokinetics in Human Performance

## Lee E. Brown, MEd, CSCS, *D
Florida Atlantic University
Davie, Florida

Editor

Human Kinetics

**Library of Congress Cataloging-in-Publication Data**

Isokinetics in human performance / Lee E. Brown, editor.
    p.   cm.
    Includes bibliographical references and index.
    ISBN 0-7360-0005-4
    1. Isokinetic exercise.    I. Brown, Lee E., 1956-   .
    QP303.I82    2000
    613.7'149--dc21                99-042887
                                     CIP

ISBN: 0-7360-0005-4

**Acquisitions Editor**: Loarn D. Robertson, PhD; **Developmental Editor**: Joanna Hatzopoulos; **Assistant Editors**: Susan C. Hagan and Chris Enstrom; **Copyeditor**: Judy Peterson; **Proofreader**: Jim Burns; **Indexer**: Nancy Ball; **Permission Manager**: Heather Munson; **Graphic Designer**: Fred Starbird; **Graphic Artist**: Sandra Meier; **Photo Editor**: Clark Brooks; **Cover Designer**: Jack W. Davis; **Illustrators**: Sharon Smith, Mac art; Tom Roberts, line drawings; **Printer**: Versa Press; **Binder**: Dekker & Sons

Printed in the United States of America

10  9  8  7  6  5  4  3  2  1

**Human Kinetics**
Web site: http://www.humankinetics.com/

*United States:* Human Kinetics
P.O. Box 5076, Champaign, IL 61825-5076
1-800-747-4457
e-mail: humank@hkusa.com

*Canada:* Human Kinetics
475 Devonshire Road Unit 100, Windsor, ON N8Y 2L5
1-800-465-7301 (in Canada only)
e-mail: humank@hkcanada.com

*Europe:* Human Kinetics
P.O. Box IW14, Leeds LS16 6TR, United Kingdom
+44 (0)113-278 1708
e-mail: humank@hke1rope.com

*Australia:* Human Kinetics
57A Price Avenue, Lower Mitcham, South Australia 5062
(08) 82771555
e-mail: liahka@senet.com.au

*New Zealand:* Human Kinetics
P.O. Box 105-231, Auckland Central
09-523-3462
e-mail: humank@hknewz.com

For Theresa,
you are so precious to me.

# Contents

## Part I  Foundations                                          1

## Part II  Limitations                                        75

# Contributors

Brooks Applegate, PhD
Western Michigan University
Kalamazoo, Michigan

Marcas M. Bamman, PhD
University of Alabama at
  Birmingham
Birmingham, Alabama

James W. Bellew, MS, PT
University of Kentucky
Lexington, Kentucky

Kristen Brinks, MS, PT, ATC
Gundersen Lutheran Sports Medicine
La Crosse, Wisconsin

Lee E. Brown, MEd, CSCS, *D
Florida Atlantic University
Davie, Florida

John C. Bruno, BS, ATC
INRTEK
Twinsburg, Ohio

John F. Caruso, PhD, CSCS
University of Nevada–Reno
Reno, Nevada

T. Jeff Chandler, EdD, CSCS, FACSM
Marshall University
Huntington, West Virginia

George J. Davies, MEd, PT, SCS,
  ATC, CSCS
University of Wisconsin–La Crosse
La Crosse, Wisconsin

Joan M. Eckerson, PhD, FACSM,
  CSCS
Creighton University
Omaha, Nebraska

Todd S. Ellenbecker, MS, PT, CSCS
Physiotherapy Associates
Scottsdale, Arizona

Steven J. Fleck, PhD, CSCS, FACSM
Colorado College
Colorado Springs, Colorado

Mark D. Grabiner, PhD, FACSM
The Cleveland Clinic Foundation
Cleveland, Ohio

Bryan Heiderscheit, MS, PT, CSCS
University of Massachusetts
Amherst, Massachusetts

Robert J. Heitman, EdD
University of South Alabama
Mobile, Alabama

William R. Holcomb, PhD, ATC,
  CSCS
University of North Florida
Jacksonville, Florida

Douglas M. Kleiner, PhD, ATC,
  FACSM, CSCS
University of North Florida
Jacksonville, Florida

Kiersten Kluckhulm, BS
University of Miami
Miami, Florida

John E. Kovaleski, PhD, ATC
University of South Alabama
Mobile, Alabama

William J. Kraemer, PhD, CSCS,
  FACSM
Ball State University
Muncie, Indiana

Terry R. Malone, EdD, PT, ATC
University of Kentucky
Lexington, Kentucky

Scott A. Mazzetti, MS,CSCS
Ball State University
Muncie, Indiana

Scott D. Minor, PhD, PT
Washington University
St. Louis, Missouri

Louis R. Osternig, PhD, FACSM
University of Oregon
Eugene, Oregon

Tammy M. Owings, MS
The Cleveland Clinic Foundation
Cleveland, Ohio

Nicholas A. Ratamess, MS, CSCS
Ball State University
Muncie, Indiana

E. Paul Roetert, PhD, FACSM
American Sport Education Program
Human Kinetics
Champaign, Illinois

Joseph F. Signorile, PhD
University of Miami
Miami, Florida

Kent E. Timm, PhD, PT, ATC,
FACSM
Covenant HealthCare System
Saginaw, Michigan

Joseph P. Weir, PhD
Des Moines University–Osteopathic
Medical Center
Des Moines, Iowa

Lawrence W. Weiss, EdD, FACSM,
FRC, CSCS
University of Memphis
Memphis, Tennessee

Michael Whitehurst, EdD
Florida Atlantic University
Davie, Florida

Tim V. Wrigley, MSc
Victoria University of Technology
Melbourne, Australia

# Preface

The purpose of this book is to bridge the gap between the clinical and applied practice of isokinetic dynamometry. This idea grew out of a symposium given by three of the chapter authors (Brown, Weiss, and Chandler) at the National Strength and Conditioning Association National Meeting in 1995. There are presently no books on the market that focus on the nonclinical aspects of isokinetic dynamometry. The currently available books cover primarily physical therapy applications with an emphasis on injury assessment and rehabilitation. However, isokinetic dynamometry has enjoyed widespread use throughout the United States and the world. With this widespread use has come a proliferation of equipment, allowing researchers and applied practitioners to exchange protocols and normative data. Furthermore, despite a paucity of nonclinical data, exercise professionals have embraced the isokinetic dynamometer as a tool to both test and train a wide range of athletic and special populations.

The collection of chapters that makes up this book will identify and define the primary factors associated with evaluation of muscular strength and power using computerized isokinetic dynamometry. Moreover, this book explores specific benefits and limitations inherent in using these devices. Our goal is to examine this topic historically as it relates to technical aspects of test interpretation and exercise prescription as well as to apply this knowledge to unique populations and situations. Assembled herein is a compilation of chapters that concentrates on singular experimental investigations resulting in unique answers to otherwise common questions involving physiological variables.

The book is organized into four major sections, each focusing on a different methodological aspect. Part I, Foundations, describes the foundation upon which isokinetic dynamometry has been built. By providing an overview of the technology and how it interacts with traditional exercise modes and evaluation, this introduction explores the evolution of isokinetics and how it has become woven into the complex fabric of test and measurement. Part II covers the limitations of the equipment and attempts to illuminate potential obstacles the reader may encounter in using this equipment. Every effort is made to expose uncertainties and inconsistencies associated with the dynamometer while offering ways in which practitioners can increase both the validity and reliability of their test results. The final two parts construct an in-depth examination of actual investigations, focusing first on the functional application of isokinetic dynamometry to broad human movement conditions and second on unique nonclinical populations.

We hope the reader benefits from the experience of the authors, who have chronicled their ongoing efforts to assess and train individuals in order to further elucidate human movement. These chapters include a wealth of practical information compiled by the authors through years of data collection and analysis. The cumulative results of these experiments, viewed through a scientist's discerning eye, shed light on the peculiar aspects of velocity-specific muscle actions. The information contained in this book has never before been available in this easy-to-use format. Detailed analysis of experimental research combined with extensive citations at the end of each chapter should make this book an indispensable reference work on isokinetic dynamometry.

# Acknowledgments

The pages of this book could not hold all the names of those who assisted in its completion. Florida Atlantic University (FAU) lab assistants, students, faculty, and staff have been immeasurably helpful in bringing together the final product. However, a few individuals do require special recognition for their exceptional support. I would like to first thank all the subjects in all the studies that make up this book. Without their tireless efforts nothing in this book could have been written. My FAU "Isokinetic Teammates" include Brian W. Findley, P. Russ Gilbert, Denise R. Groo, and Jennifer A. Ward. They always worked at maximum constant velocity. Their hard work and time spent under "Load Range" are responsible for the concepts that led to this book. I would also like to thank my parents, who always saw me in a good light even during the darkest times, and my mentor, Mike Whitehurst, who is responsible for molding me into a critical thinking professional. Finally, this work would never have materialized without the almost daily advice, direction, and encouragement of Joanna Hatzopoulos and Loarn Robertson of Human Kinetics. Thank you both for steering a novice toward the goal.

# Credits

**Figure 6.2** Reprinted, by permission, from A.M. Gordon, A.F. Huxley, and F.J. Julian, 1966, *Journal of Physiology* 184:170–92.

**Table 8.7** Reprinted, by permission, from G.J. Davies and T.S. Ellenbecker, 1998, Application of isokinetics in testing and rehabilitation. In *Physical rehabilitation of the injured athlete*, 2nd ed. Edited by Andrews, Harrelson, and Wilk (Philadelphia: W.B. Saunders), 225.

**Tables 8.9 and 8.10** Adapted, by permission, from W.J. Kraemer and S. J. Fleck, 1982, "Anaerobic metabolism and its evaluation," *National Strength and Conditioning Journal*. 4 (2): 20–21.

**Chapter 9** Extracts appearing on pages 197–98 reprinted, by permission, from A. Steindler, *Kinesiology of the human body under normal and pathological conditions*, 1955. Courtesy of Charles C. Thomas, Publisher, Springfield, Illinois.

**Figure 11.1** Reprinted, by permission, from D.H. Perrin, 1993, *Isokinetic exercise and assessment* (Champaign, IL: Human Kinetics), 64.

**Figure 11.2** Reprinted, by permission, from D.H. Perrin, 1993, *Isokinetic exercise and assessment* (Champaign, IL: Human Kinetics), 63. Data from T.W. Worrell, D.H. Perrin, B.M. Gansneder, and J.H. Gieck, 1991, "Comparison of isokinetic strength and flexibility measures between hamstring injured and non-injured athletes" *Journal of Orthopaedic and Sports Physical Therapy* 13: 118–25.

**Figure 14.6** Reprinted, by permission, from D.M. Kleiner, D.L. Blessing, W.R. Davis, and J.W. Mitchell, 1996, "Acute cardiovascular responses to various forms of resistance exercise," *Journal of Strength and Conditioning Research* 10 (1): 56–61.

**Figure 14.9** Reprinted, by permission, from D.M. Kleiner, D.L. Blessing, J.W. Mitchell, and W.R. Davis, 1999, "A description of the acute cardiovascular responses to isokinetic resistance at three different speeds," *Journal of Strength and Conditioning Research* 13 (4).

**Table 14.1** Reprinted, by permission, from D.M. Kleiner, D.L. Blessing, W.R. Davis, and J.W. Mitchell, 1996, "Acute cardiovascular responses to various forms of resistance exercise," *Journal of Strength and Conditioning Research* 10 (1): 56–61.

**Table 14.2** Reprinted, by permission, from D.M. Kleiner, D.L. Blessing, J.W. Mitchell, and W.R. Davis, 1999, "A description of the acute cardiovascular responses to isokinetic resistance at three different speeds," *Journal of Strength and Conditioning Research* 13 (4).

**Figure 19.1** Reprinted, by permission, from F.W. Jobe and B. Ling, 1986, The shoulder in sports. In *The shoulder: Surgical and son-surgical management*, edited by M. Post (Philadelphia: Lea & Febiger).

**Figure 19.2** Reprinted from C.J. Dillman, G.S. Fleisig, and J.R. Andrews, 1993, "Biomechanics of pitching with emphasis upon shoulder kinematics,"

*Journal of Orthopaedic and Sports Physical Therapy* 18 (2): 402–8, with permission of the Orthopaedic and Sports Sections of the American Physical Therapy Association.

**Table 19.1**   Adapted, by permission, from L.R. Pedegana, R.C. Elsner, D. Roberts, J. Lang, and V. Farewell, 1982, "The relationship of upper extremity strength to throwing speed," *American Journal of Sports Medicine* 10 (6): 352–54.

**Table 19.2**   Reprinted, with permission, from L.R. Bartlett, M.D. Storey, and B.D. Simons, 1989, "Measurement of upper extremity torque production and its relationship to throwing speed in the competitive athlete," *American Journal of Sports Medicine* 17 (1): 89–91.

**Tables 19.5 and 19.6**   Reprinted, with permission, from G.J. Sodenberg and M.J. Blaschak, 1987, "Shoulder internal and external rotation peak torque production through a velocity spectrum in differing positions," *Journal of Orthopaedic and Sports Physical Therapy* 8 (11): 518–24.

**Figure 20.1**   Adapted, by permission, from B. Oberg, M. Moller, J. Gillquist, and J. Ekstrand, 1986, "Isokinetic torque levels for knee extensors and knee flexors in soccer players," *International Journal of Sports Medicine* 7: 50–53.

**Figure 20.2**   Adapted, by permission, from D.G. Sale, 1991, Testing strength and power. In *Testing of the high-performance athlete*, edited by J.D. MacDougall, H.A. Wenger, and H.J. Green (Champaign, IL: Human Kinetics), 94.

**Figure 20.3**   Adapted from D.T. Kirkendall, 1985, "The applied sports science of soccer," *The Physician and Sportsmedicine* 13 (4): 53–59, with permission of McGraw-Hill, Inc.

# Part I
# Foundations

This first section is designed to lay the groundwork for the rest of the book. The following three chapters outline the foundation upon which isokinetic dynamometry now stands. This material is essential in order for the reader to understand where isokinetics fits into the realm of resistance testing and training. Chapter 1 focuses on the fundamental terms and definitions used when describing the science of isokinetics. Chapter 2 defines where isokinetic dynamometry fits into the overall scheme of exercise modes. Chapter 3 lists extensive research findings regarding the sometimes-ambiguous correlation between sport and isokinetics.

Unfortunately, the introduction and subsequent extensive use of isokinetic machines were not followed by comprehensive training in their use. Consequently, many users developed their own language and protocols, some of which were not rooted in practical science. There followed a plethora of publications, which often contained misleading advice based on anecdotal information. Recent years have seen the dynamometer move from a clinical setting to a more scientific, laboratory-based environment with concomitant publication of objective and controlled studies.

This section strives to lay the proper foundation for the rest of the book. It defines language, and places isokinetics in the proper perspective for future reading. It is essential that an accurate rationale for isokinetics be first made before exploring how the dynamometer is used in a functional manner with unique populations.

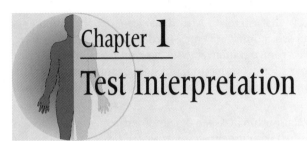

# Chapter 1
# Test Interpretation

George J. Davies, Bryan Heiderscheit,
and Kristen Brinks

Isokinetics has been used in testing and performance enhancement for over 30 years. The first articles regarding the use of isokinetic exercise were published in the late 1960s (28, 39, 50). Since that time thousands of articles have reported isokinetics as part of the testing methodology or for training. The first book devoted exclusively to isokinetics was published in 1984 (8); it went through four editions (9) before a proliferation of books in the mid '90s developed (6, 21, 43). This volume of literature devoted to the use of isokinetics demonstrates the wide use and numerous applications available for isokinetic testing and exercise.

Keating and Matyas (34) have stated that the widespread use of dynamometry is evidenced by the large number of references to dynamometric measurements in the physical therapy literature. Since 1988, 30 to 40 publications a year have reported findings based on data from electromechanical dynamometers. The machines have been used for many purposes, although data supporting these uses has not always been provided (34). Among the uses for electromechanical dynamometers that Keating and Matyas (34) found were the following:

- To collect normative values for muscles from various types of subjects

- To classify muscle performance as normal or abnormal by comparisons with the performance of contralateral muscles, with normative data, or with muscle performance in a control group

- To collect torque curves that might indicate whether pathology or characteristics specific to subject type were present

- To establish the relative efficacy of various treatment and training regimens

- To quantify exercise so that exercise regimens may be administered

- To evaluate the effects of training or testing modes (e.g., eccentric, concentric, isometric), testing or training speed, and duration of training
- To investigate factors that correlate with dynamometric measurements, including muscle cross-sectional area measured by computerized tomography, associated electromyographic activity, type or location of electrical stimulation that causes force production, physiological factors associated with muscle performance, and biomechanical factors associated with muscle performance
- To investigate the relationship between dynamometric measurements and measurements obtained with other tests
- To assess or treat persons with disabilities to determine the need for intervention, the extent of impairment, and changes in subject performance

Isokinetics reached its peak in the 1980s in the area of testing and training. Then in the '90s, everyone began emphasizing closed kinetic chain exercises. Consequently, the pendulum has swung from the use of open kinetic chain exercises to closed kinetic chain exercises. Interestingly, this trend was often based on empirical approaches rather than published research. Some research indicates that there is not a correlation between isokinetic testing and functional performance (2, 26). On the other hand, there are numerous studies that demonstrate a positive correlation between isokinetic testing and functional performance (3, 41, 45, 49, 53, 55).

Snyder-Mackler and coworkers (48) emphasized this point when they discussed the strength of the quadriceps femoris muscle and functional recovery after reconstruction of the anterior cruciate ligament.

> *Rehabilitation after reconstruction of the anterior cruciate ligament continues to be guided more by myth and fad than by science. Intensive closed-kinetic-chain (CKC) exercise has virtually replaced open-kinetic-chain (OKC) exercise of the quadriceps after a reconstruction. . . . The present study confirms the finding that the strength of the quadriceps femoris has a substantial impact on functional recovery and suggests that closed-kinetic-chain exercise alone does not provide an adequate stimulus to the quadriceps femoris to permit normal function of the knee in the stance phase in most patients in the early period after reconstruction of the anterior cruciate ligament. (p. 1, 172)*

Unfortunately, many clinicians forgot the thousands of articles that demonstrated the reliability, validity, and efficacy of using isokinetics as *one part* of the total testing and training process (12, 18, 19).

Because of the increased use of closed kinetic chain exercises in training, a dedicated dynamometer was developed to perform closed kinetic chain exercises in the supine, long sitting, or standing "squat" positions. The Linea by the Loredan Biomedical Company filled a void and provided an opportunity to perform isokinetic closed kinetic chain testing and training (see figure 1.1). Davies and Heiderscheit (14) performed a reliability study of the Lido Linea closed kinetic chain isokinetic dynamometer. They determined static calibra-

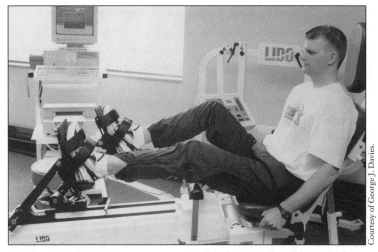

Courtesy of George J. Davies.

**Figure 1.1** Lido Linea computerized isokinetic closed kinetic chain system.

tion by using certified weights that demonstrated excellent static reliability. Furthermore, 30 subjects participated in a test-retest experimental paradigm across a velocity spectrum. Intraclass correlation coefficient values for peak force and total work ranged from .87 to .94 ($p < .05$).

A few studies (44) have demonstrated that a population produces very different findings when tested in both isokinetic OKC and CKC patterns. Isokinetic testing, whether OKC or CKC is only one part of the entire testing and training process. Therefore, we recommend a functional testing and training algorithm approach (18).

With the aforementioned comments as a backdrop, this chapter has many purposes. First we describe the commonly used terminology associated with isokinetic exercise. Next we provide rationale for testing and discuss various considerations for testing. Then we describe factors that influence isokinetic measurements and establish several components of testing protocols. Finally, we list several parameters that are commonly used in data analysis and present different methods of data interpretation. It is important that we apply critical thinking to our applications of isokinetics (12).

## Definitions of Terms

Before reading the rest of this chapter or other chapters in this book, it is important to review the vocabulary commonly used in the field of isokinetics. Therefore, we provide the definitions of relevant terms:

**isometrics:** Exercise in which muscle force development results in no change in length for the muscles and in no skeletal movement (fixed resistance and a fixed speed at 0°/s).

**isotonics:** Exercise with a fixed resistance (constant load) and a variable speed.

**variable resistance isotonics:** Exercise with a resistance that changes through the range of motion, but is consistent for all users, with a variable speed (9).

**isokinetics:** Exercise with an accommodating resistance and a fixed speed (9).

**concentric muscle action:** Development of muscle tension while the origin and insertion of the muscle approach each other, often referred to as positive work (9, 22).

**eccentric muscle action:** Development of muscle tension while the origin and insertion of the muscle move away from each other, often referred to as negative work (9, 10, 22).

**force:** A push or a pull exerted by one material object or substance on another, usually measured in units of newtons.

**torque:** A force that produces or tends to produce a rotation about a point or axis, usually measured in units of newton-meters (Nm) or foot-pounds (often used as a synonym for moment, which is the tendency or measure of tendency to produce motion, especially about a point or axis).

**work:** Force acting through a distance; that is, work = f × d, usually reported in units of newton-meters (Nm = joules).

**power:** Work per unit time; that is, power = (f × d)/t, usually reported in units of watts.

**acceleration:** The rate of change of velocity with respect to time (see, for examples of measurements, 17, 29–32, 38, 56, 57).

**rate of torque development:** The time it takes to reach (1) peak torque, (2) predetermined range of motion, or (3) predetermined torque value.

**torque acceleration energy:** A measure of the "explosiveness" of a muscle action. This is operationally defined as the total work performed in the first 1/8 of a second.

**force decay rate:** A measurement of the downslope of the torque curve. This is the force being produced at the end of a range of motion. There are no consistent, widely accepted methods to calculate this data.

**deficit:** A measured deficiency in a muscle's performance as compared to the contralateral side, to normative data, or when normalized (to the subject's body weight, etc.).

**ratio:** The relationship in quantity, amount, or size between two or more things; usually used to evaluate the relationship between the agonist and antagonist muscles or between concentric and eccentric muscle action.

**endurance testing:** Testing a subject's ability to sustain an activity by measuring the number of repetitions performed in a bilateral comparison or by comparing the total work performed at the beginning of an exercise bout (first 5 reps, or first 25%, etc.) to the total work performed at the end of the exercise bout.

**fatigue testing:** Fatigability, or the recovery rate of muscle groups, can be determined as follows. Subjects perform an endurance bout, rest, and repeat the same endurance bout. The amount of work performed in the second bout is compared to the work performed in the first endurance bout. This provides information regarding the muscle groups' rate of recovery for performing repeated bout activities (5, 9, 20).

**fatigue index:** The percent change from the beginning to the end of an endurance test bout.

**coefficient of variance:** Standard deviation expressed as a percentage of the mean; for a single set of data, a statistical measure of how closely the data points are grouped. When several repetitions are performed, there should be a consistent response with minimal variability. An often-used guideline is to require repetitions that are within 10% of one another.

# Rationale for Testing

Assessing athletes isokinetically provides valuable information that may be used for performance enhancement (6, 9, 13, 15, 19, 21, 43). Objective and quantifiable data collected during testing may be used as a baseline during preseason screening or as comparative data to evaluate the efficacy of various training regimens (24, 25, 33, 35, 52).

As previously described, with objective isokinetic testing, one can test the entire lower extremity kinetic chain or perform isolated isokinetic testing. The isolated testing allows one to identify any preexisting weaknesses that may be present, which would be missed if only closed kinetic chain testing were performed. The kinetic chain is only as strong as the weakest link (12, 44). Isokinetic testing during preseason screening can identify specific muscle weaknesses that may predispose athletes to injuries. Hamstring strains may be related to lack of flexibility, imbalance of strength and power between the quadriceps and hamstrings, or inequality of strength of the left versus the right hamstring group (bilateral comparison muscle imbalance) (25, 35, 36). Weakness and lack of endurance in rotator cuff or scapulothoracic musculature may lead to shoulder pain and instability (11). Documenting strength, power, and endurance with isokinetic testing identifies specific weaknesses and imbalances that should be addressed with strength and conditioning programs.

Performing open kinetic chain (OKC) testing allows the examiner to have significant control over the test parameters and stresses imposed on the client (see figure 1.2). In other words, the examiner controls range of motion (ROM), speeds, translational stresses (by shin pad placement), varus and valgus forces, and rotational forces. When the individual is progressed to closed kinetic chain (CKC) functional testing or exercises, the examiner has less control of such variables, which increases the potential risk to the client (9, 12, 13, 18).

## Interpretation of Test Results

Muscle performance can be classified as normal or abnormal based on isokinetic testing results. Because testing can be performed bilaterally, right and left side

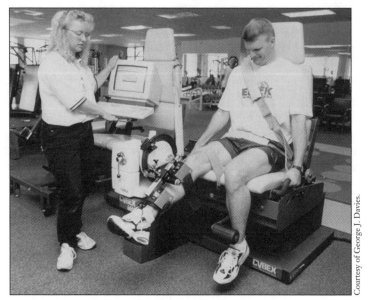

Courtesy of George J. Davies.

**Figure 1.2** Cybex computerized isokinetic open kinetic chain testing of the knee.

data can be compared to identify deficits or weakness patterns (25, 35, 36). Ratios for agonist/antagonist muscle groups like quadriceps/hamstrings or internal/external rotators of the shoulder can be evaluated for imbalances that may predispose an athlete to injury. Data can also be compared to normative data already established for different age groups and activity levels (24, 33, 51). These comparisons can facilitate the development of strength and conditioning programs to restore normal muscle balance, strength, and endurance in order to prevent injuries and enhance performance.

## Data Analysis and Program Design

Information from testing can also quantify exercise, allowing exercise regimes to be administered. Analysis of peak torque/body weight ratios, total work, average power, and torque acceleration energy can identify target areas that should be addressed. Low peak torque/body weight ratios suggest a need for more strengthening exercises, low total work values indicate endurance deficits and the need for higher repetition workouts, low average power values indicate that lifting techniques should emphasize explosive exercises and activities. Isokinetic data analysis allows for tailoring of conditioning programs to optimize muscle performance.

## Outcomes Assessment

The objectivity and reproducibility of isokinetic testing make it a valuable tool for documenting muscle performance and strength program effectiveness.

Baseline data from initial assessments can be compared to data collected during periodic testing to determine the effects of training programs and to determine and document strength gains (27). Conditioning programs can be modified if strength enhancement is not as expected. Individuals who have performed strengthening exercises using constant load free weights, variable resistance machines, or isokinetic machines can be tested to determine which strategy was most effective for improving muscle performance. Concentric and eccentric training modes as well as duration of training can also be evaluated. The shape of the torque curve may provide insights into angle-specific weaknesses or portions of the range of motion that should be targeted to improve muscle performance through the entire range of motion (9).

## Research Applications

Many researchers use isokinetic testing results (6, 9, 16, 21, 33, 43, 52). For many applications normative data for various types of subject populations has been and continues to be developed (7, 24, 51). Although most athletes do not sit flexing and extending their knees in an OKC pattern when they function, numerous studies demonstrate a correlation between OKC testing and CKC functional performance (based on a variety of functional assessment tests) (3, 41, 45, 49, 53, 55). This is an area that needs still more investigation to determine the best parameters for demonstrating the correlation. Muscle length-tension relationships and torque production can be examined by modifying the subject's position during testing to replicate performance positions of the muscles during different activities. As an example, changing the seat angle during knee testing will alter the quadriceps and hamstrings length-tension relationship. Testing the shoulder internal/external rotators in different positions, such as at the side in a modified neutral position, supine in 90°/90° or supine in the scaption position, creates different length-tension relations and resultant muscle performance values (see figure 1.3). The effect of electrical stimulation on strength gains may be explored (48). Consistent resistance training results in increased efficiency of the neuromuscular system as well as in an increase in the cross-sectional areas of specific muscle groups. Strength gains can be documented isokinetically, and correlations to muscle cross-sectional area can be performed. Research and objective measurements are necessary to validate strengthening strategies and techniques used to improve performance (33).

# Pretesting Procedures

Prior to actually performing any isokinetic testing there are a series of steps that can be followed in order to optimize the testing process and data collected.

As a first step, the examiner should establish the purpose of the testing in order to determine the specific testing protocols, the data that is to be collected, and how the data is going to be used. Once established, the examiner must educate the subject regarding the purpose of the test. It is important for

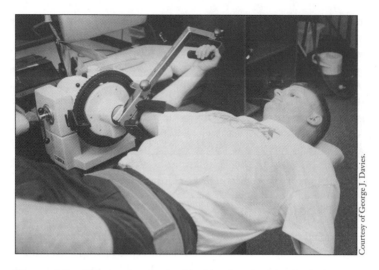

**Figure 1.3** Cybex computerized isokinetic open kinetic chain testing of the shoulder internal/external rotators.

the subject to understand the purpose of the test and how the testing will benefit the subject.

The examiner is responsible for the well-being of the subject. Thus, for the safety of the subject, the tester should have experience with the equipment, be knowledgeable about the test procedures, understand how to stabilize the subject, and be familiar with Institutional Review Board forms. The examiner must take care to use reliable equipment (9, 37, 42) that is adequately stabilized. The dynamometer should be securely anchored to the floor or wall to prevent unwanted movements and spurious data. *Equipment should be calibrated on a regular basis in accordance with the manufacturer's guidelines.*

The examiner should perform musculoskeletal screening of the subject to identify any relative or absolute contraindications for testing. Absent any contraindications for the testing, the subject may perform a general warm-up. A general warm-up is designed to use the large muscles of the body and create a systemic response to prepare the body for demands of the testing (9). The subject next performs a warm-up specific to the area being tested. A warm-up specific for the muscles to be tested prepares the muscles for the demands of testing and prevents injury (9).

The examiner must carefully document all aspects of the test. The starting position for the testing needs to be defined and replicated for repeat testing. The method used to align the anatomical axis with the joint axis must be recorded and consistently utilized. The subject must be stabilized during the testing to isolate the desired muscle group; various straps can be used to stabilize the subject to minimize any compensation during testing.

Other variables must be considered and reported. The examiner must determine the lever arm length. For consistency of testing and to increase the reliability of the measurements, it needs to remain constant when testing each individual (54). The preload or activation force can be preselected on some dynamometers. Based on each subject, the examiner may wish to vary this parameter. However, for consistency, it should remain the same on repeat testing of the same individual. With some isokinetic testing systems, the examiner may select a damp or ramp setting, and in some systems this variable is set in the computer software. Similarly, some dynamometers require a gravity correction procedure, while with some isokinetic testing systems, this is set in the computer software.

# Factors That Influence Measurements

The following factors should be considered when using isokinetics in testing and when designing programs for performance enhancement.

## Subject-Related Factors

Each individual is unique, and therefore each will yield unique results in testing and training. The examiner should keep in mind the following subject-related factors and research conclusions.

### Age

Although there is little consistency in the literature regarding test protocols or details of the testing, one consistent theme is generally demonstrated—torque, work, or power decreases with increasing age. Of the many factors that influence age-related changes, probably the most important influence is a decrease in the activity level of the older individual. Nevertheless, there is a need for research in this area to evaluate performance capabilities. This area of research will become even more important as more individuals live longer and maintain more active lifestyles. With masters category competitions increasing each year, more and more individuals will seek advice and techniques to enhance performance.

### Weight

Since the late 1970s, we have advocated normalizing a subject's test results to his or her body weight. This keys performance to body weight and individualizes the client's test performance to his or her size. Although there is some discrepancy in the literature regarding the application of normalization to body weight, the senior author (GJD) has used isokinetics in screening and performance testing for over 25 years and still thinks this is one of the most important ways to interpret isokinetic performance (9).

### Gender

Research consistently demonstrates that male subjects generally exceed forces generated by female subjects, when subjects are matched for age and activity level. Therefore, descriptive normative data should not mix the genders but be specific to the population.

## Athletic Background

Results reported in the literature indicate that participation in athletics influences force production so the participants are generally stronger and have more power and better endurance. Of course, specificity of sport participation will influence test results even more. Consequently, it is not appropriate to compare normative data on an athletic population to that of a nonathletic population.

## Height

The relationship between the height of subjects and their isokinetic performance is inconclusive.

## Presence of Impairment

Much isokinetic literature has addressed this topic. The uninvolved side is often compared to the side with the impairment by means of bilateral comparisons and comparisons to descriptive normative data. Many studies demonstrate that deficits do exist, but oftentimes the research methodology describing the results is too incomplete for replication and application for others to readily use.

## Limb Dominance

Most research does not demonstrate a significant difference in the lower extremities of subjects who participate in symmetric activities. However, if a subject is involved in a sport like high jumping in which one limb is unilaterally dominant, one would expect that the push off/jumping leg would have increased power. To the contrary, more literature indicates an asymmetry in the upper extremities. The reason is a matter of use. Whether one is involved in a sport that involves one dominant extremity movement pattern or not, through activities of daily living, most individuals have a dominant extremity that is more often used. Therefore, when performing a bilateral comparison on the upper extremities, these activities and usage patterns need to be taken into consideration.

# Movement-Related Factors

The following movement-related items should be considered when testing and interpreting data.

## Joint Angle

Because of the length-tension relationship and the biomechanics of a joint, force production is angle specific. One of the unique characteristics of isokinetics is accommodating resistance, which permits maximal dynamic loading through the range of motion. Each degree through the range of motion has the capacity to develop different amounts of force production based on the aforementioned criteria.

### Muscle Action (Concentric, Eccentric)

The primary muscle actions tested with isokinetic equipment are concentric or eccentric (although there are other variations that have been tested, such as isoacceleration). Most of the literature demonstrates an increased force production with eccentric muscle actions because both contractile and non-contractile tissue (elastic components) contribute to force production, whereas with concentric muscle actions, there is only the contractile unit that can contribute to force development.

### Mode of Testing (Isometric, Constant Load, Isokinetic)

It is beyond the scope of this chapter to discuss all the variations and modes of testing, but we point out that muscle performance can be assessed in numerous ways (6, 9, 21, 43).

# Components of Testing Protocols

Basic mechanics should be developed and followed when testing. Examples of some are described below.

## Test Speeds

The examiner selects a test speed, or angular velocity, after determining which speeds will provide the most useful information. As a general recommendation, we suggest sampling the muscle force-producing abilities across a velocity spectrum. Oftentimes, subjects will have a lot of strength at slower speeds, but they cannot produce the force quickly at the faster speeds. These results would then allow one to tailor a strength and conditioning program predicated on the test results. If a subject has a particular pathology, then it is even more important to perform velocity spectrum testing (9), because there are particular pathologies that manifest deficits more at different speeds.

## Test Repetitions

The number of repetitions depends on the purpose of the test. Researchers recommend that a subject perform at least five repetitions and that the test data is not taken from the first repetition if one is evaluating peak torque. If one is evaluating muscular power, fewer repetitions will be used (< 10), whereas if one is evaluating the muscle group for muscular endurance, more repetitions are going to be used (i.e., > 20) (5, 9, 20).

## Rest Intervals During Testing

We believe that the optimum rest interval between each set of repetitions is 90 seconds. However, although this is the optimum rest interval, it may not be appropriate because of the time lapse between bouts or sets. If power profile testing is performed, then we recommend that the rest interval be three minutes.

## Joint Angle or Range of Motion

Most testing will perform full range of motion testing limited by interfacing the client on the test equipment and the limitations of the technology. However, there may be instances where it is important to evaluate muscle performance in a limited arc of motion, for example, to replicate a specific sport or a part of the range of motion that is particularly important for performance.

## Consistent Feedback

It has been documented that providing feedback to the subject (verbal, visual, etc.) enhances performance. Therefore, the examiner should be consistent in either providing feedback or not when performing the testing. This is particularly importantly when there will be follow-up testing performed, rather then a one-time screening.

## Test Position

As previously mentioned, the position of the subject is important relative to muscle performance. If possible, the subject should be positioned as closely to sport performance positions as possible. We must recognize that altering the position of the subject alters factors such as the muscle length-tension relationship and the kinesthetic input into the joint.

## Joint-Specific Direction

The direction of the movement and functionally oriented testing, such as looking at eccentric/concentric ratios at end range of motion, are important. By being aware of joint-specific direction, the subject can mimic muscle performance in functional movement patterns.

## Testing the Uninvolved Side First

It is important to test the uninvolved side first for two reasons. First, it allows the subject to understand and perform the movement that is to be completed and decreases any apprehension. Second, it provides data for a bilateral comparison, unilateral ratios, and the like.

## Minimum and Maximum Force or Torque Limits

These limits are determined by the examiner based on the particular subjects tested. For human performance testing, generally the upper limits of the isokinetic dynamometer threshold would probably be necessary and desired.

## Skill and Training of the Tester

Because of the many factors that can influence the test results—such as proper positioning and stabilization, various computer settings, feedback to the subject—it is preferred to have a skilled experienced tester perform the testing.

For consistency with repeated testing, the same examiner should also perform subsequent testing.

# Data Analysis

Each isokinetic system has its own particular format for data collection and reporting. Examples of both graphic and numeric computerized printouts of Cybex isokinetic open kinetic chain tests and Lido Linea isokinetic closed kinetic chain tests are illustrated (see figures 1.4–1.7).

Following are common parameters for data analysis.

• *Peak torque.* This is the most commonly reported parameter with isokinetic testing that is used in the literature. This represents the single highest point on the torque curve.

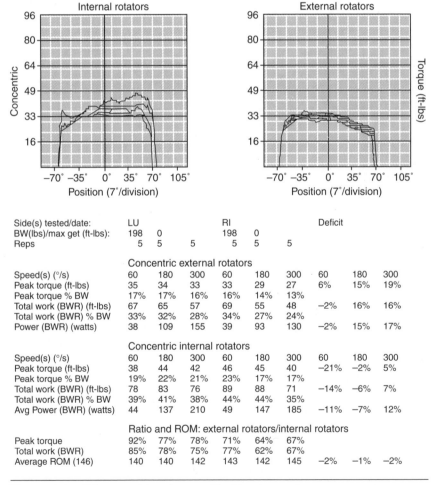

| Side(s) tested/date: | LU | | | RI | | | Deficit | | |
|---|---|---|---|---|---|---|---|---|---|
| BW(lbs)/max get (ft-lbs): | 198 | 0 | | 198 | 0 | | | | |
| Reps | 5 | 5 | 5 | 5 | 5 | 5 | | | |

| Concentric external rotators | | | | | | | | | |
|---|---|---|---|---|---|---|---|---|---|
| Speed(s) (°/s) | 60 | 180 | 300 | 60 | 180 | 300 | 60 | 180 | 300 |
| Peak torque (ft-lbs) | 35 | 34 | 33 | 33 | 29 | 27 | 6% | 15% | 19% |
| Peak torque % BW | 17% | 17% | 16% | 16% | 14% | 13% | | | |
| Total work (BWR) (ft-lbs) | 67 | 65 | 57 | 69 | 55 | 48 | −2% | 16% | 16% |
| Total work (BWR) % BW | 33% | 32% | 28% | 34% | 27% | 24% | | | |
| Power (BWR) (watts) | 38 | 109 | 155 | 39 | 93 | 130 | −2% | 15% | 17% |

| Concentric internal rotators | | | | | | | | | |
|---|---|---|---|---|---|---|---|---|---|
| Speed(s) (°/s) | 60 | 180 | 300 | 60 | 180 | 300 | 60 | 180 | 300 |
| Peak torque (ft-lbs) | 38 | 44 | 42 | 46 | 45 | 40 | −21% | −2% | 5% |
| Peak torque % BW | 19% | 22% | 21% | 23% | 17% | 17% | | | |
| Total work (BWR) (ft-lbs) | 78 | 83 | 76 | 89 | 88 | 71 | −14% | −6% | 7% |
| Total work (BWR) % BW | 39% | 41% | 38% | 44% | 44% | 35% | | | |
| Avg Power (BWR) (watts) | 44 | 137 | 210 | 49 | 147 | 185 | −11% | −7% | 12% |

| Ratio and ROM: external rotators/internal rotators | | | | | | | | | |
|---|---|---|---|---|---|---|---|---|---|
| Peak torque | 92% | 77% | 78% | 71% | 64% | 67% | | | |
| Total work (BWR) | 85% | 78% | 75% | 77% | 62% | 67% | | | |
| Average ROM (146) | 140 | 140 | 142 | 143 | 142 | 145 | −2% | −1% | −2% |

**Figure 1.4** Cybex graphic printout of isokinetic test data.

| Side(s) tested/date: | LU | | | RI | | | Deficit | | |
|---|---|---|---|---|---|---|---|---|---|
| BW(lbs)/max get (ft-lbs): | 198 | 0 | | 198 | 0 | | | | |
| Reps | 5 | 5 | 5 | 5 | 5 | 5 | | | |

**Concentric external rotators**

| | | | | | | | | | |
|---|---|---|---|---|---|---|---|---|---|
| Speed(s) (deg/sec) | 60 | 180 | 300 | 60 | 180 | 300 | 60 | 180 | 300 |
| Peak torque (ft-lbs) | 35 | 34 | 33 | 33 | 29 | 27 | 6% | 15% | 19% |
| Peak torque % BW | 17% | 17% | 16% | 16% | 14% | 13% | | | |
| Angle of peak torque | −32 | −31 | −37 | −39 | −30 | −37 | | | |
| Accel time (s) | 0.02 | 0.04 | 0.06 | 0.03 | 0.07 | 0.06 | | | |
| Total work (BWR) (ft-lbs) | 67 | 65 | 57 | 69 | 55 | 48 | −2% | 16% | 16% |
| Total work (BWR) % BW | 33% | 32% | 28% | 34% | 27% | 24% | | | |
| Power (BWR) (watts) | 38 | 109 | 155 | 39 | 93 | 130 | −2% | 15% | 17% |
| Power (BWR) % BW | 19% | 55% | 78% | 19% | 46% | 65% | | | |
| TAE (ft-lbs) | 3.0 | 10.9 | 18.3 | 3.2 | 10.1 | 15.3 | −7% | 7% | 16% |
| ASD (ft-lbs) | 2 | 1 | 2 | 1 | 1 | 0 | | | |
| Set Total work (ft-lbs) | 317 | 321 | 261 | 329 | 258 | 235 | −3% | 20% | 10% |
| Endurance ratio | | | | | | | | | |
| 50% Fatigue work (ft-lbs) | | | | | | | | | |
| 50% Fatigue time (sec) | | | | | | | | | |
| 50% Fatigue reps | | | | | | | | | |
| Work recovery ratio | | | | | | | | | |

**Concentric internal rotators**

| | | | | | | | | | |
|---|---|---|---|---|---|---|---|---|---|
| Speed(s) (deg/sec) | 60 | 180 | 300 | 60 | 180 | 300 | 60 | 180 | 300 |
| Peak torque (ft-lbs) | 38 | 44 | 42 | 46 | 45 | 40 | −21% | −2% | 5% |
| Peak torque % BW | 19% | 22% | 21% | 23% | 22% | 20% | | | |
| Angle of peak torque | 28 | 36 | 41 | 49 | 30 | 23 | | | |
| Accel time (s) | 0.02 | 0.06 | 0.02 | 0.02 | 0.05 | 0.07 | | | |
| Total work (BWR) (ft-lbs) | 78 | 83 | 76 | 89 | 88 | 71 | −14% | −6% | 7% |
| Total work (BWR) % BW | 39% | 41% | 38% | 44% | 44% | 35% | | | |
| Avg. Power (BWR) (watts) | 44 | 137 | 210 | 49 | 147 | 185 | −11% | −7% | 12% |
| Avg. Power (BWR) % BW | 22% | 69% | 106% | 24% | 74% | 93% | | | |
| TAE (ft-lbs) | 0.5 | 13.7 | 22.3 | 4.5 | 14.2 | 22.4 | −29% | −4% | 0% |
| ASD (ft-lbs) | 1 | 2 | 5 | 1 | 5 | 2 | | | |
| Set Total work (ft-lbs) | 372 | 391 | 337 | 413 | 352 | 320 | −11% | 10% | 6% |
| Endurance ratio | | | | | | | | | |
| 50% Fatigue work (ft-lbs) | | | | | | | | | |
| 50% Fatigue time (sec) | | | | | | | | | |
| 50% Fatigue reps | | | | | | | | | |
| Work recovery ratio | | | | | | | | | |

**Ratio and ROM: external rotators/internal rotators**

| | | | | | | | | | |
|---|---|---|---|---|---|---|---|---|---|
| Peak torque | 92% | 77% | 78% | 71% | 64% | 67% | | | |
| Total work (BWR) | 85% | 78% | 75% | 77% | 62% | 67% | | | |
| Avg. Power (BWR) | 86% | 79% | 73% | 79% | 63% | 70% | | | |
| Set Total work | 85% | 82% | 77% | 79% | 73% | 73% | | | |
| Average ROM (146) | 140 | 140 | 142 | 143 | 142 | 145 | | | |
| | | | | | | | −2% | −1% | −2% |

**Figure 1.5** Cybex numeric printout of isokinetic test data.

- *Average peak torque.* This averages the peak torque of each repetition to more accurately indicate the average of the test values.

- *Angle-specific torque.* This value represents the specific torque at a particular point in the range of motion.

- *Peak torque to body weight.* Normalization of the data compared to the subject's size allows the data to be individualized (9).

- *Total work.* This is the total amount of work that is produced based on the number of repetitions (9).

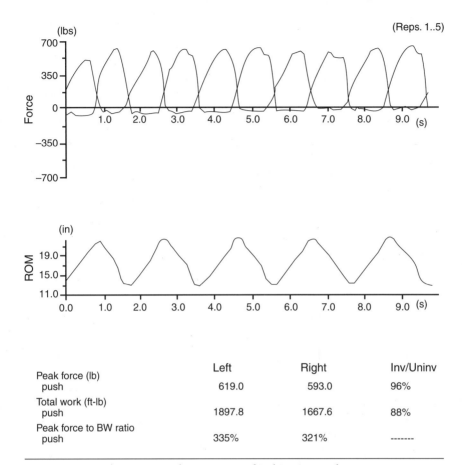

**Figure 1.6** Lido Linea graphic printout of isokinetic test data.

- *Average power.* This is the total work divided by the time it takes to perform the work (9).
- *Peak power.* Peak power is the maximum product of the velocity times its peak torque. The points may be plotted on a graph, which allows one to determine the optimum velocities where the subject can produce his or her maximum forces and would be an indication of where in the velocity spectrum optimum training can occur (9).
- *Torque acceleration energy (TAE).* This is the amount of work performed in the first 1/8 of a second. We feel that this is probably one of the more important parameters to evaluate when analyzing isokinetic data. Several studies have demonstrated TAE deficits associated with various pathologies (17, 29–32, 56, 57). Furthermore, Manske and Davies (38) have recently reported that TAE can be improved and normalized to within 10% of the uninvolved side through training.
- *Acceleration time.* This is the time to a predetermined variable, such as peak torque or a specific angle in the range of motion.

| | Left | Right | (Reps. 1..5) Inv/Uninv |
|---|---|---|---|
| Peak force push (lb) | 619.0 | 593.0 | 96% |
| Peak force position push (in) | 17.6 | 18.9 | ------- |
| Average peak force push (lb) | 594.7 | 570.3 | 96% |
| Average peak force position push (in) | 16.7 | 19.4 | ------- |
| Average work push (ft-lb) | 379.6 | 333.5 | 88% |
| Average power push (ft-lbs/s) | 402.1 | 336.9 | 84% |
| Average extreme ROM inner (in) outer (in) | 12.8 22.3 | 12.9 22.2 | ------- ------- |
| Peak force to BW ratio push | 335% | 321% | ------- |
| Average peak force to BW ratio push | 321% | 308% | ------- |
| Total work push (ft-lb) | 1897.8 | 1667.6 | 88% |
| Fatigue index push | 96% | 117% | ------- |
| (CV Reps. 1..5) push | 6% | 8% | ------- |

**Figure 1.7**    Lido Linea numeric printout of isokinetic test data.

• *Average points variance.* When evaluating several repetitions on test performance, there should be a consistent response. A guideline is that high and low values should be within 10% of the average. More than a 10% average points variance indicates an inconsistent test performance.

• *Speed-specific data.* This is the subject's force-producing capability at different velocities. Because of the force-velocity curve, as velocity increases with concentric isokinetics, force decreases. However, with eccentric isokinetics there is an opposite response. As the velocity increases with eccentric actions, the force increases. This increase varies, but some literature (10) indicates that at approximately 100°/s, the force plateaus.

• *Time rate of torque development (time to peak torque).* This is similar to acceleration time, or the amount of time it takes to reach a predetermined parameter.

• *Torque/velocity ratio.* Because of the force-velocity relation, there will be a change in the force production with change in velocity. This is also discussed under speed-specific data.

• *Endurance ratios and indexes.* These values assess the total work performance capabilities of the muscles. A variety of endurance testing protocols is used to determine these ratios. For example, the subject may be asked to perform·maximum volitional repetitions until a predetermined percentage drop in work is noted. A common protocol terminates the test when the muscle torque drops below 50% peak torque. A bilateral comparison is performed on each leg to determine endurance capabilities. Another commonly used protocol is to use a preset number of repetitions and calculate the total amount of work that can be performed. Once again a bilateral comparison, unilateral ratios, or comparison to sport-specific normative data can be used to interpret the results (5, 20).

• *Force decay rate.* This is the downslope of the torque curve. It is reflective of the subject's ability to continue to produce force through the range of motion until the end.

• *Reciprocal innervation time.* This is the time between the agonist muscle action and the antagonist muscle action. This is usually delayed if various pathologies are present.

• *Windowing of data.* When testing with isokinetics, there are parts of the range of motion where free limb acceleration and free limb deceleration occur. Acceleration, of course, is not a fixed velocity and therefore cannot be isokinetic. The faster the isokinetic angular velocity, the more free limb acceleration and deceleration occurs. Consequently, some researchers recommend windowing the data, to select for analysis data only from the "pure" isokinetic portion of the range of motion (load range).

• *Isomap procedure.* This is a relatively new procedure developed by Biodex for computerized data analysis through multidimensional analysis.

# Data Interpretation

There are many ways to analyze and interpret isokinetic data to use it as the basis for designing or altering a conditioning or performance enhancement exercise program. The following are some of the more commonly used examples of data interpretation and their application to designing exercise programs.

• *Bilateral comparison* (25, 35, 36). Evaluating one extremity in relation to the other is probably the most common comparison used in data analysis. Values differing by 10 to 15% are usually considered to be sensitive for significant asymmetry. More of a deficit indicates a muscle imbalance, which may predispose the subject for possible muscle-related injuries such as strains and tendinitis. However, this single parameter, used by itself, has limitations.

• *Unilateral ratios (agonist/antagonist ratios)* (1, 9, 33, 47). Comparing the relationship between the agonist and the antagonist muscles may identify weaknesses in certain muscle groups. This parameter is particularly important to assess when doing velocity spectrum testing because the percentage relationship of the muscles changes with changing speeds in many muscle groups. Application of this information may be important for athletes who need the advantage of muscular cocontractions with various activities. There may also be instances where it is preferred to have a dominant muscle group to enhance performance.

- *Eccentric/concentric ratios* (1, 47). Many functional activities use this muscle action pattern. In throwing, there is an eccentric action followed immediately by a concentric action of the glenohumeral internal rotators. This occurs in the cocking phase to acceleration phase of throwing.

- *Peak torque to body weight (normalized data)* (9). Comparing torque to body weight (BW) adds another dimension in interpreting test results. Oftentimes, even though a subject has bilateral symmetry and normal unilateral ratios, the torque/body weight ratio is altered. The various norms for muscle groups will be included in the chapters throughout this book. We evaluate torque to body weight rather than to lean body weight because an individual must function with the total BW and not just lean BW.

- *Parameter/body weight to normalize the data.* Other test data can also be normalized to the subject's body weight to normalize the data to the individual.

- *Total leg strength (TLS).* Nicholas and coworkers (40), Gleim and associates (23), and Boltz and Davies (4) have published information on the concept of total leg strength. To calculate total leg strength, several isolated tests of lower extremity muscles are performed and the data is summated to develop a composite score. This allows one to evaluate the entire lower extremity as a total kinetic chain unit and, at the same time, to evaluate each of the links of the kinetic chain. This same concept should also be applied to the upper extremity, but there is less research on total arm strength (TAS) (46). As previously mentioned, oftentimes the entire lower extremity composite test performance may be symmetric from side to side, but the symmetry may be due to specific muscles compensating for a weaker muscle (44). If only the entire kinetic chain score is assessed, then the weak link may never be identified. If a weak link is not discovered, then it can't be addressed in the strength and conditioning program.

- *Endurance ratios.* The fatigability and recovery rate of a muscle group can be evaluated by using any of a variety of endurance test protocols.

- *Comparisons to descriptive normative data.* Although the use of normative data is controversial, if it is used properly relative to the specific population, then it can be used as a guideline for testing and developing strength and conditioning programs (7, 24, 51).

## Summary

This chapter introduced various concepts about isokinetic testing and its application to human performance. It presented information on terminology commonly used with isokinetic exercise, provided a rationale for isokinetic testing, discussed various considerations for testing, described factors that influence isokinetic measurements, established several components of testing protocols, listed several parameters that are commonly used in data analysis, and presented different methods of data analysis.

# References

1. Aagaard, P, Simonsen, EB, Magnusson, P, et al. 1998. A new concept for isokinetic hamstring/quadriceps muscle strength ratios. *Am J Sports Med* 26: 231–37.

2. Anderson, MA, Gieck, JH, Perrin, D, Weltman, A, Ruth, R, Denegar, C. 1991. The relationship among isometric, isotonic, and isokinetic concentric and eccentric quadriceps and hamstring force and three components of athletic performance. *J Orthop Sports Phys Ther* 14: 114–20.

3. Barber, SD, Noyes, FR, Mangine, RE, et al. 1990. Quantitative assessment of functional limitations in normal and anterior cruciate ligament-deficient knees. *Clin Orthop* 255: 204–14.

4. Boltz, S, Davies, GJ. 1984. Leg length differences and correlation with total leg strength. *J Orthop Sports Phys Ther* 6: 123–29.

5. Burdett, RG, VanSwearingen, J. 1987. Reliability of isokinetic muscle endurance tests. *J Orthop Sports Phys Ther* 8: 484–88.

6. Chan, KM, Maffulli, N, ed. 1996. *Principles and practice of isokinetics in sports medicine and rehabilitation*. Baltimore: Williams & Wilkins.

7. Davies, GJ, Gould, J. 1982. Trunk testing using a prototype Cybex II isokinetic dynamometer stabilization system. *J Orthop Sports Phys Ther* 3: 164–70.

8. Davies, GJ. 1984. *A compendium of isokinetics in clinical usage.* Onalaska, WI: S & S.

9. Davies, GJ. 1992. *A compendium of isokinetics in clinical usage*, 4th ed. Onalaska, WI: S & S.

10. Davies, GJ, Ellenbecker, TS. 1992. Eccentric isokinetics. *Orthop Clin No Am* 1: 297–336.

11. Davies, GJ, Dickoff-Hoffman, SD. 1993. Neuromuscular testing and rehabilitation of the shoulder complex. *J Orthop Sports Phys Ther* 18: 449–58.

12. Davies, GJ. 1995. The need for critical thinking in rehabilitation. *J Sport Rehab* 4: 1–22.

13. Davies, GJ, Heiderscheit, BC, Clark, M. 1995. Open kinetic chain assessment and rehabilitation. *Ath Train: Sports Health Care Perspective* 1: 347–70.

14. Davies, GJ, Heiderscheit, BC. 1997. Reliability of the Lido Linea closed kinetic chain isokinetic dynamometer. *J Orthop Sports Phys Ther* 25: 133–36.

15. Davies, GJ, Wilk, K, Ellenbecker, TS. 1997. Assessment of strength. In *Orthopaedic and Sports Physical Therapy*, 3d ed. Ed. Malone, TR, McPoil, T, Nitz, AJ, 225–57. St. Louis: Mosby.

16. Davies, GJ, Ellenbecker, TS. 1988. Application of isokinetic testing and rehabilitation. In *Physical rehabilitation of the injured athlete*, ed. Andrews, JR, Harrelson, GL, Wilk, KE, 219–60. Philadelphia: Saunders.

17. Davies, GJ, Manske, R. In review. The evaluation of torque acceleration energy (TAE) in 110 patients with shoulder conditions.

18. Davies, GJ, Zillmer, DA. 1999. Functional progression of exercise during rehabilitation. In *Knee ligament rehabilitation*, ed. Ellenbecker, TS. New York: Churchill Livingstone.

19. Davies, GJ, Heiderscheit, BC, Clark, M. 1999. The scientific and clinical rationale for the use of open and closed kinetic chain exercises in rehabilitation. In *Knee ligament rehabilitation*, ed. Ellenbecker, TS. New York: Churchill Livingstone.

20. DeNuccio, D, Davies, GJ, Rowinski, M. 1991. Comparison of quadriceps isokinetic eccentric and isokinetic concentric data using a standard fatigue protocol. *Isok Exerc Sci* 1: 81–86.

21. Dvir, Z. 1995. *Isokinetics: Muscle testing, interpretation, and clinical applications.* New York: Churchill Livingstone.

22. Ellenbecker, TS, Davies, GJ, Rowinski, M. 1988. Concentric vs. eccentric isokinetic strengthening of the rotator cuff: Objective data vs. functional test. *Am J Sports Med* 16: 64–69.

23. Gleim, GW, Nicholas, JA, Webb, JN. 1978. Isokinetic evaluation following leg injuries. *Phys Sports Med* 6: 74–82.

24. Goslin, BR, Chateris, J. 1979. Isokinetic dynamometry: Normative data for clinical use in lower extremity (knee) cases. *Scand J Rehabil Med* 11: 105–9.

25. Grace, TG, Sweetser, ER, Nelson, MA, et al. 1984. Isokinetic muscle imbalance and knee joint injuries. *J Bone Joint Surg* 66A: 734–40.

26. Greenberger, HB, Paterno, MV. 1995. Relationship of knee extensor strength and hopping test performance in the assessment of lower extremity function. *J Orthop Sports Phys Ther* 22: 202–6.

27. Heiderscheit, B, Palmer-Mclean, K, Davies, GJ. 1996. The effects of isokinetic versus plyometric training of the shoulder internal rotators. *J Orthop Sports Phys Ther* 23: 125–33.

28. Hislop, HJ, Perrine, JJ. 1967. The isokinetic concept of exercise. *Phys Ther* 47: 114–17.

29. Huston, LM, Wojtys, EM. 1996. Neuromuscular performance in elite women athletes. *Am J Sports Med* 24: 427–36.

30. Kannus, P, Jarvinen, M. 1989. Prediction of torque acceleration energy and power of thigh muscles from peak torque. *Med Sci Sports Exerc* 21: 304–7.

31. Kannus, P, Latvala, K. 1989. Torque acceleration energy, power, and peak torque in thigh muscles after knee sprain. *Canadian J Sports Sci* 14: 102–6.

32. Kannus, P. 1992. Normality, variability, and predictability of work, power, and torque acceleration energy with respect to peak torque in isokinetic muscle testing. *Int J Sports Med* 133: 249–56.

33. Kannus, P. 1994. Isokinetic evaluation of muscular performance: Implications for muscle testing and rehabilitation. *Int J Sports Med* 15(Suppl): S11–18.

34. Keating, JL, Matyas, TA. 1996. The influence of subject and test design on dynamometric measurements of extremity muscles. *Phys Ther* 76: 866–89.

35. Knapik, JJ, Bauman, CL, Jones, BH, et al. 1991. Preseason strength and flexibility imbalances associated with athletic injuries in female collegiate athletes. *Am J Sports Med* 19: 76–81.

36. Knight, KL. 1980. Strength imbalance and knee injury. *Phys Sports Med* 8: 140.

37. Madsen, OR. 1996. Torque, total work, power, torque acceleration energy, and acceleration time assessed on a dynamometer: Reliability of knee and elbow extensor and flexor strength measurements. *Eur J App Physiol* 74: 206–10.

38. Manske, R, Davies, GJ. In review. The effects of rehabilitation on torque acceleration energy (TAE) in 60 patients with TAE deficits on the index test.

39. Moffroid, M, Whipple, R, Hofkosh, J, Lowman, E, Thistle, H. 1969. A study of isokinetic exercise. *Phys Ther* 49: 735–44.

40. Nicholas, JA, Strizak, AM, Veras, G. 1976. A study of thigh muscle weakness in different pathological states of the lower extremity. *Am J Sports Med* 4: 241–48.

41. Noyes, FR, Barber, SD, Mangine, RE. 1991. Abnormal lower limb symmetry determined by functional hop test after anterior cruciate ligament rupture. *Am J Sports Med* 19: 513–18.

42. Perrin, DH. 1986. Reliability of isokinetic measures. *Ath Training* 21: 319–94.

43. Perrin, DH. 1993. *Isokinetic exercise and assessment.* Champaign, IL: Human Kinetics.

44. Rosenthal, MD, Aer, LL, Griffith, PP, et al. 1994. Comparability of work output measures as determined by isokinetic dynamometry and a closed kinetic chain exercise. *J Sports Rehab* 3: 218–27.

45. Sachs, RA, Adniel, DM, Stone, ML, Carfein, FR. 1989. Patellofemoral problems after anterior cruciate ligament reconstruction. *Am J Sports Med* 17: 760–65.

46. Schexneider, MA, Catlin, PA, Davies, GJ, Mattson, PA. 1991. An isokinetic estimation of total arm strength. *Isok Exerc Sci* 1: 117–21.

47. Scoville, CR, Arciero, RA, Taylor, DC, et al. 1997. End range eccentric antagonistic/concentric agonist strength ratios: A new perspective in shoulder strength assessment. *J Orthop Sports Phys Ther* 25: 203–7.

48. Snyder-Mackler, L, Delitto, A, Bailey, SL, et al. 1995. Strength of the quadriceps femoris muscle and functional recovery after reconstruction of the anterior cruciate ligament. *J Bone Joint Surg* 77A: 1166–73.

49. Tegner, Y, Lysholm, J, Lysholm, M, Gilquist, J. 1986. A performance test to monitor rehabilitation and evaluate anterior cruciate ligament injuries. *Am J Sports Med* 14: 156–59.

50. Thistle, HG, Hislop, HJ, Moffroid, M, Lowman, EW. 1967. Isokinetic contractions: A new concept of resistive exercise. *Arch Phys Med Rehabil* 6: 279–82.

51. Thompson, NN, Gould, JA, Davies, GJ. 1985. Descriptive measures of isokinetic trunk testing. *J Orthop Sports Phys Ther* 7: 43–49.

52. Timm, KE. 1988. Postsurgical knee rehabilitation: A five-year study of four methods and 5,381 patients. *Am J Sports Med* 16: 463–68.

53. Wiklander, J, Lysholm, J. 1987. Simple tests for surveying muscle strength and muscle stiffness in sportsmen. *Int J Sports Med* 8: 50–54.

54. Wilk, KE, Andrews, JR. 1993. The effects of pad placement and angular velocity on tibial displacement during isokinetic exercise. *J Orthop Sports Phys Ther* 17: 223–30.

55. Wilk, KE, Romanillo, WT, Soscia, SM, et al. 1994. The relationship between subjective knee scores, isokinetic testing, and functional testing in the ACL-reconstructed knee. *J Orthop Sports Phys Ther* 20: 60–73.

56. Wojtys, EM, Huston, LJ. 1994. Neuromuscular performance in normal and anterior cruciate ligament-deficient lower extremities. *Am J Sports Med* 22: 89–104.

57. Wojtys, EM, Huston, LJ, Taylor, PD, et al. 1996. Neuromuscular adaptations in isokinetic, isotonic, and agility training programs. *Am J Sports Med* 4: 187–92.

# Chapter 2

# Specificity of Training Modes

William J. Kraemer, Scott A. Mazzetti,
Nicholas A. Ratamess, and Steven J. Fleck

**S**ince the development of the isokinetic modality over 30 years ago, its benefits have been touted in athletic, fitness, and rehabilitative scenarios. As with any other resistance training tool, it has specific characteristics that make it the optimal choice for some training goals but not for others. The advent of computer interfaces, which allow the collection of force production output, made it an attractive high-tech instrument for many not familiar with resistance training, whether it was appropriate or not for the job to be done. The development of isokinetic dynamometers with eccentric force capabilities expanded the potential for use in fields outside of rehabilitation. Some abstracted biomechanical preliminary research has indicated that it may be possible for even lower cost equipment to maintain an isokinetic velocity over a limited range of speeds (e.g., Nordic Flex Gold), which could present an isokinetic stimulus.

Since an isokinetic muscle action is performed at constant angular limb velocity, it is unlike other types of resistance exercise choices in that there is no set resistance to meet; rather, the velocity of movement is controlled. The resistance offered by the isokinetic machine cannot be accelerated since any force applied against the equipment results in an equal reaction force. The reaction force mirrors the force applied to the equipment throughout the range of movement of an exercise, making it theoretically possible for the muscle(s) to exert a continual, maximal force through the full range of motion. The more expensive isokinetic machines allow the user to perform both concentric and eccentric actions. However, most equipment found in resistance training facilities allows only concentric actions. Be that as it may, concentric-only isokinetic training has been shown to increase eccentric isokinetic strength (44). Thus the effects of concentric-only isokinetic training will be reviewed here.

Advocates of isokinetic training believe that the ability to exert maximal force throughout the range of motion leads to optimal strength increases.

However, a key factor appears to be the ability, which would be otherwise limited with the use of resistances that have an accelerating mass (e.g., free weights or stack plate machines), to train single joints for speed development. Furthermore, sport-specific exercise requires training that develops specific neuromuscular attributes most needed to perform a particular task. With free weights and stack plate machines energy is only partially absorbed and the remainder is dissipated with accelerations in the exercise motion. Conversely, with isokinetic exercise, energy cannot be dissipated by acceleration because this is mechanically prevented by the device (22). Another advantage with isokinetic training has been minimal muscle and joint soreness following a workout after a base level of training exposure has been completed (two to four workouts). However, isokinetic eccentric protocols have been used in muscle-damage studies in untrained subjects to study delayed onset muscle soreness (16).

# Strength Changes With Isokinetic Training

The vast majority of studies examining concentric-only isokinetic training have been of short duration (i.e., 3–16 weeks) and have tested for strength gains using isometric, constant external resistance, and concentric-only isokinetic tests.

## Training Velocities and Repetitions

Programs of one set at various velocities of movement and numbers of repetitions cause significant increases in strength: 1 set of 15 repetitions at either 60 or 240°/s (1 × 15 at 60 and 1 × 15 at 240) (24); 1 × 20 at 60°/s and 1 × 20 at 180°/s (28); 1 × 30 at 22.5°/s (31); 1 × 50 at 30°/s (26); and 1 × 65 at 120°/s (34). Two set programs also result in increased strength: 2 × 12 at 60°/s (19); 2 × 10 at 60°/s for four weeks, followed by 2 × 15 at 90°/s for four additional weeks (18). A variety of three set programs also results in increased strength: 3 × 8 at 60°/s and 3 × 20 at 240°/s (14); 3 × 10 at 100°/s (44); 3 × 15 at 90°/s (17); 3 × 15 at 60°/s (17); and 3 sets of 1 × 10 at 60°/s, 1 × 30 at 179°/s, and 1 × 50 at 299°/s (25). Multiple set programs of greater than three sets also result in increased strength: 4 or 5 × 12 at 60°/s (8); 5 × 6 at 60°/s or 5 × 12 at 300°/s (11); 6 sets of 3 × 6 at 60°/s followed by 3 × 12 at 300°/s (11); 5 × 5 at 60°/s (7); 5 × 10 at 120°/s (36); 6 × 25 at 240°/s or 5 × 15 at 60°/s (30); 6 × 10 at 120°/s (23); 6 × 5 at 90°/s (10); 6 × 10 at 120°/s (33); and 5 × 5 at 60°/s or 15 × 10 at 60°/s (7).

## Training at Velocity With Repetitions/Time

Gains in strength have also been achieved by performing as many repetitions as possible in set periods of time. Examples of this approach include 1 set of 6 or 30 s at 180°/s (1 × 6 s at 180°/s, 1 × 30 s at 180°/s) (29); 2 × 20 s at 180°/s (5, 35); 2 × 30 s at 60°/s (4); 2 × 30 s at 120°/s or 2 × 30 s at 300°/s (3); and

1 × 60 s at 36°/s or 1 × 60 s at 108°/s (40). Increases in strength have also been achieved by performing 1 set of voluntary maximal contractions until a peak force of at least 60, 75, or 90% could no longer be generated at each velocity of 30, 60, and 90°/s (15), and until 50% of peak force could no longer be maintained during slow speed training (1 set at each velocity of 30, 60, and 90°/s) or fast speed training (1 set at each velocity of 180, 240, and 300°/s) (41). Table 2.1 includes reports of changes in strength in the bench press and leg press due to isokinetic training. It is apparent that many combinations of sets and repetitions of concentric-only isokinetic training can cause increases in force production.

## Other Testing Methods

Isokinetic training has also been shown to result in increased strength when tested by other modes. The studies in table 2.1 also indicate that concentric isokinetic training can result in significant increases in strength when isometric, isotonic, and variable resistance testing procedures are used. Examples include statistically significant increases of up to 80% in isometric strength (26), 15% increases in constant external resistance strength after 12 weeks of study (8), and 18% increases in variable resistance strength after 8 weeks of study (18). These studies clearly indicate that concentric isokinetic training does result in significant increases in strength no matter what the testing mode used to determine strength.

# Optimal Number of Sets and Repetitions

Despite the vast quantity of research concerning the effects of concentric-only isokinetic training, few studies have investigated the optimal number of sets and repetitions. One study (29) shows no difference in gains of peak torque between 10 sets of 6-second duration, performing as many repetitions as possible (i.e., about 3), and 2 sets of 30-second duration, performing as many repetitions as possible (i.e., about 10). Both groups trained at 180°/s four times a week for seven weeks. Another study compared all combinations of 5, 10, and 15 repetitions along with slow, intermediate, and fast velocities of movement. After training three days per week for nine weeks no significant differences existed in strength among any of the groups (12). Five sets of 5 repetitions and 15 sets of 10 repetitions have also been compared (7). In this study both groups trained at 60°/s, three times per week for 16 weeks. Peak torque was tested at eight velocities ranging from 0 to 300°/s. Both groups improved significantly at all testing velocities; only one significant difference existed between the two: at 30°/s the 15-set group showed greater gains than the 5-set group. All three of these studies agree on at least one point: The number of repetitions performed appears to have little impact on increases in peak torque. (Note that the minimal number of repetitions performed per set in these studies was three.)

**Table 2.1 Comparative Strength Increases**

| Reference | Gender of subject | Length of training (weeks) | Days of training /week | Sets, reps | Knee movement trained | % Increase isokinetic | Comparative test type | % Increase |
|---|---|---|---|---|---|---|---|---|
| Thistle et al. 1967 | M & F | 8 | 4 | IK<br>IS | Extension<br>Flexion | 47%<br>29% | | |
| Moffroid et al. 1969 | M & F | 4 | 7 | IK 30 contractions<br><br>IS 3x10 RM | Extension @ 22.5°/s<br>Flexion @ 22.5°/s<br>Extension @ 22.5°/s<br>Flexion @ 22.5°/s | 14%*<br>11%<br>-2%<br>4%<br>(IK group did increase total work) | IM knee extension<br>IM knee flexion<br>IM knee extension<br>IM knee flexion | 24%*<br>19%*<br>13%*<br>1% |
| Pearson & Costill 1988 | M | 8 | 3 | IK 6x10 – 11 @ 120°/s<br><br>IS 3x6 @ 70% IRM<br>3x4 @ 80% IRM<br>3x2 @ 90% IRM | Extension @ 60°/s<br>Extension @ 180°/s<br>Extension @ 240°/s<br>Extension @ 60°/s<br>Extension @ 180°/s<br>Extension @ 240°/s | 12%*<br>7%*<br>10%*<br>8%<br>5%<br>1% | IS IRM<br><br><br>IS IRM | 4%<br><br><br>32%* |
| Smith & Melton 1981 | M | 3 | 3 | IK 30, 60 & 90°/s until 50% fatigued | Extension @ 60°/s<br>Extension @ 240°/s<br>Flexion @ 60°/s<br>Flexion @ 240°/s | 21%**<br>25%***<br>17%***<br>10%*** | IM knee extension<br>IM knee extension<br>IS leg press | 1%**<br>16%***<br>10%*** |
| | M | 3 | 3 | IK 180, 240 & 300°/s until 50% fatigued | Extension @ 60°/s<br>Extension @ 240°/s<br>Flexion @ 60°/s<br>Flexion @ 240°/s | 3%**<br>61%***<br>17%***<br>10%*** | IM knee extension<br>IM knee flexion<br>IS leg press | 7%**<br>9%***<br>7%** |
| | M | 3 | 3 | VR 3x10 @ 80% IRM | Extension @ 60°/s<br>Extension @ 240°/s<br>Flexion @ 60°/s<br>Flexion @ 240°/s | 1%*<br>7%*<br>15%*<br>14% | IM knee extension<br>IM knee flexion<br>IS leg press | 15%*<br>11%*<br>11%* |

** = no statistics run; * = significant increase; IK = isokinetic; IS = isotonic; IM = isometric.

# Rest Periods During Isokinetic Training

The amount of rest between sets is also an important variable when designing a resistance training program. In general, longer rest periods are used for optimal strength and power development, whereas short rest periods are used for improving muscular endurance and hypertrophy (16). A recent study has examined the effect of different rest period lengths on muscular strength during isokinetic training. Pincivero, Lephart, and Karunakara (37) had subjects train three days per week for four weeks using either a short rest period (40 s) or a long rest period (160 s) (37). The results showed that the group using a long rest period increased peak hamstring torque significantly more than the group using a short rest period. Thus, rest period length can significantly affect the magnitude of strength changes associated with isokinetic resistance training, and as with other training modalities, longer rest periods may optimize strength improvements.

# Optimal Training Velocity

Previously cited studies firmly support the idea that isokinetic training can result in increased strength. Two questions inherent to isokinetic training have yet to be given unequivocal answers. What is the optimal training speed: fast or slow? Do strength increases obtained at a particular training speed carry over to speeds above and below the training speed? Several studies have investigated the first of these questions; however, no conclusive answer has emerged. A velocity of training that is superior to another would result in greater strength gains not just at one velocity but over a greater range of movement velocities. Moffroid and Whipple (32) compared training at 36 and 108°/s and determined that training at 108°/s was superior to training at 36°/s. Alternatively, slow speed training—4 s to complete one leg press repetition—has been shown to result in greater strength increases than fast speed training—2 s to complete one leg press repetition (45).

Some research indicates that there is no evidence to favor a particular speed when considering gains in peak torque. Training at 60 or 180°/s results in equal gains in peak torque at 60, 120, 180, and 240°/s (3, 21, 27, 28). Training at 60 or 240°/s results in equal gains in isometric strength (30). Other factors impede any conclusions favoring slow or fast speed training. All of the above projects covered a short duration of no more than 16 weeks, making conclusions concerning long-term training difficult. Because the majority of these studies experimented with such slow speeds, in general, any comparison between slow and fast speeds based on these studies is artificial.

Several studies do, however, provide some insight into the question of fast versus slow velocity. Jenkins, Thackaberry, and Killian (24) trained groups at 60 and 240°/s three times per week for six weeks. Both groups trained with one set of 15 repetitions per training session. Peak torque test results show the group trained at 60°/s improved at all but the 30 and 300°/s velocities, while the group trained at 240°/s improved at all test velocities from 30 to 300°/s. No significant difference between the two training groups was shown in peak torque improvement. However, due to the nonsignificant improvement at the 30 and 300°/s test velocities by the group trained at 60°/s, it could be theorized that training at 240°/s resulted in better overall gains in strength at a variety of velocities.

Another study examined changes in peak torque at 60, 180, and 240°/s between two groups: a slow speed group, which performed three sets of 8 repetitions at 60°/s and a fast speed group, which performed three sets of 20 repetitions at 240°/s (14). The isokinetic training regimen included three sessions per week for 10 weeks. The results indicated that the peak torque of the slow speed group increased significantly at 60 and 180°/s (8.5 and 10.9%, respectively), and the peak torque of the fast speed group increased significantly at 180 and 240°/s (17.5 and 19.7%, respectively). Coyle and colleagues (11) also utilized three groups: a slow speed group trained at 60°/s with five sets of six maximal contractions; a fast speed group trained at 300°/s with five sets of 12 maximal contractions; and a group using a combination of slow and fast speeds trained with two or three sets of six repetitions at 60°/s and two or three sets of 12 repetitions at 300°/s. Each group showed its greatest gains at its specific training velocity, suggesting that the velocity of training should be determined by the velocity of desired peak torque increases (see figure 2.1).

Collectively, these studies indicate that if gains in strength over a wide range of velocities are desired, then training should be performed at a velocity of somewhere between 180 and 240°/s. However, if the goal of training is to maximally increase strength at a specific velocity, then training should be performed at that velocity.

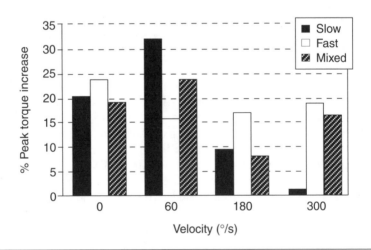

**Figure 2.1**   The effect of isokinetic training at slow (60°/s), fast (300°/s), and mixed (60 and 300°/s) velocities on peak torque (%).

Data adapted from Coyle et al. (11).

# Velocity and Strength Carryover

The second question concerning concentric-only isokinetic training is to what magnitude do increases in torque carry over to velocities other than the training velocity? Moffroid and Whipple (32) compared training at 36 and 108°/s and found that increases in peak torque only carried over to speeds of movement below the training velocity (32). Other studies using training velocities of 60 and 240°/s and testing at velocities of 30 to 300°/s (24) or 60 to 240°/s (14) suggest there is carryover of peak torque gains at velocities above and below the training velocity. The carryover may be as great as 210°/s below the training velocity and up to 180°/s above the training velocity. Studies of training at 60 or 180°/s indicate that significant gains in peak torque are made at all velocities from 60 to 240°/s (3, 28).

Collectively these studies indicate that gains in peak torque may occur above and below the training velocity except when the training velocity is very slow (30°/s). In general, fast velocity training (108 up to 240°/s) causes significant increases in torque below the training velocity and in some cases above the training velocity, but the amount of carryover may decrease as the difference between the training and testing velocity increases. Differences in the amount (significant or insignificant) of carryover to other velocities may in part be attributed to the velocities that were defined as fast (108 up to 240°/s). With slow velocity training (36 up to 96°/s), all studies also indicate that significant carryover in torque below and above the training velocity does occur. Interestingly, the aforementioned studies all determined peak torque irrespective of the joint angle at which peak torque occurred. It might be questioned whether the torque was actually increased at a specific joint angle and therefore at a specific muscle length, which would indicate that the mechanisms controlling muscle tension at that length have been altered.

# Power

In trying to answer questions related to strength, many may have forgotten the impact of isokinetic training on power production at higher movement speeds. Strength has been defined as the maximum force a muscle or muscle group can generate (48). Power, on the other hand, is defined as force × distance/time, which makes the rate of force development very important to many everyday activities and athletic events. For example, if two individuals can each power clean 250 lb moving the weight the same distance, but one can do it in half the time, that person has more power than the other lifter. Developing power is thus an aspect of strength and is crucial to athletic performance.

To develop power while strength training, one must attempt to contract the muscle as fast as possible even when using heavy weights. Trainers have thus suggested that persons lessen the weight they normally use and move the bar faster. There are several problems with this approach. First, not all exercises can be performed using what is called speed reps, because some exercises are not designed for this type of movement. For example, performing arm curls as fast as you can would, over time, cause soreness and possible injury to the elbow joint. In addition, rapid flexing of the elbow joint would cause the resistance to bump up against the upper arm and chest, possibly resulting in injury. Furthermore, for most of the movement your body would be trying to decelerate or inhibit the movement to prevent the resistance momentum from carrying the load into the joint end point just described. The use of an isokinetic form of resistance would be more helpful in developing this type of power or so-called speed strength for single joint movements. Thus, isokinetic exercise allows for high velocity movement to be performed without the fear of having to decelerate a mass at the end of the range of motion for the joint. Thus, speed strength can be developed for some exercise movements in a resistance exercise training program.

Consideration must also be given to the optimal training velocity for power development. Kanehisa and Miyashita (25) trained three groups at specified velocities of 60, 179, and 300°/s, six times per week for eight weeks (25). The 60°/s training was 10 voluntary maximal contractions per session. The 179 and 300°/s training was 30 and 50 repetitions per training session, respectively. All were tested for peak torque at 60, 119, 179, 239, and 300°/s both before and after the training program. Training at 60 and 179°/s increased average power of a repetition significantly at all test speeds. Training at 300°/s increased average power of a repetition significantly only at the fastest test speeds (239 and 300°/s). In addition, training at 179 and 300°/s resulted in a significantly greater increase in average power of a repetition at the test speeds of 239 and 300°/s than training at 60°/s. The fact that this study varied the number of repetitions limits general conclusions. However, from the results it appears that an intermediate speed (about 179°/s) is the most advantageous for gains across velocities of movement in average power.

# Athletic Performance

Although most people have within their mind a definition of athletic performance and a picture of what an athletic individual looks like, defining athletic performance is not as simple as it might seem. The Olympic decathlon champion is often labeled "the best all-around athlete in the world." The decathlon is an event composed of 10 separate contests involving jumping, sprinting, running, hurdling, and throwing. Many individuals define athletic ability as the ability to run, jump, and throw. However, in some sports, such as basketball, the person who is the best runner, jumper, and thrower may not be the best all-around athlete. In other sports, such as archery and rifle shooting, the participants may not be better than average in running, jumping, and throwing tasks. However, they are very good at their chosen discipline. Thus, there are many components that could make up what is termed "athletic ability." Athletic ability is the composite physiological integration for a skill. Many factors related to the neuromuscular system's ability to properly activate muscle, fitness characteristics of the muscles activated, and temporal integration of the force production patterns all contribute to measurement of whole body skills such as running and jumping abilities.

## Choice of Training Speed

Most motor performance tests and actions normally thought to be athletic are performed at a fast speed. Thus, control of speed with training helps simulate athletic performance. Isokinetic training enables the athlete to select speeds ranging from 0 to 500°/s, which, more so than conventional resistance training modalities, can be used to simulate the types of muscle actions employed in his or her athletic activities (46). Furthermore, proponents of plyometrics (i.e., exercises that enable a muscle to develop maximal force in as short a time as possible, usually used by athletes to improve sport-specific power capabilities) believe that performance of fast speed actions is necessary to promote maximal increases in athletic performance. On the other hand, performance of conventional resistance training, meaning a slow or very controlled movement speed, can also result in increased motor performance. However, long-term performance of conventional resistance training may actually change the ratio of strength at a fast speed of movement (300°/s) compared to a slower speed of movement (180°/s) (6). This means that more strength was gained at the slower speed of movement as compared to the strength gained at the faster speed of movement. Over time this could result in less improvement in athletic performance than if strength was increased to a greater extent at faster speeds of movement. Isokinetic training at a fast speed of movement, on the other hand, results in increased strength at a fast speed of movement to a greater extent than training at a slow speed of movement (2). Because most motor performance tests require force output at high velocities of movement, increasing strength at high velocities of movement should result in increased athletic performance. Thus, over a long training period, performance of fast speed muscle actions, as can be performed using isokinetics, may be needed to elicit maximal gains of motor performance.

## Improvement in Performance With Training

Previous studies have shown that improved athletic performance occurs following isokinetic training. Weltman and coworkers (47) demonstrated a 10% increase in the vertical jump after 14 weeks of training three days a week for three 30-second bouts (47). Ellenbecker, Davies, and Rowinski (13) demonstrated an 11% increase in tennis serve velocity after only six weeks of study, training twice per week. Smith and Melton (41) demonstrated a variety of improvements including 4% and 5% in the vertical jump, depending upon the isokinetic group. Pipes and Wilmore (38) also demonstrated significant improvement in performance in events such as the vertical jump, 40-yard dash, and softball throw. Improvement occurred in both slow (24°/s) and fast (136°/s) groups. It is important to note that several of the studies used already well-trained athletes as subjects. This is an important consideration, because it is more difficult to induce a change in a well-trained individual than in an individual who is untrained.

# Body Composition

Both no significant change (8–10) and significant increases (11, 14) in muscle fiber area have been reported due to concentric-only isokinetic training. Increases in muscle cross-sectional area determined by computerized tomography or magnetic resonance imaging have been demonstrated following concentric-only isokinetic training (5, 23, 33). Increases in cross-sectional area in one muscle group (quadriceps) and not another (hamstrings) due to the same training program have also been shown (36). Thus, concentric-only isokinetic training can result in increased muscle fiber and muscle cross-sectional areas, resulting in increased lean body mass. These compositional changes, including increases in lean body mass and decreases in percent fat, are of the same magnitude as those induced by other types of training.

## Muscle Hypertrophy

Narici and coworkers (33) utilized magnetic resonance imaging (MRI) to demonstrate significant increases in quadriceps muscle CSA following concentric-only isokinetic training. The training included six sets of 10 repetitions of dominant leg extension at 120°/s, four times per week for 60 days. Seven axial scans were carried out on each subject before and after training to determine the changes in CSA for each muscle. These scans were taken at 2/10, 3/10, 4/10, 5/10, 6/10, 7/10, and 8/10 of the length of the femur. The results of the study indicated that significant hypertrophy (5 to 21%) occurred at various percentages of femur length for each muscle of the quadriceps femoris muscle group. In order to assess the kinetics of hypertrophy, the maximal CSA of the quadriceps group as a whole was measured at 4/10 of the length of the femur every 20th day of training. Results of statistical analysis indicated that the CSA at the maximal CSA of the quadriceps femoris increased at a rate of 0.14% per day. The study by Narici and associates (33) was a landmark investigation into the subject of isokinetic training and muscle hypertrophy.

## Training for Increased CSA

In a study reported in 1981 the authors reported a significant increase (11%) in the mean fiber area of type II muscle fibers in a group of subjects performing five sets of 12 repetitions of leg extension at 300°/s, three times per week for six weeks using concentric-only isokinetic training (11). Coyle and coworkers (11) also reported significant increases (15–24%) in strength at all velocities tested (0, 60, 180, and 300°/s). Another study trained 13 males isokinetically (concentric only) three times per week for eight weeks (23). The subjects performed six sets of 10 repetitions at a speed of contraction of 120°/s. The training involved the triceps, biceps, quadriceps, and hamstrings muscle groups. The cross-sectional areas of the triceps and biceps muscle groups as well as the individual muscles of quadriceps and hamstrings were determined using MRI. Standardized MRI scans were taken prior to and following the training at three levels (proximal, middle, and distal) of each muscle group. The results indicated that for the nondominant (trained) limbs, the training resulted in statistically significant ($p < .0008$) increases in cross-sectional areas for the arm muscles (triceps and biceps groups) ranging from 11.0% to 17.7%. For the trained thigh muscles (extensors = vastus intermedius, vastus lateralis, vastus medialis, and rectus femoris; flexors = long head of the biceps femoris, semitendinosus, and semimembranosus) there were statistically significant ($p < .0008$) increases in the cross-sectional areas, ranging from 8.0% to 34.4% (23). These results demonstrate that concentric isokinetic resistance training can lead to increased muscular hypertrophy. The statistical procedures used in the present study were very conservative, and, therefore, one can be confident that the statistically significant increases in muscle cross-sectional area and strength were not due to chance.

## Other Considerations

There are other factors to examine when considering isokinetic training. Training isokinetically has been reported to cause minimal muscular soreness (1). Because neither a free weight nor a weight stack has to be lifted in isokinetic training, the possibility of injury is minimal and no spotter is required. It is, however, difficult to judge an individual's effort unless the machine has an accurate feedback system of either the force generated or the actual work performed. Furthermore, motivation is a problem with some trainees because most equipment lacks visible movement of a weight or weight stack. Some equipment does have a monitor that displays such things as force for each repetition. Presently, this type of equipment is not widely available.

## Isokinetic Versus Dynamic Constant Resistance

Dynamic constant resistance training refers to training where the weight or resistance being lifted is constant and both lifting (concentric) and lowering (eccentric) phases occur during each repetition (16). Traditionally, isotonic training (where the muscle applies a constant tension) has been used to describe resistance training performed on free weights and various weight-training machines. However, the force exerted during such exercises varies with the joint angle and the muscle length of the movement (16). Dynamic constant resistance (DCR), therefore, will be used here to describe the aforementioned types of conventional weight-training exercises.

Certain advantages of isokinetic exercise over DCR exercise have been reported in the literature. One advantage is that with isokinetics one exercises the muscle closer to maximum through the entire range of motion of the joint.

Specifically, isokinetic exercise facilitates maximal muscle contraction at each point in a joint's available range of motion (22, 43). Conversely, because DCR exercise may place maximum demand on the muscle only during a limited portion of any range of motion (extreme of the exercise motion pattern), the total work done may be suboptimal (43). Therefore, by providing a maximal load to the active muscles during the entire range of motion with isokinetic exercise, it is possible to perform more work in the same period of time than can be accomplished with either constant resistance or variable resistance exercise (41).

In a study at Texas Women's University, muscle action potential (related to strength) was found to be "significantly greater" for isokinetic actions of the biceps muscle than for DCR actions of the same muscle (39). This seems logical because, in comparison to DCR exercises, isokinetic work is not affected by the factor of inertia, as is DCR work. Muscle length-tension curves during isometric, concentric, or eccentric muscle actions (DCR exercise) demonstrate that muscular force generated through a range of motion is not constant. With the isokinetic system, a muscle or muscle group can work maximally through the full arc of motion, resulting in superior strength gains. This optimization of strength performance with isokinetic exercise has been attributed to the accommodating contraction enabling one to do more work in the same period of time than is possible in DCR exercise (41, 46). In a 5-year study comparing isokinetics and DCR exercise, it was reported that isokinetics produces substantially better results in short- and long-term knee rehabilitation (43). The rehabilitation success over the 5-year period for the isokinetic program was a 61% success rate as compared to 7%, 0%, and 0% for DCR, home exercise, and no exercise programs, respectively. The isokinetic program had an 84% success rate in follow-up treatment over 3 years, versus 41% for the DCR exercise program (43). Pearson testing was used to correlate the rehabilitation method to the overall success rate within the 5-year study period, and the results demonstrated a significant correlation between the isokinetic exercise program and postsurgical success at the $p = .05$ significance level, whereas the no exercise, home exercise, and DCR exercise programs yielded relationships that were not significantly correlated with success (43).

In addition to allowing the muscle to work near maximal levels throughout the full range of motion, the ability to control the speed of movement with isokinetics also offers other advantages during exercise. As a rehabilitating patient progresses through his or her program, the speed of exercising can be increased above initially slow rates in accordance with neuromuscular improvement until rates simulating functional activity have been attained. Also, previous studies have shown that there is a tendency for an increase in the mean muscle fiber areas and relative muscle fiber areas, especially of type IIA fibers, which is in agreement with the recruitment and, thus, training of type II fibers at heavy dynamic (isokinetic) exercises (20).

Few studies have compared the effects of isokinetic concentric-only training and DCR training. The specificity of testing phenomenon is apparent in several of these studies, with the isokinetic training resulting in greater increases in isokinetic strength than DCR training, and the DCR training resulting in greater increases of DCR strength than the isokinetic training. However, Moffroid and associates (31) showed that it is possible for isokinetic training to result in greater increases in isometric strength than DCR training. An isokinetic group increased isometric knee extensions by 24% as compared to the DCR group's increase of 13%. The isokinetic group increased isometric knee flexion strength by 19% as compared to the DCR group's increase of 1%. It is important to note that when isometric testing is used to evaluate gains brought about by isokinetic or DCR training, testing specificity is not a concern. In addition, Pipes and Wilmore (38) also found that a 136°/s isokinetic group outperformed a DCR group when tested with DCR. While the DCR group outperformed the slow speed (24°/s) isokinetic group when tested with DCR, the slow speed isokinetic group in turn outperformed the DCR group when tested for static strength, a nontraining-specific testing mode. Another study that lends support to testing specificity between dynamic constant external resistance and isokinetic training used eight weeks of DCR or isokinetic training (34). Results from this study showed that the DCR and isokinetic training resulted in 32% and 4% increases in 1 RM strength when tested using DCR, and 8% and 12% increases in isokinetic force at 60°/s and 1% and 10% increases at 240°/s, respectively, indicating testing specificity.

Gettman, Cutler, and Strathman (19) compared changes in lean body weight and strength (as well as $\dot{V}O_2$max, body weight, and skinfold thickness) following a 20-week program of either DCR or isokinetic circuit training. The DCR group performed the following exercises using Nautilus equipment: pullover, hip and back, chest bench press, chest pull, knee extension, leg press, biceps curl, triceps curl, and leg curl. The isokinetic group performed the following exercises utilizing Cybex equipment: shoulder press, shoulder pull down, knee extension, bench press, leg press, biceps curl, triceps pull down, knee flexion, rowing push, and rowing pull. The training regimen involved three workouts per week of approximately 20 to 30 minutes per workout. Each workout involved the completion of two circuits of the exercises. Twelve repetitions of each exercise were performed at each workstation, and workstations were separated by 30-seconds rest. Subjects in the Nautilus group trained at 50% of their maximum lifting capacity at each station, and subjects in the isokinetic group trained at 60°/s. The results indicated that both the Nautilus and isokinetics group had significant increases (1.61 kg or 2.52% and 2.13 kg or 3.22% increases, respectively) in lean body weight (19). With regard to strength changes, the Nautilus group significantly increased in isotonic 1 RM leg press strength by 17.6%, whereas the isokinetic group had a 9.7% increase in DCR 1 RM leg press strength that was not statistically significant (19). Conversely, the isokinetic group showed a 41.9% increase in isokinetic leg press strength compared to no significant changes in the isokinetic leg press strength by the Nautilus group (19).

Studies comparing these two types of training indicate no clear superiority of either type over the other. After eight weeks of training, the knee extensors of an isokinetically trained group increased 47.2% in isokinetic torque, whereas a DCR group increased by 28.6% (42). Daily training of the knee extensors and flexors for four weeks shows that isokinetic training (22.5°/s) is superior to DCR training in isokinetic and isometric strength increases (31). The isokinetic and DCR groups exhibited increases in isometric knee extension force of 24% and 13%, respectively, and 19% and 1%, respectively, in isometric knee flexion force. Isokinetic peak torque at 22.5°/s of the isokinetic and DCR groups increased 11% and 3%, respectively, in knee extension and 16% and 1%, respectively, in knee flexion.

## Isokinetic Versus Variable Resistance Training

Variable resistance training uses equipment (lever arm, cam, or pulley operated) that tries to mimic the changes in strength (strength curve) throughout the range of motion of an exercise (16). By matching an exercise's strength curve, a muscle, or group of muscles, would be maximally activated throughout the entire range of motion. The efficacy with which variable resistance machines accomplish this, however, has been suggested to be quite inadequate (16).

Comparisons of isokinetic and variable resistance training also demonstrate a test specificity phenomenon. Slow and fast speed isokinetic training has been compared with variable resistance training (41). Slow speed isokinetic training consisted of one set until peak torque declined to 50% at the velocities of 30, 60, and 90°/s. Fast speed isokinetic training followed the same format as slow speed training except the velocities trained at were 180, 240, and 300°/s. Variable resistance training initially consisted of 3 sets of 10 repetitions at 80% of a 10 RM; once all sets could be completed, more resistance was added. All groups performed knee extensions and flexions only. In measures of strength the isokinetic groups demonstrated a relatively consistent pattern of test speed specificity. The variable resistance group demonstrated consistent increases in knee flexion, regardless of the test criterion, but knee extension showed large increases in isometric force only. Another study involving changes in leg press strength also supports a test specificity phenomenon between these two types of training (19). These results attest to the difficulty in identifying which type of training possesses superiority with regard to strength increases.

## Summary

Isokinetic resistance training is a viable choice of exercise to accomplish specific tasks related to motor unit recruitment, especially in upper body musculature, in speed and power development, while playing a classic role in rehabilitation. Its use as a measurement tool remains more in question as studies start to show that the high amount of specificity to the mode of training and testing are sensitive to differences between the two. Speed training in closed kinetic chain exercises may also be of benefit with this exercise modality. The proper use of this tool can augment the training of human musculature for physiological gains in muscle size and specific strength on the force-velocity curve. More research is needed to better understand this modality for use in training programs beyond its conventional use in rehabilitation from injury and in clinical assessments.

# References

1. Atha, J. 1981. Strengthening muscle. *Exerc. Sport Sci. Rev.* 9: 1–73.

2. Behm, D.G., and D.G. Sale. 1993. Intended rather than actual movement velocity determines velocity-specific training response. *Sports Med.* 15: 374–88.

3. Bell, G.J., G.D. Snydmiller, J.P. Beary, and H.A. Quinney. 1989. The effect of high and low velocity resistance training on anaerobic power output in cyclists. *J. Hum. Mov. Studies* 16: 173–81.

4. Bell, G.J., S.R. Petersen, J. Wessel, K. Bagnall, and H.A. Quinney. 1991. Adaptations to endurance and low velocity resistance training performed in sequence. *Can. J. Sport Sci.* 16: 186–92.

5. Bell, G.J., and H. Wenger. 1992. Physiological adaptations to velocity controlled resistance training. *Sports Med.* 13(4): 234–44.

6. Bell, G.J., and I. Jacobs. 1992. Velocity specificity of training in bodybuilders. *Can. J. Sports Sci.* 17: 28–33.

7. Ciriello, V.M., W.C. Holden, and W.J. Evans. 1983. The effects of two isokinetic training regimens on muscle strength and fiber composition. In *Biochemistry exercise*, ed. Knuttgen, H., Vogel, J., and Poortmans, J. 787–93. Champaign, IL: Human Kinetics.

8. Colliander, E.B., and P.A. Tesch. 1990. Effects of eccentric and concentric muscle actions in resistance training. *Acta Physiol. Scand.* 140: 31–39.

9. Costill, D.L., E.F. Coyle, W.F. Fink, G.R. Lesmes, and F.A. Witzmann. 1979. Adaptations in skeletal muscle following strength training. *J. Appl. Phys.* 46: 96–99.

10. Cote, C., J. Simoneau, P. Lagasse, M. Boulay, M. Thibault, M. Marcotte, and C. Bouchard. 1988. Isokinetic strength-training protocols: Do they induce skeletal muscle fiber hypertrophy? *Arch. Phys. Med. Rehab.* 69: 281–85.

11. Coyle, E., D.C. Feiring, T.C. Rotkis, R.W. Cote, F.B. Roby, W. Lee, and J.H. Wilmore. 1981. Specificity of power improvements through slow and fast isokinetic training. *J. Appl. Phys.* 51: 1437–42.

12. Davies, A.H. 1977. Chronic effects of isokinetic and allokinetic training on muscle force, endurance, and muscular hypertrophy. *Dissertation Abstracts International.* 38: 153A.

13. Ellenbecker, T.S., G.J. Davies, and M.J. Rowinski. 1988. Concentric versus eccentric isokinetic strengthening of the rotator cuff. *Am. J. Sports Med.* 16(1): 64–69.

14. Ewing, J.L., D.R. Wolfe, M.A. Rogers, M.L. Amundson, and G.A. Stull. 1990. Effects of velocity of isokinetic training on strength, power, and quadriceps muscle fiber characteristics. *Eur. J. Appl. Phys.* 61: 159–62.

15. Fleck, S.J. 1979. Varying frequency and intensity of isokinetic strength training. *Dissertation Abstracts International.* 39: 2126A.

16. Fleck, S.J., and W.J. Kraemer. 1997. *Designing resistance training programs.* 2d ed. Champaign, IL: Human Kinetics.

17. Gettman, L.R., J.J. Ayres, M.L. Pollock, and A. Jackson. 1978. The effect of circuit training on strength, cardiorespiratory function, and body composition of adult men. *Med. Sci. Sports* 10: 171–76.

18. Gettman, L.R., J.J. Ayres, M.L. Pollock, J.C. Durstine, and W. Grantham. 1979. Physiological effects on adult men of circuit strength training and jogging. *Arch. Phys. Med. Rehab.* 60: 115–20.

19. Gettman, L.R., L.A. Cutler, and T. Strathman. 1980. Physiological changes after 20 weeks of isotonic vs. isokinetic circuit training. *J. Sports Med. Phys. Fit.* 20: 265–74.

20. Grimby, G., and O. Hook. 1979. Rehabilitation medicine in Sweden. Part 2: Education and research. *Int. Rehab. Med.* 1(4): 213–15.

21. Hinson, M., and J. Rosentswieg. 1973. Comparative electromyographic values of isometric, isotonic, and isokinetic contraction. *Res. Quart.* 44(1): 71–78.

22. Hislop, H., and J. Perrine. 1967. The isokinetic concept of exercise. *Phys. Ther.* 47: 114–17.

23. Housh, D.J., T.J. Housh, G.O. Johnson, and W.K. Chu. 1992. Hypertrophic response to unilateral concentric isokinetic training. *J. Appl. Phys.* 73(1): 65–70.

24. Jenkins, W.L., M. Thackaberry, and C. Killian. 1984. Speed-specific isokinetic training. *J. Orth. Sports Phys. Ther.* 6: 181–83.

25. Kanehisa, H., and M. Miyashita. 1983. Effect of isometric and isokinetic muscle training on static strength and dynamic power. *Eur. J. Appl. Phys.* 50: 365–71.

26. Knapik, J.J., J.E. Wright, R.H. Mawdsley, and J. Braun. 1983. Isometric, isotonic, and isokinetic torque variations in four muscle groups through a range of joint motion. *Phys. Ther.* 63: 938–47.

27. Lander, J.E., B.T. Bates, J.A. Sawhill, and J.A. Hamill. 1985. Comparison between free weight and isokinetic bench pressing. *Med. Sci. Sports Exerc.* 17(3): 344–53.

28. Lacerte, M., B.J. deLateur, A.D. Alquist, and K.A. Questad. 1992. Concentric versus combined concentric-eccentric isokinetic training programs: Effect on peak torque of human quadriceps femoris muscle. *Arch. Phys. Med. Rehab.* 73: 1059–62.

29. Lesmes, G.R., D.L. Costill, E.F. Coyle, and W.J. Fink. 1978. Muscle strength and power changes during maximal isokinetic training. *Med. Sci. Sports* 4: 266–69.

30. Mannion, A.F., P.M. Jakeman, and P.L.T. Willan. 1992. Effect of isokinetic training of the knee extensors on isokinetic strength and peak power output during cycling. *Eur. J. Appl. Phys.* 65: 370–75.

31. Moffroid, M.A., R.H. Whipple, J. Hofkosh, E. Lowman, and H. Thistle. 1969. A study of isokinetic exercise. *Phys. Ther.* 49: 735–47.

32. Moffroid, M.A., and R.H. Whipple. 1970. Specificity of speed of exercise. *Phys. Ther.* 50: 1693–99.

33. Narici, M.V., G.S. Roi, L. Landoni, A.E. Minetti, and P. Cerretelli. 1989. Changes in force, cross-sectional area, and neural activation during strength training and detraining of the human quadriceps. *Eur J. App. Phys.* 59: 310–19.

34. Pearson, D.R., and D.L. Costill. 1988. The effects of constant external resistance exercise and isokinetic exercise training on work induced hypertrophy. *J. Appl. Sport Sci. Res.* 3: 39–41.

35. Petersen, S.R., G.D. Miller, H.A. Quinney, and H.A. Wenger. 1987. The effectiveness of a mini-cycle on velocity-specific strength acquisition. *J. Orth. Sports Phys. Ther.* 9: 156–59.

36. Petersen, S., J. Wessel, K. Bagnall, H. Wilkens, A. Quenney, and H. Wenger. 1990. Influence of concentric resistance training on concentric and eccentric strength. *Arch. Phys. Med. Rehab.* 71: 101–5.

37. Pincivero, D.M., S.M. Lephart, and R.G. Karunakara. 1997. Effects of rest interval on isokinetic strength and functional performance after short term high intensity training. *Brit. J. Sports Med.* 31: 229–34.

38. Pipes, T.V., and J.H. Wilmore. 1975. Isokinetic vs. isotonic strength training in adult men. *Med. Sci. Sports* 7(4): 262–74.

39. Rosentswieg, J., and M. Hinson. 1972. Comparison of isometric, isotonic, and isokinetic exercises by electomyography. *Arch. Phys. Med. Rehab.* 53: 249–52.

40. Seaborne, D., and A.W. Taylor. 1984. The effects of speed of isokinetic exercise on training transfer to isometric strength in the quadriceps. *J. Sports Med.* 24: 183–88.

41. Smith, M.J., and P. Melton. 1981. Isokinetic versus isotonic variable resistance training. *Am. J. Sports Med.* 9(4): 275–79.

42. Thistle, H.G., H.J. Hislop, M. Moffroid, and E.W. Lowman. 1967. Isokinetic contraction: A new concept in resistive exercise. *Arch. Phys. Med. Rehab.* 48: 279–82.

43. Timm, K. 1985. Postsurgical knee rehabilitation. *Am. J. Sports Med.* 16(5): 463–68.

44. Tomberline, J.P., J.R. Basford, E.E. Schwen, P.A. Orte, S.C. Scott, R.K. Laughman, and D.M. Ilstrud. 1991. Comparative study of isokinetic eccentric and concentric quadriceps training. *J. Orth. Sports Phys. Ther.* 14: 31–36.

45. Van Oteghen, S. 1975. Two speeds of isokinetic exercise as related to the vertical jump performance of women. *Res. Quart.* 46(1): 78–84.

46. Watkins, M., and B. Harris. 1983. Evaluation of isokinetic muscle performance. *Clin. Sports Med.* 2(1): 37–53.

47. Weltman, A., C. Janney, C. Rians, K. Strand, B. Berg, S. Tippit, J. Wise, B. Cahill, and F. Katch. 1986. The effects of hydraulic resistance strength training in prepubertal males. *Med. Sci. Sports Exerc.* 18: 629–38.

48. Wilmore, J.H., and D.L. Costill. 1994. *Physiology of sport and exercise.* Champaign, IL: Human Kinetics.

# Chapter 3

# Correlations With Athletic Performance

Tim V. Wrigley

**W**hile isokinetic dynamometry is widely used, it has been believed in some quarters that it is not "specific" to athletic performance. This contention usually stems from a face-validity position: How can movements performed at relatively slow, constant angular velocities—usually at single joints—be closely related to the performance of athletic activities that involve high, nonconstant velocities, and usually involve movement at multiple joints?

On first inspection, this would appear to be a relatively clear-cut case. But as Rothstein (203) has warned, "Face validity is the lowest form of validity because it reflects only whether a test *appears* to do what it is supposed to do" [emphasis added] (p. 17). In contrast, the strongest form of validity, *criterion-related validity*, is assessed by directly testing the relationship between scores on the test whose validity is in question (i.e., isokinetic dynamometry) and by direct measures of the characteristics of interest (i.e., various athletic performances) (146).

Therefore, the main focus of this chapter is the criterion-related validity of isokinetic dynamometry. It is not widely known that a substantial number of research studies exist on this issue—mainly for jumping, sprinting, throwing, kicking, swimming, and cycling—but they have never been reviewed in totality before.

The chapter first considers in general terms the role of strength in different sports. Then, the published experimental research evidence for the relationship between isokinetic measures and various athletic performances, that is, criterion-related validity, is reviewed. Many of the issues that must be considered in interpreting this evidence are briefly outlined. Next, explanations for the conclusions that emerge from the research evidence are considered, in terms of the biomechanics and neuromuscular physiology of isokinetic and athletic movements. Finally, potential ways in which the relationship between isokinetic dynamometry and athletic performance might be improved are canvassed.

# The Role of Strength in Athletic Performance

The relative importance of strength in relation to other factors varies among sports. Different sports can be considered as lying on a continuum. At one extreme are sports for which strength is critical—these may be termed *strength-limited* or *strength-dependent* sports. At the other extreme are *strength-independent* sports, for which strength is of minor or no importance. Between these two extremes are *strength-related* sports, for which strength is important but not critical to performance success.

The determination of the relevance of strength for a given sport should be based on the correlation between strength measures (isokinetic or otherwise) and performance and the ability of such measures to discriminate between elite and subelite performers.

Correlation between strength and athletic performance will be most readily demonstrated for strength-limited sports. High correlation will be more difficult to demonstrate for strength-related sports, as elite athletes in such sports may demonstrate exceptional levels of either strength, endurance, speed, or skill (or combinations thereof), each of which may be compatible with elite performance. However, there may still be particular tasks within these sports that are strength limited. A broader range of strength and task performance scores may be found among athletes in these strength-limited sports, however, again because exceptional performance on all such tasks may not be necessary for elite performance.

The *lack* of a measured correlation between a given strength assessment and performance for a particular sport may indicate

- a lack of relevance of strength to that performance,
- the insensitivity of the strength assessment methods to performance-specific strength,
- a requirement for only a threshold level of strength (above which increased strength does not correlate with increased performance), or
- problems with the strength or athletic performance measurement (e.g., poor test-retest reliability).

In the elite athlete context, it is likely that differences in actual competition performance levels, as determined by physiological and biomechanical measures, may be relatively small among athletes. This can make it difficult to demonstrate correlation between any physiological or biomechanical parameter and athletic performance (e.g., 68, 70, 215, 253).

Before focusing on the major issues of this chapter, two points need to be made. First, note that no dichotomous distinction between strength and power is made in this chapter. Muscle force—and thus joint torque—can be developed across the entire concentric/eccentric force-velocity (and torque-velocity) continuum. Performance of particular athletic tasks may depend on an athlete's abilities in certain regions of this continuum (e.g., high force/low velocity, or high velocity/low concentric force). It is unrealistic to narrow the focus to simple notions of strength and power; nor is it the aim to delve into definitional issues in relation to these terms (262). Therefore, for the purposes of this chapter, the term strength is used generically to refer to the generation of force by muscle and the application of that force—via muscle-joint systems—in an athletic context. When the velocity at which strength must be exerted is significant in a particular instance, that will be noted.

Second, note that the term specificity is used in several different ways in exercise science. In physiological testing, specificity typically refers to the use of testing methods that bear a close *physical resemblance* to the movement patterns and intensity of the sporting activity. It is assumed—and sometimes actually known from research evidence—that such methods also bear a close relationship to the *physiological* requirements of the sport. The ultimate proof of such specificity is a high correlation between test performance and athletic performance. This is the criterion for specificity that is used in this chapter.

# Correlation With Athletic Performance

At the time of writing, there are over sixty studies that have demonstrated a correlation between isokinetic strength and athletic performance. Most of these studies cover five categories of athletic performances:

- jumping (11, 12, 29, 35, 77, 88, 103, 139, 144, 161, 167, 169, 174, 181, 183, 185, 186, 197, 198, 230, 255, 258, 265)
- sprinting (7, 9, 20, 24, 52, 76, 90, 92, 103, 106, 116, 153, 159, 176, 181, 218)
- throwing (17, 66, 123, 172, 179, 180, 202, 251, 254)
- kicking (35, 56, 154, 158, 188)
- swimming (18, 39, 122, 153, 155, 171)
- other performances (43, 74, 144, 184, 220, 223)

All of the above studies have reported correlations of 0.5 or higher (most substantially higher) between an isokinetic measure and an athletic performance measure; 0.5 was chosen in light of the many issues related to the level and interpretation of correlation coefficients, as discussed in the following sections. A more extensive review of the above studies had to be omitted due to space constraints. There is also a large number of studies that have addressed the correlation between isokinetic measures and cycling performance in cycle ergometry; these are also discussed below.

The number of known studies that have been unable to find a correlation between isokinetic strength and athletic performance are relatively few (63, 65, 101, 148, 150, 243). In some cases, explanations for such findings are obvious; for example, Housh and coworkers (101) did not find an isokinetic correlation with an athletic performance—middle distance running—that is unlikely to be strength limited. In the studies that have found substantial correlation between athletic performance and a particular isokinetic parameter, other isokinetic parameters investigated within these studies have not necessarily yielded good correlations (e.g., 7). Therefore, it is possible that the studies that did not find good correlations might have done so had the choice of isokinetic measurement parameters or muscle group(s) been different.

The way in which the isokinetic data is handled, such as whether strength is expressed relative to body mass or not, may affect the strength of the correlation between isokinetic measures and athletic performance. For example, Farrar and Thorland (65) failed to find an association between absolute isokinetic strength and sprint performance. A failure to scale the torque data for differences in body mass is likely to explain the lack of a substantial correlation, especially given the other studies of sprinting that have found such a correlation when body mass differences were accounted for, such as those listed above.

Since sprinting requires that the athlete's body mass be moved by muscle action, it makes sense that a relative strength expression rather than absolute strength should correlate with performance. For other athletic performances, absolute strength may be the appropriate expression. For example, Cohen and associates (43) found that tennis service velocity was more closely related to absolute strength, presumably because racket velocity is enhanced by greater absolute strength and not limited by body mass. Such issues are discussed further under Body Mass, Isokinetic Strength, and Athletic Performance.

# Correlation Between Isokinetic Dynamometry and Anaerobic Ergometry

Cycle ergometry is the most common laboratory test of anaerobic power and endurance of athletes. In such tests, maximum, all-out efforts are performed on a cycle ergometer (*not* usually a constant velocity ergometer) over a short time period, from as short as 10 seconds to as long as 60 seconds. Many studies have demonstrated relatively high correlations between isokinetic parameters and cycle ergometer anaerobic test results (15, 31, 51, 67, 106, 138, 157, 176, 177, 219, 221, 242, 261). Good correlations have also been found between isokinetic measures and the results of other common anaerobic ergometry tests (19, 29, 138, 139, 198). Few studies have not found such correlations (132, 133).

# Interpretation of Correlation Coefficients

When interpreting the magnitude of a Pearson product moment correlation coefficient between strength (the predictor) and athletic performance (the criterion), phenomena that may artificially raise or lower a correlation should also be borne in mind:

   • The effective upper limit on the correlation coefficient is the square root of the test-retest reliability coefficient (57). For example, a variable with a test-retest reliability of .80 cannot have a correlation with another variable of greater than .91. The reliability of isokinetic dynamometry has generally been found to be high (84, 163), albeit having been studied mainly with nonathletes. However, the reliability of the criterion athletic performances against which isokinetic strength has been correlated has rarely been considered; there is some evidence to suggest that such performances are subject to varying levels of reliability, which are sometimes poor (e.g., 97).

• The interpretation of $r^2$—the coefficient of determination—as the proportion of variance in the predicted variable (e.g., athletic performance) explained by the predictor variable (e.g., isokinetic strength) may underestimate this explained variance (170, 173).

• A lack of statistical significance, while suggesting some caution in the interpretation of the correlation coefficient, should not preclude consideration of the "practical" significance of the correlation, as large sample sizes are necessary to achieve statistical significance for even relatively low correlations (212, 215).

• The correlation coefficient may be inflated or deflated by unrealistic heterogeneity or homogeneity in the data (99, 206).

## Multifactorial Nature of Athletic Performance

When interpreting the importance of a correlation between a single measure of strength and a measure of athletic performance, it is important to remember that athletic performance success is, more often than not, multifactorial. Strength may be required in combination in particular muscle groups, for particular muscle actions, and at particular joints, positions, and angular velocities. In this light, to expect a single strength measure to explain all athletic performance variance is unreasonable.

Multiple regression studies would thus be expected to yield higher correlation coefficients when individual isokinetic variables (which may have yielded only moderate univariate correlations) are combined. However, relatively few such studies have been performed. An example of such studies is that of isokinetic strength and sprint time among elite Canadian sprinters by Alexander (7), which yielded an $r^2$ of .99 for the females and .67 for the males; the $r^2$s for the univariate correlations of individual isokinetic measures were below .5. High multivariate correlations between isokinetic measures and sprint performance have been found in other studies (9, 20, 76), again where the univariate correlations were often much lower.

In these multivariate studies and the univariate correlation studies of sprint performance, a range of isokinetic parameters has been found to correlate with sprint performance. This suggests that different isokinetic measures may be sensitive to different elements of sprint-related strength. The work of Delecluse and associates (52) has provided further explanation for the variation in correlated parameters across these studies. By measuring sprint performance at

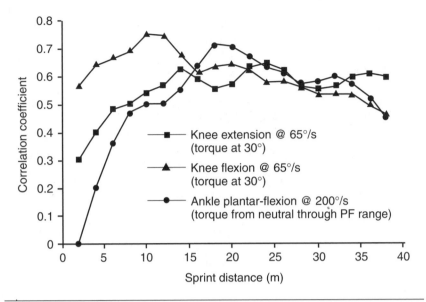

**Figure 3.1**   Correlation between three isokinetic measurement parameters and sprint velocities, at 2-meter intervals over a 40-meter sprint.

Modified from Delecluse et al. (52).

2-meter intervals over a 40-meter distance, these authors were able to show how the correlation of sprint performance with different knee and ankle isokinetic strength parameters varied with distance (see figure 3.1). Some knee and ankle isokinetic parameters appeared to be more closely associated with performance during the acceleration phase, while others correlated more highly with performance once sprint velocity had begun to level out.

Thus while some sports are clearly multifactorial, others may not always appear to be so. Studies such as that of Delecluse and associates (52) are important in highlighting the fact that while a sport may have a single, ultimate performance criterion (e.g., sprint time), the achievement of this ultimate criterion may occur only by satisfying a number of performance requirements, which may be related or may be quite dissimilar. Thus, more sophisticated measurement and statistical models may be required to delineate the important factors in athletic performance.

## Isokinetic Discrimination Between Athletes

Many studies have found isokinetic dynamometry to discriminate among:

- athletes in different sports (10, 58, 78, 83, 86, 95, 104, 105, 112, 119, 126, 130, 135, 141, 151, 192, 193, 206, 219, 224, 231, 232, 233, 236, 237, 242, 247, 259, 264), and

- different competition levels or positional roles within a single sport (3, 14, 34, 37, 40, 45, 48, 49, 65, 74, 82, 83, 85, 92, 93, 108, 119, 120, 121, 131, 134, 136, 147, 152, 156, 165, 166, 167, 182, 200, 209, 210, 217, 222, 249, 260, 264).

Discrimination between athletes and nonathletes has been demonstrated in other studies but is not considered relevant here.

The isokinetic test results in a relatively small number of studies have been unable to discriminate among athletes of different performance abilities (73, 195, 196, 199), positional roles (4, 5, 6, 50, 168), or between different sports (114, 192). Such results may indeed be a reflection of poor discriminating ability of isokinetic testing for these athletic groups. Alternatively, factors such as sample homogeneity or sample size may have confounded the results of these studies, or the isokinetic parameters chosen may not have been the most appropriate. Tesch (237) reported that while some isokinetic parameters discriminated between elite skiers, others did not. Similarly, Imwold and coworkers (105) found that some parameters discriminated between female college basketball and track athletes, while others did not.

However, perhaps the most likely explanation for the lack of discrimination in some studies stems from the fact that one should not automatically assume that the strength requirements of different sports, performance levels, or positional roles are in fact markedly different. For example, the absence of a relationship between lower limb isokinetic strength and provincial ranking among middle distance runners in Ready (195) is hardly remarkable. Regarding differences between sports, one would not expect to find such differences between sports that are strength independent or only strength related (e.g., 192). Also, strength-limited sports with similar requirements for strength, or similar strength training regimes, might fail to exhibit differences in isokinetic strength; for example, Johnson and associates (114) did not find differences between female bodybuilders and power lifters.

Figure 3.2 shows torque/body mass ratios for concentric knee extension peak torque at 60, 180, and 300°/s, recorded by a wide range of male American college athletes (192). While some interesting patterns are apparent, it would appear that the means and standard deviations for many sports are similar. As such, the knee extension torque/body mass ratio may not clearly discriminate between many sports. This suggests that a similar type of relative strength is required for success in these sports. However, the evidence from the correlation studies would suggest that *within* many of these sports, performance success for various athletic tasks is closely related to isokinetic strength.

Reilly and coworkers (196) did not find a difference in isokinetic shoulder strength between high and low speed male collegiate freestyle swimmers. An interesting but speculative explanation for a similar finding of no correlation between swim bench strength, or power, and swim performance among elite swimmers was put forward by Sharp (216) and may have broader relevance. Sharp suggested that the wide spread of power scores (albeit nonisokinetic)

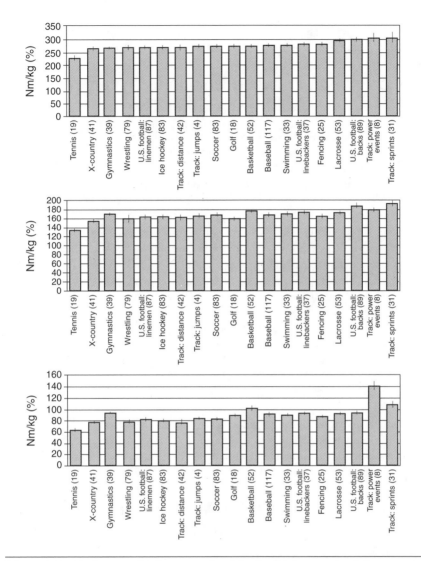

**Figure 3.2** Peak torque/body mass ratios (Nm/kg %) for concentric knee extension at 60 (top), 180 (middle), and 300 (bottom) °/s, from a range of male American college athletes.

Data from Rankin and Thompson (192).

among elite competitors might be explained by an increased need for power by inefficient swimmers with body types creating increased drag forces, while swimmers with efficient strokes and body types might require less power. This would indicate that strength or power might be vital for elite swim performance, but only in some athletes. Thus the same event may be strength- or power-*limited* for some athletes, but only strength- or power-*related* for others.

Such speculations raise the possibility that the relationship between strength and performance may be more complex than has often been assumed.

## Correlation Between Isokinetic Dynamometry and Muscle Fiber Type

Isokinetic dynamometry has been the standard tool used by physiologists to investigate dynamic human muscle function of single muscle groups for over two decades. Among their findings that bear on the question of the relationship between isokinetic measures and muscle performance, there is a substantial body of evidence supporting the relationship between isokinetic measures and muscle fiber type. This lends support to the notion that isokinetic dynamometry assesses "'generic" characteristics of muscle. Furthermore, these fiber type characteristics are known to be important factors in the athletic performances requiring either high speed or endurance (208). Thus, the sensitivity of isokinetic measures to these performance determinants helps to explain the positive findings in the studies of the correlation between isokinetic measures and athletic performance.

Numerous studies have demonstrated an association of muscle fiber composition or relative area with high velocity concentric isokinetic performance, mainly for the knee extensors (28, 42, 46, 78, 79, 89, 106, 107, 112, 136, 137, 142, 164, 204, 205, 219, 225, 234, 241, 244, 245, 247, 250, 263). A relatively small number of studies have not found such correlations (41, 71, 75, 207, 211).

While most studies have found muscle fiber composition to correlate with higher velocity isokinetic strength, findings on the correlation with lower velocity isokinetic and isometric performance present a more equivocal picture (see, for example, the review in 124).

## Isokinetic Anaerobic Muscular Endurance, Fiber Type, and Athletic Performance

Just as some sports are strength-limited, some sports are *anaerobic endurance-limited*. For example, Haymes and Dickinson (93) found a good correlation (.80 for males, .78 for females) between the international ranking of elite slalom skiers and their concentric isokinetic knee extensor endurance at 180°/s.

A correlation between muscle fiber composition and concentric isokinetic endurance has been found in many studies—a high proportion of fast twitch fibers, or equivalently a low proportion of slow twitch fibers, has been found to be associated with a more rapid decline in concentric torque generation over the duration of a test consisting of multiple, continuous, maximum effort repetitions, usually 20 or more (44, 109, 117, 125, 141, 162, 225, 234, 235, 239, 241, 246, 250). Thus, sprint athletes will generally exhibit a more rapid fatigue than endurance athletes (111, 141). A small number of studies have not found a correlation between muscle fiber type and isokinetic endurance (41, 42, 240).

Interestingly, the strongest athletes tend to show the greatest concentric fatigue (e.g., 41, 42, 80, 115, 178). This finding possibly reflects a greater proportion of fast twitch fibers in such athletes, which confers greater strength at slow velocities (via the typically greater cross-sectional area of fast twitch fibers) and at fast velocities (due to the faster cross-bridge cycling time of fast twitch fibers) but also greater fatigability due to the metabolic profile of fast twitch fibers. Inbar, Kaiser, and Tesch (106), for example, found a significant correlation between vastus lateralis fast twitch fiber percentage and both (1) knee extension peak torque and (2) percent decline in peak torque over 50 repetitions at 180°/s.

Eccentric isokinetic endurance has only rarely been assessed, and its significance is uncertain. Eccentric fatigue occurs at a much slower rate than concentric fatigue for the same muscle group (55, 64, 87, 145, 238). Johansson (111) presented a case study that suggested that eccentric isokinetic endurance testing in runners might reveal information not apparent from concentric testing. While there was little evidence to suggest that such findings might discriminate between athletes of different performance abilities, the recent study of Westblad, Svedenhag, and Rolf (256) has raised this possibility. These authors found good correlations (up to .77) between physiological measures of treadmill performance in elite 800- to 5000-meter runners and eccentric isokinetic endurance.

# Seasonal Changes in Isokinetic Strength

Foster, Thompson, and Snyder (70) argued that a vital criterion for an athlete assessment methodology is that it can track longitudinal changes. A number of studies have shown isokinetic dynamometry to be sensitive to seasonal changes in athletic strength, presumably reflecting an athlete's overall training and competition intensity, in-season strength training, and possibly also overtraining (8, 36, 62, 69, 72, 81, 91, 96, 100, 113, 127–129, 143, 187, 194, 201; see figure 3.35 in 206).

# Summary of Correlation Evidence

As noted in the chapter introduction, it has been thought in some quarters that isokinetic dynamometry is not specific to athletic performance, because constant velocity movements are rarely found in sports, and because the maximum velocities of isokinetic dynamometers do not approach the velocities often observed in the actual athletic performances. These essentially theoretical, face-validity challenges to the specificity of isokinetic dynamometry would seem to have been seriously questioned by the positive evidence of criterion-related validity offered by the correlation studies.

Isokinetic dynamometry has been shown to correlate with athletic performances that do not occur at constant velocity; hence the imposition of constant velocity in a strength assessment does not appear to be of any great importance in terms of the mechanical output (257). Furthermore, the correlations have been demonstrated at angular velocities often well below peak velocities observed during the athletic performances. The assertion that the range of angular velocities at which isokinetic dynamometers operate is deficient appears to reflect an overly simplistic understanding of the generation of high velocities during athletic movements.

The "high" velocity movements assessed by isokinetic dynamometry are almost always single-joint movements. The maximum isokinetic test angular velocity for most dynamometers is in the range of 300 to 500°/s. By comparison, the maximum unloaded, peak angular velocity for isolated knee extension, for example, is of the order of 500 to 700°/s (27, 102, 245). As for how this compares to functional sporting activities, the knee may reach a peak extension velocity of around 2000°/s during a punt kick, for example (189). The maximum velocities in sporting movements such as these usually occur at distal joints in a multijoint kinematic chain (38, 190), after acceleration across several joints, and often over a large range of motion. Thus peak velocities seen in multijoint sporting movements may be at least several times greater than the maximum velocity that can be achieved for isolated movement at the same joint.

When high velocities are observed during sporting activities, they typically occur during ballistic movements. Such movements are the result of a large burst of agonist muscle activity at the beginning of the movement that accelerates the limb segment in the desired direction. This often occurs in the concentric phase of an eccentric/concentric, stretch-shortening cycle, with the muscle in a high state of activation as a result of the preceding eccentric muscle action. Thus the concentric phase of the movement commences from zero velocity, in the transition between movement directions (which corresponds approximately to the transition from eccentric to concentric muscle action). As such, much of the muscle activation during movement is associated with limb acceleration over a range of relatively slow velocities that increase from zero velocity. Very high velocities are typically not reached until well into the range of motion. Therefore, much of the movement will be over a range of velocities that increases from zero through the velocity range offered by isokinetic dynamometers.

Furthermore, *any* addition of resistance—such as that applied and measured by an isokinetic dynamometer—must reduce the maximum angular velocity at which an isolated joint can be moved (e.g., 1). Even just the weight of the limb and dynamometer lever arm limit the velocity that can be achieved. For example, when isokinetic knee extension measurements have been attempted at a velocity of 600°/s, many subjects were unable to move the limb and lever arm fast enough to reach this preset velocity (47). Taylor and coworkers (231) found that knee extensor tests at a nominal velocity of 450°/s involved very little time actually spent at this velocity, due to the relatively large proportion of the range of motion needed by subjects to accelerate the limb and lever arm up to that velocity and to decelerate as the end of the range of motion was approached. Brown and associates (32) found that none of their elite male junior tennis players was able to move the limb and lever arm fast enough to reach 450°/s for shoulder internal and external rotation.

In summary, maximum isokinetic test angular velocities are less than maximum, single, unloaded, isolated joint angular velocities by a relatively small margin that is consistent with the effect of adding resistance to movement, as must occur with any form of strength assessment. Furthermore, these isokinetic angular velocities are less than *functional* peak velocities by virtue of restricting the movement to a single joint. As such, the maximum velocities of isokinetic dynamometers do not represent a limitation of the dynamometers but are an obligatory reflection of the physics involved.

Indeed, if the above explanations were not the case, isokinetic dynamometry could not have been found to be sensitive to muscle fiber type differences, at isolated joint isokinetic velocities well below the functional athletic performance velocities at which athletes with higher fast twitch fiber composition show superiority in athletic performance. Similarly, correlations between isokinetic performances and high velocity athletic performances could not have been found at isokinetic velocities well below the maximum velocities that are seen during such athletic performances.

# Improving the Correlation Between Isokinetic Dynamometry and Athletic Performance

The evidence from the correlation studies suggests that isokinetic dynamometry is sensitive to some of the important characteristics of a range of athletic performances. However, if we are to improve the ability of isokinetic dynamometry to discriminate performance-related strength, particularly in strength-limited sports, we must ask where there might be room for improvement in the conduct of isokinetic dynamometry.

The majority of the correlation studies have investigated only concentric isokinetic performance, usually employing reciprocal or single muscle actions. Despite this, correlations have been found with athletic performances that involve eccentric muscle actions and particular muscle action sequences, such as eccentric/concentric, stretch-shortening cycles. However, better correlations may result if isokinetic dynamometry is adapted to measure the most relevant muscle actions and sequences and the most critical ranges of motion. Our knowledge of exactly what are these most critical performance determinants is not well developed. More precise isokinetic and performance assessment methods, often combined with muscle modeling, will hopefully refine our judgments regarding the most appropriate assessment techniques. For example, the work of Bobbert and van Ingen Schenau (25, 26) has highlighted the importance of early muscle activation to jumping performance. They found that a faster activation rate in isokinetic plantarflexion more closely approximated that seen during jumping.

It is important to note that there is very little evidence to suggest that agonist/antagonist muscle group strength ratios, such as the concentric hamstring/quadriceps torque ratio, bear any relationship to performance success for any athletic performance. There are a number of possible reasons for this. First, relatively few studies have investigated this issue. Of the more commonly calculated isokinetic muscle group strength ratios, the shoulder internal/external rotation peak torque ratio is among the very few that have been found to relate to an athletic performance. Cohen and associates (43) found this ratio to be predictive of tennis serve velocity among elite male players. A higher ratio was associated with greater serve velocity. Fleck and coworkers (66) found that the horizontal shoulder adduction/abduction concentric peak torque ratio at 300°/s correlated with handball throwing velocity in U.S. squad members.

Second, one can question the logic behind some apparently popular muscle group strength ratios. For example, while the concentric hamstring/quadriceps ratio was measured from the early days of isokinetic dynamometry because it *could* be measured (while the ability to measure eccentric muscle actions came later), it is not clear that the justified interest in hamstring strength should be pursued by relating concentric hamstring strength to concentric quadriceps strength. More recent efforts have been directed toward devising ratios that relate more closely to the way in which the hamstrings are employed during functional activities (e.g., 2, 30, 59, 61).

The development of isokinetic test protocols to assess the important stretch-shortening cycle (23, 94, 226, 227) should allow investigation of this important element of many athletic performances. In some strength-limited sports with specific, clearly defined strength tasks, some efforts have been directed toward designing specific configurations of isokinetic dynamometers that attempt to mimic athletic tasks more closely (e.g., 16, 60, 74, 118, 122, 191, 219, 252). Also, isokinetic dynamometers allowing multijoint movements are now commercially available (e.g., 12, 98, 110).

The possible inadequacy of univariate correlation, in relation to multifactorial athletic performance, has already been raised. The use of multiple regression, including regression diagnostics (e.g., 144) and more sophisticated mathematical models should improve the understanding of the important factors in the relationship between strength and athletic performance. In most cases, where athletic performance is multijoint rather than single joint, such models should allow consideration of the isokinetic strength about all relevant joints.

In addition to the potential for improvement in the measurement of the isokinetic variable, part of the difficulty in achieving higher correlations with athletic performance may lie with the variability of the criterion athletic performance itself (e.g., 97), as noted previously. Therefore, correlation studies must test the reliability of these performance parameters and only utilize reliable parameters.

# Body Mass, Isokinetic Strength, and Athletic Performance

Use of relative strength indexes such as the torque/body mass ratio is assumed to facilitate interindividual comparisons between athletes, by *appropriately* scaling absolute strength measures for differences in body mass. There is good evidence for the correlation of torque/body mass ratios and various athletic performances among the correlation studies reviewed in this chapter. However, it has rarely been questioned whether the use of body mass in this way is indeed the most appropriate approach.

Some authors have suggested that without a strong statistical correlation between torque and body mass, the use of torque/body mass ratios is not justified (33, 53, 54). While there is usually a substantial correlation between torque and body mass among athletes, this statistical criterion does not provide a convincing, rigorous approach to this issue.

One or both of two assumptions are probably implicitly being made when practitioners choose to use the simple torque/body mass ratio (262):

1. Functional sporting performance is limited by body mass and, therefore, the torque/body mass ratio expresses strength relative to this limitation.

2. Body mass is a reflection of muscle mass and, therefore, is an appropriate means of controlling for differences in force generating "potential" between athletes.

Regarding the first of these assumptions, approaches to discerning the exact nature of body mass limitations on various athletic performances are not straightforward. One cannot simply assume that if the athlete's body mass must be supported, then it is reasonable to express strength relative to body mass (to the power of 1). More precise determination of the way in which body mass limits athletic performance should be based on detailed biomechanical and physiological studies of the athletic performances in question (e.g., 21, 22, 160, 175, 214, 228, 229, 248).

Regarding the second assumption, "allometry" provides a more direct means to determine how torque production is related to body mass. Allometry is the study of changes in biological processes associated with changes or differences in body size. Human bodies are generally deemed to obey geometric similarity, that is, differences in body size do not generally involve changes in shape: a large body is just a scaling up of a small body and vice versa (13, 149, 213). Under this principle, it is possible to discern theoretically how strength—measured as joint torque—should relate to body mass, for example. A full discussion of allometric scaling of strength is beyond the scope of this chapter, but a brief introduction will highlight its importance in understanding the interrelationships of isokinetic strength, body mass, and athletic performance.

Under geometric similarity, linear dimensions (L) in two bodies scale in direct proportion to each other. Consequently, areas (A) in two such bodies will be related by a ratio of the respective linear dimensions raised to the power of two $(A:L^2)$ and volumes (V) will be related by a ratio of the linear dimensions raised to the third power $(V:L^3)$. Since muscle force (F) is directly related to its cross-sectional area, this force should scale with linear dimensions (e.g., stature, limb length) to the second power (i.e., $F:A:L^2$).

The torque (T) that can be generated at a joint by a muscle is given by the muscle force (F) multiplied by the moment arm (r) of the muscle. So while force should scale with linear dimensions squared $(F:L^2)$ under geometric similarity, the moment arm length should scale with linear dimensions to the power of 1 $(r:L^1)$. Thus torque, being the product of these two, should scale with linear dimensions to the power of 3 $(T:L^3)$. As indicated above, volume, and therefore mass (density is generally size independent), also scale with linear dimensions to the power of three in geometrically similar bodies. Therefore, torque should scale with body mass (M) in such bodies $(T:L^3:M)$.

The use of the simple torque/body mass ratio assumes that torque scales with body mass (to the power of 1); thus, geometric similarity supports the use of this scaling inherent in the torque/body mass ratio. However, strength is usually applied as force at the end of a limb. Under geometric similarity, this force scales with body mass to the power of 2/3. For example, weightlifting records correspond closely to the competitors' mass raised to this power (e.g., 140). These theoretical implications of geometric similarity for torque and force development can be tested using real isokinetic, body mass, and athletic performance data, as has been done for other physiological and biomechanical measures (e.g., 160). Such analyses should lead to more rigorous approaches to assessing strength in relation to athletic performance.

## Summary

In this chapter, the research that establishes an association between isokinetic measures and various athletic performances has been reviewed. On the basis of this evidence, the previous theoretical challenges to the specificity of isokinetic dynamometry in relation to athletic performance have been seriously questioned. The characteristics of muscle and joint function that are measured during the muscle actions that occur in isokinetic strength assessments would appear to clearly relate to the muscle and joint characteristics required for athletic performance. This would suggest that isokinetic measures *reflect*, and athletic performances are *governed by*, characteristics of muscle and joint function that are "generic" to a significant extent, rather than unique to the circumstances under which they are measured.

Having established that an association exists between many isokinetic measures and athletic performance, the challenge is now to improve this association by adapting isokinetic protocols to measure the most appropriate strength characteristics, and by appropriate scaling of isokinetic data for body size differences, according to the way in which size is related to strength and also limits athletic performance.

# References

1. Aagaard, P., E.B. Simonsen, M. Trolle, J. Bangsbo, and K. Klausen. 1994. Moment and power generation during maximal knee extensions performed at low and high speeds. *European Journal of Applied Physiology* 69: 376–81.

2. Aagaard, P., E.B. Simonsen, M. Trolle, J. Bangsbo, and K. Klausen. 1995. Isokinetic hamstring/quadriceps strength ratio: Influence from joint angular velocity, gravity correction, and contraction mode. *Acta Physiologica Scandinavica* 154: 421–27.

3. Abe, T., Y. Kawakami, S. Ikegawa, H. Kanehisa, and T. Fukunaga. 1992. Isometric and isokinetic knee joint performance in Japanese alpine ski racers. *Journal of Sports Medicine and Physical Fitness* 32(4): 353–57.

4. Agre, J.C., and T.L. Baxter. 1987. Musculoskeletal profile of male collegiate soccer players. *Archives of Physical Medicine and Rehabilitation* 68: 147–50.

5. Agre, J.C., T.L. Baxter, D.C. Casal, A.S. Leon, M.C. McNally, and R.C. Serfass. 1987. Musculoskeletal characteristics of professional ice hockey players. *Canadian Journal of Sport Science* 12(4): 202–6.

6. Agre, J.C., D.C. Casal, A.S. Leon, C. McNally, T.L. Baxter, and R.C. Serfass. 1988. Professional ice hockey players: Physiologic, anthropometric, and musculoskeletal characteristics. *Archives of Physical Medicine and Rehabilitation* 69: 188–92.

7. Alexander, M.J.L. 1989. The relationship between muscle strength and sprint kinematics in elite sprinters. *Canadian Journal of Sports Science* 14: 148–57.

8. Alexander, M.J.L. 1991. Physiological characteristics of top ranked rhythmic gymnasts over three years. *Journal of Human Movement Studies* 21: 99–127.

9. Anderson, M.A., J.H. Gieck, D. Perrin, A. Weltman, R. Rutt, and C. Denegar. 1991. The relationships among isometric, isotonic, and isokinetic concentric and eccentric quadriceps and hamstring force and three components of athletic performance. *Journal of Orthopaedic and Sports Physical Therapy* 14(3): 114–20.

10. Appen, L., and P.W. Duncan. 1986. Strength relationship of the knee musculature: Effects of gravity and sport. *Journal of Orthopaedic and Sports Physical Therapy* 7(5): 232–35.

11. Appling, S.A., and L.W. Weiss. 1993. The association of jump performance with quadriceps muscle function and body composition in women [Abstract]. *Physical Therapy* 73(6): S13.

12. Ashley, C.D., and L.W. Weiss. 1994. Vertical jump performance and selected physiological characteristics of women. *Journal of Strength and Conditioning Research* 8: 5–11.

13. Astrand, P-O., and K. Rodahl. 1977. Body dimensions and muscular work. In *Textbook of work physiology*, ed. Astrand, P-O. and Rodahl, K. 369–88. New York: McGraw-Hill.

14. Atwater, A.E., F.B. Roby, K. Huey, J.L. Puhl, and M. Tucker. 1991. Absolute and relative isokinetic shoulder strength in elite synchronized swimmers [Abstract]. Proceedings of the 2d World Congress on Sport Sciences, 297–98. Barcelona: COOB '92.

15. Baltzopoulos, V., R.G. Eston, and D. MacLaren. 1988. A comparison of power outputs on the Wingate test and on a test using an isokinetic device. *Ergonomics* 31(11): 1693–99.

16. Barra, A. 1985. A class act. *Sports Fitness* 1(6): 37–40, 112.

17. Bartlett, L.R., M.D. Storey, and B.D. Simons. 1989. Measurement of upper extremity torque production and its relationship to throwing speed in the competitive athlete. *American Journal of Sports Medicine* 17(1): 89–91.

18. Beam, W.C., R.A. Axtell, and R.L. Bartels. 1986. The relationship of strength, stroke mechanics, and VO2 max to swimming performance in college females [Abstract]. *Medicine and Science in Sports and Exercise* 18(2, Suppl.): S77–78.

19. Bell, G.J., S.R. Petersen, H.A. Quinney, and H.A. Wenger. 1989. The effect of velocity-specific strength training on peak torque and anaerobic rowing power. *Journal of Sport Science* 7: 205–14.

20. Berg, K., M. Miller, and L. Stephens. 1986. Determinants of 30-meter sprint time in pubescent males. *Journal of Sports Medicine and Physical Fitness* 26: 225–31.

21. Bergh, U. 1987. The influence of body mass in cross-country skiing. *Medicine and Science in Sports and Exercise* 19(4): 324–31.

22. Bergh, U., and A. Forsberg. 1992. Influence of body mass on cross-country ski racing performance. *Medicine and Science in Sports and Exercise* 24(9): 1033–39.

23. Blanpied, P., J-A. Levins, and E. Murphy. 1995. The effects of different stretch velocities on average force of the shortening phase in the stretch-shortening cycle. *Journal of Orthopaedic and Sports Physical Therapy* 21(6): 345–53.

24. Blazevich, A.J., and D.G. Jenkins. 1998. Predicting sprint running times from isokinetic and squat lift tests: A regression analysis. *Journal of Strength and Conditioning Research* 12(2): 101–3.

25. Bobbert, M.F., and G.J. van Ingen Schenau. 1990. Mechanical output about the ankle joint in isokinetic plantarflexion and jumping. *Medicine and Science in Sports and Exercise* 22(5): 660–68.

26. Bobbert, M.F., and G.J. van Ingen Schenau. 1990. Isokinetic plantarflexion: Experimental results and model calculations. *Journal of Biomechanics* 23(2): 105–19.

27. Bober, T., C.A. Putnam, and G.G. Woodworth. 1987. Factors influencing the angular velocity of a human limb segment. *Journal of Biomechanics* 20(5): 511–21.

28. Borges, O., and B. Essen-Gustavsson. 1989. Enzyme activities in type I and II muscle fibers of human skeletal muscle in relation to age and torque development. *Acta Physiologica Scandinavica* 136: 29–36.

29. Bosco, C., P. Mognoni, and P. Luhtanen. 1983. Relationship between isokinetic performance and ballistic movement. *European Journal of Applied Physiology* 51: 357–64.

30. Brady, E.C., M. O'Regan, and B. McCormack. 1993. Isokinetic assessment of uninjured soccer players. In *Science and football II*, ed. T. Rielly, J. Clarys, and A. Stibbe, 351–56. London: Spon.

31. Brown, L.E., M. Whitehurst, and D.N. Buchalter. 1994. Comparison of bilateral isokinetic knee extension/flexion and cycle ergometry tests of power. *Journal of Strength and Conditioning Research* 8(3): 139–43.

32. Brown, L.E., M. Whitehurst, B.W. Findley, R. Gilbert, and D.N. Buchalter. 1995. Isokinetic load range during shoulder rotation exercise in elite male junior tennis players. *Journal of Strength and Conditioning Research* 9(3): 160–64.

33. Brown, M., W.M. Kohrt, and A. Delitto. 1991. Peak torque/body weight ratios in older adults: A reexamination. *Physiotherapy Canada* 43: 7–11.

34. Brown, S.L., and J.G. Wilkinson. 1983. Characteristics of national, divisional, and club male alpine ski racers. *Medicine and Science in Sports and Exercise* 15(6): 491–95.

35. Cabri, J., E. DeProft, W. Dufour, and J.P. Clarys. 1988. The relation between muscular strength and kick performance. In *Science and football*, ed. T. Reilly, A. Lees, K. Davids, and W.J. Murphy, 186–93. London: Spon.

36. Callister, R., R.J. Callister, S.J. Fleck, and G.A. Dudley. 1990. Physiological and performance responses to overtraining in elite judo athletes. *Medicine and Science in Sports and Exercise* 22: 816–24.

37. Callister, R., R.J. Callister, R.S. Staron, S.J. Fleck, P. Tesch, and G.A. Dudley. 1991. Physiological characteristics of elite judo athletes. *International Journal of Sports Medicine* 12(2): 196–203.

38. Chapman, A.E., and D.J. Sanderson. 1990. Muscular coordination in sporting skills. In *Multiple muscle systems: Biomechanics and movement organization*, ed. J.M. Winters and S.L-Y. Woo, 608–20. New York: Springer-Verlag.

39. Ciccone, C.D., and C.M. Lyons. 1987. Relationship of upper extremity strength and swimming stroke technique on competitive freestyle swimming performance. *Journal of Human Movement Studies* 13: 143–50.

40. Cisar, C.J., G.O. Johnson, A.C. Fry, T.J. Housh, R.A. Hughes, A.J. Ryan, and W.G. Thorland. 1987. Preseason body composition, build, and strength as predictors of high school wrestling success. *Journal of Applied Sport Science Research* 1(4): 66–70.

41. Clarkson, P.M., J. Johnson, D. Dextraeur, W. Leszczynski, J. Wai, and A. Melchionda. 1982. The relationship among isokinetic endurance, initial strength level, and fiber type. *Research Quarterly* 53(1): 15–19.

42. Clarkson, P.M., W. Kroll, and A.M. Melchionda. 1982. Isokinetic strength, endurance, and fiber type composition in elite American paddlers. *European Journal of Applied Physiology* 48(1): 67–76.

43. Cohen, D.B., M.A. Mont, K.R. Campbell, B.N. Vogelstein, and J.W. Loewy. 1994. Upper extremity physical factors affecting tennis serve velocity. *American Journal of Sports Medicine* 22(6): 746–50.

44. Colliander, E.B., G.A. Dudley, and P.A. Tesch. 1988. Skeletal muscle fiber type composition and performance during repeated bouts of maximal, concentric contractions. *European Journal of Applied Physiology* 58: 81–86.

45. Cordill, M.R., M.C. Meyers, H.H. Erickson, L. Noble, and J. Rudy. 1995. Isokinetic quadriceps/hamstring torque and power production in collegiate lacrosse athletes [Abstract]. *Medicine and Science in Sports and Exercise* 27(5, Suppl.): S25.

46. Coyle, E.F., D.L. Costill, and G.R. Lesmes. 1979. Leg extension power and muscle fiber composition. *Medicine and Science in Sports and Exercise* 11: 12–15.

47. Davies, G.J. 1992. A descriptive study of isokinetic knee flexion extension testing at 300 to 600°/s. Paper presented at the 67th Annual Conference of the American Physical Therapy Association, Denver.

48. Davies, G.J., D.T. Kirkendall, D.H. Leigh, M.L. Lui, T.R. Reinbold, and P.K. Wilson. 1981. Isokinetic characteristics of professional football players: I. Normative relationships between quadriceps and hamstring muscle groups and relative to body weight [Abstract]. *Medicine and Science in Sports and Exercise* 13(2): 76–77.

49. Davis, J.A., J. Brewer, and D. Atkin. 1992. Preseason physiological characteristics of English first and second division soccer players. *Journal of Sports Sciences* 10: 541–47.

50. Davis, J.A., J. Brewer, and D. Atkin. 1994. A physiological comparison of first class male batsmen and bowlers [Abstract]. *Journal of Sports Science* 12(2): 159.

51. Davy, K.P., M. Kent, J. Shorten, and J.H. Williams. 1992. Relationship between power output during cycle ergometry and isokinetic testing [Abstract]. *Medicine and Science in Sports and Exercise* 24(5, Suppl.): S75.

52. Delecluse, C., M. Van Leemputte, E. Willems, R. Diels, R. Andries, and H. Van Coppenolle. 1995. Study of performance-related strength tests for competition level sprinters. In *Biomechanics in sports*, vol. XII, ed. A. Barabas and G. Fabian, 347–50. Budapest: ISBS.

53. Delitto, A. 1990. Trunk strength testing. In *Muscle strength testing. Instrumented and noninstrumented approaches*, ed. L.R. Amundsen, 151–62. New York: Churchill Livingstone.

54. Delitto, A., C.E. Crandell, and S.J. Rose. 1989. Peak torque/body weight ratios in the trunk: A critical analysis. *Physical Therapy* 69(2): 138–43.

55. DeNuccio, D.K., G.J. Davies, and M.J. Rowinski. 1991. Comparison of quadriceps isokinetic eccentric and isokinetic concentric data using a standard fatigue protocol. *Isokinetics and Exercise Science* 1(2): 81–86.

56. DeProft, E., J. Cabri, W. Dufour, and J.P. Clarys. 1988. Strength training and kick performance in soccer players. In *Science and football*, ed. T. Reilly, A. Lees, K. Davids, and W.J. Murphy, 108–13. London: Spon.

57. Dick, W., and N. Haggerty. 1971. *Topics in measurement: Reliability and validity*, 137. New York: McGraw-Hill.

58. Doherty, M., S.J.E. Humphrey, and E.M. Winter. 1994. Scaling knee extension peak torque for differences in body mass in male endurance and explosive athletes [Abstract]. *Journal of Sports Science* 12(2): 159–60.

59. Dvir, Z. 1991. Clinical applicability of isokinetics: A review. *Clinical Biomechanics* 6: 133–44.

60. Dvir, Z. 1996. An isokinetic study of combined activity of the hip and knee extensors. *Clinical Biomechanics* 11(3): 135–38.

61. Dvir, Z., G. Eger, N. Halperin, and A. Shklar. 1989. Thigh muscle activity and anterior cruciate ligament insufficiency. *Clinical Biomechanics* 4: 87–91.

62. Eckerson, J.M., D.J. Housh, T.J. Housh, and G.O. Johnson. 1994. Seasonal changes in body composition, strength, and muscular power in high school wrestlers. *Pediatric Exercise Science* 6: 39–52.

63. Ellenbecker, T.S. 1991. A total arm strength isokinetic profile of highly skilled tennis players. *Isokinetics and Exercise Science* 1(1): 9–21.

64. Emery, L., M. Sitler, and J. Ryan. 1994. Mode of action and angular velocity fatigue response of the hamstrings and quadriceps. *Isokinetics and Exercise Science* 4(3): 91–95.

65. Farrar, M., and W. Thorland. 1987. Relationship between isokinetic strength and sprint times in college age men. *Journal of Sports Medicine and Physical Fitness* 27: 368–72.

66. Fleck, S.J., S.L. Smith, M.W. Craib, T. Denahan, R.W. Snow, and M.L. Mitchell. 1992. Upper extremity isokinetic torque and throwing velocity in team handball. *Journal of Applied Sport Science Research* 6(2): 120–24.

67. Floros, N., A. Kiousis, A. Giavroglou, and L. Tsarouchas. 1994. Muscle power output during maximal short-term cycling exercise and isokinetic repeated knee extensions in elite soccer players. In *Abstracts of the XIIth International Symposium on Biomechanics in Sports*, ed. A. Barabas and G. Fabian. Budapest: ISBS.

68. Foster, C. 1989. Physiologic testing: Does it help the athlete? *Physician and Sports Medicine* 17(10): 103–10.

69. Foster, C., and N.N. Thompson. 1990. The physiology of speed skating. In *Winter sports medicine*, ed. M.J. Casey, C. Foster, and E.G. Hixson, 221–40. Philadelphia: Davis.

70. Foster, C., N.N. Thompson, and A.C. Snyder. 1993. Ergometric studies with speed skaters: Evolution of laboratory methods. *Journal of Strength and Conditioning Research* 7(4): 193–200.

71. Froese, E.A., and M.E. Houston. 1985. Torque-velocity characteristics and muscle fiber type in human vastus lateralis. *Journal of Applied Physiology* 59(2): 309–14.

72. Fry, A.C., W.J. Kraemer, F. van Borselen, J.M. Lynch, J.L. Marsit, E.P. Roy, N.T. Triplett, and H.G. Knuttgen. 1994. Performance decrements with high-intensity resistance exercise overtraining. *Medicine and Science in Sports and Exercise* 26(9): 1165–73.

73. Fry, A., W.J. Kraemer, C.A. Weseman, B.P. Conroy, S.E. Gordon, J.R. Hoffman, and C.M. Maresh. 1991. The effects of off-season strength and conditioning program on starters and nonstarters in women's intercollegiate volleyball. *Journal of Applied Sports Science Research* 5: 174–81.

74. Fry, R.W., and A.R. Morton. 1991. Physiological and kinanthropometric attributes of elite flatwater kayakers. *Medicine and Science in Sports and Exercise* 23(11): 1297–301.

75. Fugl-Meyer, A.R., M. Sjostrom, and L. Wahlby. 1979. Human plantarflexion strength and structure. *Acta Physiologica Scandinavica* 107: 47–56.

76. Galbreath, R.W., F.L. Goss, R.J. Robertson, K.F. Metz, and R. Burdett. 1989. The relationship between selected isokinetic variables and sprint times [Abstract]. *Medicine and Science in Sports and Exercise* 21(1, Suppl.): S51.

77. Genuario, S.E., and F.A. Dolgener. 1980. The relationship of isokinetic torque at two speeds to the vertical jump. *Research Quarterly for Exercise and Sport* 51(4): 593–98.

78. Gerard, E.S., V.J. Caiozzo, B.D. Rubin, C.A. Prietto, and O.M. Davidson. 1986. Skeletal muscle profiles among elite long, middle, and short distance swimmers. *American Journal of Sports Medicine* 14(1): 77–82.

79. Gerard, E.S., V.J. Caiozzo, B.D. Rubin, C.A. Prietto, and O.M. Davidson. 1987. Skeletal muscle profiles in elite springboard and platform divers. *American Journal of Sports Medicine* 15(2): 125–28.

80. Gerdle, B., C. Johansson, and R. Lorentzon. 1988. Relationship between work and electromyographic activity during repeated leg muscle contractions in orienteerers. *European Journal of Applied Physiology* 58: 8–12.

81. Gibala, M.J., and J.D. MacDougall. 1993. The effects of tapering on strength performance in trained athletes (Abstract). *Medicine and Science in Sports and Exercise* 25(5, Suppl.): S47.

82. Gilliam, T.B., S.P. Sady, P.S. Freedson, and J. Villanacci. 1979. Isokinetic torque levels for high school football players. *Archives of Physical Medicine and Rehabilitation* 60: 110–14.

83. Gioux, M., P. Arne, M. Dogui, and C. Bensch. 1984. Biomechanical and electromyographic characteristics of the human quadriceps in relation with sports performance. In *Current topics in sports medicine*. Proceedings of the World Congress of Sports Medicine, Vienna, 1982, ed. N. Bachl, L. Prokop, and R. Suckert, 699–705. Vienna: Urban & Schwarzenberg.

84. Gleeson, N.P., and T.H. Mercer. 1996. The utility of isokinetic dynamometry in the assessment of human muscle function. *Sports Medicine* 21(1): 18–34.

85. Gleim, G.W. 1984. The profiling of professional football players. *Clinics in Sports Medicine* 3(1): 185–97.

86. Gleim, G.W., M. Marino, L. Best, M. Fingerhood, P. Rosenthal, and J.A. Nicholas. 1982. Pro sports profiling by discriminant analysis [Abstract]. *Medicine and Science in Sports and Exercise* 14(2): 151.

87. Gray, J.C., and J.M. Chandler. 1989. Percent decline in peak torque production during repeated concentric and eccentric contractions of the quadriceps femoris muscle. *Journal of Orthopaedic and Sports Physical Therapy* 10(8): 309–14.

88. Greenberger, H.B., and M.V. Paterno. 1995. Relationship between knee extensor strength and hopping test performance in the assessment of lower extremity function. *Journal of Orthopaedic and Sports Physical Therapy* 22(5): 202–6.

89. Gregor, R.J., V.R. Edgerton, J.J. Perrine, D.S. Campion, and C. DeBus. 1979. Torque-velocity relationships and muscle fiber composition in elite female athletes. *Journal of Applied Physiology* 47: 388–92.

90. Guskiewicz, K., S. Lephart, and R. Burkholder. 1993. The relationship between sprint speed and hip flexion/extension strength in collegiate athletes. *Isokinetics and Exercise Science* 3(2): 111–16.

91. Hagerman, F.C., and R.S. Staron. 1983. Seasonal variations among physiological variables in elite oarsmen. *Canadian Journal of Applied Sport Science* 8(3): 143–48.

92. Harman, E., P. Frykman, M. Rosenstein, M. Johnson, and R. Rosenstein. 1990. The relationship of individual torque-velocity curve shapes to sprint running performance [Abstract]. *Medicine and Science in Sports and Exercise* 22(2): S8.

93. Haymes, E.M., and A.L. Dickinson. 1980. Characteristics of elite male and female ski racers. *Medicine and Science in Sports and Exercise* 12(3): 153–58.

94. Helgeson, K., and R.L. Gajdosik. 1993. The stretch-shortening cycle of the quadriceps femoris muscle group measured by isokinetic dynamometry. *Journal of Orthopaedic and Sports Physical Therapy* 17(1): 17–23.

95. Herzog, W., A.C. Guimaraes, M.G. Anton, and K.A. Carter-Erdman. 1991. Moment-length relations of rectus femoris muscles of speed skaters/cyclists and runners. *Medicine and Science in Sports and Exercise* 23(11): 1289–96.

96. Hoffman, J.R., A.C. Fry, R. Howard, C.M. Maresh, and W.J. Kraemer. 1991. Strength, speed, and endurance changes during the course of a Division I basketball season. *Journal of Applied Sport Science Research* 5(3): 144–49.

97. Hopkins, W.G., and D.J. Hewson. 1993. Reliability of competitive performance in cycling, running, swimming, and golf [Abstract]. *Medicine and Science in Sports and Exercise* 25(5, Suppl.): S171.

98. Hortobagyi, T., F.I. Katch, and P.F. LaChance. 1989. Interrelationships among various measures of upper body strength assessed by different contraction modes: Evidence of a general strength component. *European Journal of Applied Physiology* 58: 749–55.

99. Hortobagyi, T., F.I. Katch, V.L. Katch, P.F. LaChance, and A.R. Behnke. 1990. Relationships of body size, segmental dimensions, and ponderal equivalents to muscular strength in high strength and low strength subjects. *International Journal of Sports Medicine* 11(5): 349–56.

100. Housh, T.J., G.O. Johnson, R.A. Hughes, C.J. Cisar, and W.G. Thorland. 1988. Yearly changes in the body composition and muscular strength of high school wrestlers. *Research Quarterly for Exercise and Sport* 59(3): 240–43.

101. Housh, T.J., W.G. Thorland, G.O. Johnson, R.A. Hughes, and C.J. Cisar. 1988. The contribution of selected physiological variables to middle distance running performance. *Journal of Sports Medicine and Physical Fitness* 28(1): 20–26.

102. Houston, M.E., R.W. Norman, and E.A. Froese. 1988. Mechanical measures during maximal velocity knee extension exercise and their relation to fiber composition of the human vastus lateralis muscle. *European Journal of Applied Physiology* 58: 1–7.

103. Hrysomallis, C., R. Koski, M. McCoy, and T. Wrigley. In review. Correlations between field and laboratory tests of strength, power and muscular endurance for elite Australian Rules footballers.

104. Huesner, W. 1980. *The theory of strength development.* Application Note ASPL-25. Albany, CA: Isokinetics.

105. Imwold, C.H., R.A. Rider, E.M. Haymes, and K.D. Green. 1983. Isokinetic torque differences between college female varsity basketball and track athletes. *Journal of Sports Medicine and Physical Fitness* 23(2): 67–73.

106. Inbar, O., P. Kaiser, and P. Tesch. 1981. Relationships between leg muscle fiber type distribution and leg exercise performance. *International Journal of Sports Medicine* 2(3): 154–59.

107. Ivy, J.L., R.T. Withers, G. Brose, B.D. Maxwell, and D.L. Costill. 1981. Isokinetic contractile properties of the quadriceps with relation to fiber type. *European Journal of Applied Physiology* 47: 247–55.

108. Jackson, D.L., and J. Nyland. 1990. Club lacrosse: A physiological and injury profile. *Annals of Sports Medicine* 5: 114–17.

109. Jacobs, I. 1981. Lactate, muscle glycogen, and exercise performance in man. *Acta Physiologica Scandinavica* Suppl.: 495.

110. Jacobs, I., and J. Pope. 1986. A computerized system for muscle strength evaluation: Measurement reproducibility, validity, and some normative data. *National Strength and Conditioning Association Journal* 8(3): 28–33.

111. Johansson, C. 1992. Knee extensor performance in runners: Differences between specific athletes and implications for injury prevention. *Sports Medicine* 14(2): 75–81.

112. Johansson, C., R. Lorentzon, M. Fagerlund, M. Sjostrom, and A.R. Fugl-Meyer. 1987. Sprinters and marathon runners: Does isokinetic knee extensor performance reflect muscle size and structure? *Acta Physiologica Scandinavica* 130: 663–69.

113. Johansson, C., R. Lorentzon, S. Rasmuson, S. Reiz, S. Haggmark, H. Nyman, and A.R. Fugl-Meyer. 1988. Peak torque and OBLA running capacity in male orienteerers. *Acta Physiologica Scandinavica* 132: 525–30.

114. Johnson, G.O., T.J. Housh, D.R. Powell, and C.J. Ansorge. 1990. A physiological comparison of female bodybuilders and power lifters. *Journal of Sports Medicine and Physical Fitness* 30(4): 361–64.

115. Kanehisa, H., S. Ikegawa, T. Fukunaga. 1997. Force-velocity relationships and fatigability of strength and endurance-trained subjects. *International Journal of Sports Medicine* 18(2): 106–12.

116. Kano, Y., H. Takahashi, Y. Morioka, H. Akima, K. Miyashita, S. Kuno, and S. Katsuta. 1997. Relationship between the morphological features of thigh muscles and sprinting performance. *Medicine and Science in Sports and Exercise* 29(5, Suppl.): S220.

117. Karlsson, J. 1979. Localized muscular fatigue: Role of muscle metabolism and substrate depletion. In *Exercise and sport science reviews*, vol. 7, ed. R.S. Hutton and D.I. Miller, 1–42. Philadelphia: Franklin Institute.

118. Katch, F.I., W.D. McArdle, G.S. Pechar, and J.J. Perrine. 1974. Measuring leg force-output capacity with an isokinetic dynamometer-bicycle ergometer. *Research Quarterly* 45(1): 86–91.

119. Kirkendall, D.T. 1979. Comparison of isokinetic power-velocity profiles in various classes of American athletes. PhD diss., Ohio State University. Michigan: University Microfilms.

120. Kirkendall, D.T. 1985. The applied sport science of soccer. *Physician and Sports Medicine* 13(4): 53–59.

121. Kirkendall, D.T., G.J. Davies, D.H. Leigh, M.L. Lui, T.R. Reinbold, and P.K. Wilson. 1981. Isokinetic characteristics of professional football players. II. Absolute and relative power-velocity relationships [Abstract]. *Medicine and Science in Sports and Exercise* 13(2): 77.

122. Klentrou, P.P., and R.R. Montpetit. 1991. Physiological and physical correlates of swimming performance. *Journal of Swimming Research* 7(1): 13–18.

123. Kluckhuhn, K.L., J.F. Signorile, P.C. Miller, B.C. Webber, and M. Garcia. 1997. An analysis of high speed isokinetics and pitching [Abstract]. *Medicine and Science in Sports and Exercise* 29(5, Suppl.): S222.

124. Komi, P.V. 1984. Physiological and biomechanical correlates of muscle function: Effects of muscle structure and stretch-shortening cycle on force and speed. In *Exercise and sport sciences reviews*, vol. 12, ed. R.L. Terjung, 81–121. Lexington, MA: Collamore.

125. Komi, P.V., and P. Tesch. 1979. EMG frequency spectrum, muscle structure, and fatigue in man. *European Journal of Applied Physiology* 42: 41–50.

126. Kort, H.D., and E.R.H.A. Hendriks. 1992. A comparison of selected isokinetic trunk strength parameters of elite male judo competitors and cyclists. *Journal of Orthopaedic and Sports Physical Therapy* 16(2): 92–96.

127. Koutedakis, Y., C. Boreham, C. Kabitsis, and N.C.C. Sharp. 1992. Seasonal deterioration of selected physiological variables in elite male skiers. *International Journal of Sports Medicine* 13: 548–51.

128.Koutedakis, Y., R. Frischknecht, G. Vrbova, N.C. Sharp, and R. Budgett. 1995. Maximal voluntary quadriceps strength patterns in Olympic overtrained athletes. *Medicine and Science in Sports and Exercise* 27(4): 566–72.

129.Koutedakis, Y., P.J. Pacy, R.M. Quevedo, D.J. Millward, R. Hesp, C. Boreham, and N.C.C. Sharp. 1994. The effects of two different periods of weight reduction on selected performance parameters in elite lightweight oarswomen. *International Journal of Sports Medicine* 15(8): 472–77.

130.Kovaleski, J.E., R.J. Heitman, and M.H. Ficca. 1994. Eccentric and concentric torque production of the knee extensors in endurance runners and cyclists. *Isokinetics and Exercise Science* 4(3): 104–7.

131.Kramer, J.F., and A. Leger. 1991. Oarside and nonoarside torques of the knee extensors and flexors in lightweight and heavyweight sweep oarsmen. *Physiotherapy Canada* 43(3):23–27.

132.Kramer, J.F., A. Leger, and A. Morrow. 1991. Oarside and nonoarside knee extensor strength measures and their relationship to rowing ergometer performance. *Journal of Orthopaedic and Sports Physical Therapy* 14(5): 213–19.

133.Kramer, J.F., A. Leger, D.H. Paterson, and A. Morrow. 1994. Rowing performance and selected descriptive, field, and laboratory variables. *Canadian Journal of Applied Physiology* 19(2): 174–84.

134.Kramer, J.F., A. Morrow, and A. Leger. 1993. Changes in rowing ergometer, weightlifting, vertical jump and isokinetic performance in response to standard plus plyometric training programs. *International Journal of Sports Medicine* 14: 449–54.

135.Kuhn, S., A. Gallagher, and T. Malone. 1991. Comparison of peak torque and hamstring/quadriceps femoris ratios during high velocity isokinetic exercise in sprinters, cross-country runners, and normal males. *Isokinetics and Exercise Science* 1(3): 138–45.

136.Larsson, L., and A. Forsberg. 1980. Morphological muscle characteristics in rowers. *Canadian Journal of Applied Sport Science* 5: 239–44.

137.Larsson, L., G. Grimby, and J. Karlsson. 1979. Muscle strength and speed of movement in relation to age and muscle morphology. *Journal of Applied Physiology* 46(3): 451–56.

138.Latin, R.W. 1992. The relationship between isokinetic power and selected anaerobic power tests. *Isokinetics and Exercise Science* 2(2): 56–59.

139.Lephart, S.M., D.H. Perrin, J.M. Manning, J.H. Gieck, F.C. McCue, and E.N. Saliba. 1987. Torque acceleration energy as an alternative predictor of anaerobic power [Abstract]. *Medicine and Science in Sports and Exercise* 19(2, Suppl.): S59.

140.Lietzke, M.H. 1956. Relation between weightlifting totals and body weight. *Science* 124: 486–87.

141.Lorentzon, R., C. Johansson, M. Sjostrom, M. Fagerlund, and A.R Fugl-Meyer. 1988. Fatigue during dynamic muscle contractions in male sprinters and marathon runners: Relationships between performance, electromyographic activity, muscle cross-sectional area, and morphology. *Acta Physiologica Scandinavica* 132: 531–36.

142.MacIntosh, B.R., W. Herzog, E. Suter, J.P. Wiley, and J. Sokolosky. 1993. Human skeletal muscle fiber types and force-velocity properties. *European Journal of Applied Physiology* 67: 499–506.

143. Martin, D.T., J.C. Scifres, S.D. Zimmerman, and J.G. Wilkinson. 1994. Effects of interval training and a taper on cycling performance and isokinetic leg strength. *International Journal of Sports Medicine* 15: 485–91.

144. Mascaro, T., B.L. Seaver, and L. Swanson. 1992. Prediction of skating speed with off-ice testing in professional hockey players. *Journal of Orthopaedic and Sports Physical Therapy* 15(2): 92–98.

145. Mathiassen, S.E. 1989. Influence of angular velocity and movement frequency on development of fatigue in repeated isokinetic knee extensions. *European Journal of Applied Physiology* 59: 80–88.

146. Mayhew, T.P., and J.M. Rothstein. 1985. Measurement of muscle performance with instruments. In *Measurement in physical therapy*, ed. J.M. Rothstein, 57–102. New York: Churchill Livingstone.

147. McHugh, M.P., G.W. Gleim, S.P. Magnusson, and J.A. Nicholas. 1993. A cross-sectional study of age-related musculoskeletal and physiological changes in soccer players. *Medicine, Exercise, Nutrition, and Health* 2: 261–68.

148. McLean, B.D., and D.McA. Tumilty. 1993. Left-right asymmetry in two types of soccer kick. *British Journal of Sports Medicine* 27(4): 260–62.

149. McMahon, T.A., and J.T. Bonner. 1983. *On size and life.* New York: Scientific American.

150. Mikesky, A.E., J.E. Edwards, J.K. Wigglesworth, and S. Kunkel. 1995. Eccentric and concentric strength of the shoulder and arm musculature in collegiate baseball pitchers. *American Journal of Sports Medicine* 23(5): 638–42.

151. Mikesky, A.E., J.K. Wigglesworth, J.E. Edwards, and E.P. Roetert. 1993. Comparison of rotational shoulder strength between baseball pitchers and tennis players [Abstract]. *Medicine and Science in Sports and Exercise* 25(5, Suppl.): S171.

152. Minkoff, J. 1982. Evaluating parameters of a professional hockey team. *American Journal of Sports Medicine* 10(5): 285–92.

153. Miyashita, M., and H. Kanehisa. 1979. Dynamic peak torque related to age, sex, and performance. *Research Quarterly* 50(2): 249–55.

154. Mognoni, P., M.V. Narici, M.D. Sirtori, and F. Lorenzelli. 1994. Isokinetic torques and kicking maximal velocity in young soccer players. *Journal of Sports Medicine and Physical Fitness* 34(4): 357–61.

155. Mookerjee, S., K.W. Bibi, G.A. Kenney, and L. Cohen. 1995. Relationship between isokinetic strength, flexibility, and flutter kicking speed in female collegiate swimmers. *Journal of Strength and Conditioning Research* 9(2): 71–74.

156. Morrow, J.R., A.S. Jackson, W.W. Hosler, and J.K. Kachurik. 1979. The importance of strength, speed, and body size for team success in women's intercollegiate volleyball. *Research Quarterly* 50(3): 429–37.

157. Murphy, A.J., and G.J. Wilson. 1997. The ability of tests of muscular function to reflect training-induced changes in performance. *Journal of Sports Sciences* 15: 191–200.

158. Narici, M.V., M.D. Sirtori, and P. Mognoni. 1988. Maximal ball velocity and peak torques of hip flexor and knee extensor muscles. In *Science and football*, ed. T. Reilly, A. Lees, K. Davids, and W.J. Murphy, 429–33. London: Spon.

159. Nesser, T.W., R.W. Latin, K. Berg, and E. Prentice. 1996. Physiological determinants of 40-meter sprint performance in young male athletes. *Journal of Strength and Conditioning Research* 10(4): 263–67.

160. Nevill, A.M., R. Ramsbottom, and C. Williams. 1992. Scaling measurements in physiology and medicine for individuals of different size. *European Journal of Applied Physiology* 64: 419–25.

161. Newberry, J.E., A. DeLeon, P.J. Merriman, and E.K. Castillo. 1997. Relationship of isokinetic knee extensor strength and closed kinetic chain functional ability [Abstract]. *Medicine and Science in Sports and Exercise* 29(54, Suppl.): S9.

162. Nilsson, J., P. Tesch, and A. Thorstensson. 1977. Fatigue and EMG of repeated fast voluntary contractions in man. *Acta Physiologica Scandinavica* 101: 194–98.

163. Nitschke, J.E. 1992. Reliability of isokinetic torque measurements: A review of the literature. *Australian Journal of Physiotherapy* 38(2): 125–34.

164. Nygaard, E., M. Houston, M. Suzuki, Y. Jorgenson, and B. Saltin. 1983. Morphology of the brachial biceps muscle and elbow flexion in man. *Acta Physiologica Scandinavica* 117: 287–92.

165. Oberg, B., J. Ekstrand, M. Moller, and J. Gillquist. 1984. Muscle strength and flexibility in different positions of soccer players. *International Journal of Sports Medicine* 5: 213–16.

166. Oberg, B., M. Moller, J. Gillquist, and J. Ekstrand. 1986. Isokinetic torque levels for knee extensors and knee flexors in soccer players. *International Journal of Sports Medicine* 7: 50–53.

167. Oberg, B., P. Odenrick, and H. Tropp. 1985. Muscle strength and jump performance in soccer players. *Abstract book*, 311. 10th International Congress of Biomechanics, Umea.

168. O'Connor, D. 1997. Fitness profile of professional rugby league players. In *Science and football III*, ed. T. Reilly, J. Bangsbo, and M. Hughes, 11–15. London: Spon.

169. Oddsson, L.I.E., and S.H. Westing. 1991. Jumping height can be accurately predicted from selected measurements of muscle strength and biomechanical parameters. In *Proceedings of 9th ISBS Symposium*, ed. C. Tant, P. Patterson, and S. York, 29–33. Ames, Iowa: ISBS.

170. O'Grady, K.E. 1982. Measures of explained variance: Cautions and limitations. *Psychological Bulletin* 92(3): 766–77.

171. Olbrecht, J., B. Underechts, B. Robben, A. Mader, and W. Hollman. 1992. Relation between metabolic performance capacity and test results on isokinetic movements by fin swimmers. In *Biomechanics and medicine in swimming: Swimming science VI*, ed. D. MacLaren, T. Reilly, and A. Lees, 307-311. London: Spon.

172. Olsen, C., and A. Harris. 1986. Relationship of rotator cuff strength components to throwing velocity in collegiate students [Abstract]. *Physical Therapy* 66(5): 772.

173. Ozer, D.J. 1985. Correlation and the coefficient of determination. *Psychological Bulletin* 97(2): 307–15.

174. Paasuke, M., J. Ereline, and H. Gapeyeva. 1997. Comparison of dynamic and isometric knee extensor muscles strength and power output in Nordic combined athletes. In *Book of abstracts*. XVIth International Society of Biomechanics Congress, ed. Organizing and Program Committee, 380. Tokyo: University of Tokyo.

175. Pate, R.R., C.A. Macera, S.P. Bailey, W.P. Bartoli, and K.E. Powell. 1992. Physiological, anthropometric, and training correlates of running economy. *Medicine and Science in Sports and Exercise* 24(1): 1128–33.

176. Patton, J.F., and A. Duggan. 1987. An evaluation of tests of anaerobic power. *Aviation, Space and Environmental Medicine* 58: 237–42.

177. Patton, J.F., W.J. Kraemer, H.G. Knuttgen, and E.A. Harman. 1990. Factors in maximal power production and in exercise endurance relative to maximal power. *European Journal of Applied Physiology* 60: 222–27.

178. Patton, R.W., M.M. Hinson, B.R. Arnold, and B. Lessard. 1978. Fatigue curves of isokinetic contractions. *Archives of Physical Medicine and Rehabilitation* 59: 507–9.

179. Pawlowski, D., and D.H. Perrin. 1989. Relationship between shoulder and elbow isokinetic peak torque, torque acceleration energy, average power, and total work and throwing velocity in intercollegiate pitchers. *Athletic Training* 24(2): 129–32.

180. Pedegana, L.R., R.C. Elsner, D. Roberts, J. Lang, and V. Farewell. 1982. The relationship of upper extremity strength to throwing speed. *American Journal of Sports Medicine* 10(6): 352–54.

181. Perrine, J.J., and V.R. Edgerton. 1975. Isokinetic anaerobic ergometry [Abstract]. *Medicine and Science in Sports* 7(1): 78.

182. Phillips, C.M., C.J. Cisar, and W.P. Russum. 1989. Physiological determinants of triathlon performance [Abstract]. *Medicine and Science in Sports and Exercise* 21(2, Suppl.): S7.

183. Piastra, G., R. Capanna, and P. Greco. 1990. Dinamometria isocinetica e forza esplosiva. Confronto tra due gruppi di pallavoliste di differente livello agonistico (Isokinetic dynamometry and explosive force. Comparison between groups of volleyball players of different level). *Medicina Dello Sport* 43(4): 297–301 (in Italian with English abstract).

184. Picconatto, W., N. Greer, R. Serfass, and J. Blatherwick. 1989. Relationship between isokinetic leg strength and skating performance in bantam ice hockey players [Abstract]. *Medicine and Science in Sports and Exercise* 21(2, Suppl.): S79.

185. Pincivero, D.M., S.M. Lephart, and R.G. Karunakara. 1997. Relation between open and closed kinetic chain assessment of knee strength and functional performance. *Clinical Journal of Sports Medicine* 7(1): 11–16.

186. Podolsky, A., K.R. Kaufman, T.D. Cahalan, S.Y. Aleshinsky, and E.Y.S. Chao. 1990. The relationship of strength and jump height in figure skaters. *American Journal of Sports Medicine* 18(4): 400–5.

187. Posch, E., Y. Haglund, and E. Eriksson. 1989. Prospective study of concentric and eccentric leg muscle torques, flexibility, physical conditioning, and variation of injury rates during one season of amateur ice hockey. *International Journal of Sports Medicine* 10(2): 113–17.

188. Poulmedis, P., G. Rondoyannis, A. Mitsou, and E. Tsarouchas. 1988. The influence of isokinetic muscle torque exerted in various speeds on soccer ball velocity. *Journal of Orthopaedic and Sports Physical Therapy* 10: 93–96.

189. Putnam, C.A. 1983. Interaction between segments during a kicking motion. In *Biomechanics* VIII-B, ed. H. Matsui, and K. Kobayashi, 688–94. Champaign, IL: Human Kinetics.

190. Putnam, C.A. 1993. Sequential motions of body segments in striking and throwing skills: Descriptions and explanations. *Journal of Biomechanics* 26(Suppl. 1): 125–35.

191. Pyke, F.S., B.R. Minikin, L.R. Woodman, A.D. Roberts, and T.G. Wright. 1979. Isokinetic strength and maximal oxygen uptake of trained oarsmen. *Canadian Journal of Applied Sports Science* 4(4): 277–79.

192. Rankin, J.M., and C.B. Thompson. 1983. Isokinetic evaluation of quadriceps and hamstrings function: Normative data concerning body weight and sport. *Athletic Training* 18(Summer): 110–14.

193. Read, M.T.F., and M.J. Bellamy. 1990. Comparison of hamstring/quadriceps isokinetic strength ratios and power in tennis, squash, and track athletes. *British Journal of Sports Medicine* 24(3): 178–82.

194. Ready, A.E. 1982. Seasonal evaluation of isokinetic strength, power, and endurance of middle distance runners [Abstract]. *Canadian Journal of Applied Sport Sciences* 7(4): 238.

195. Ready, A.E. 1984. Physiological characteristics of male and female middle distance runners. *Canadian Journal of Applied Sport Science* 9(2): 70–77.

196. Reilly, M.F., V.D. Kame, B. Termin, M.E. Tedesco, and D.R. Pendergast. 1990. Relationship between freestyle swimming speed and stroke mechanics to isokinetic muscle function. *Journal of Swimming Research* 6(3): 16–21.

197. Reilly, T., G. Atkinson, and A. Coldwells. 1991. Isokinetic strength and standing broad jump performance [Abstract]. *Perceptual and Motor Skills* 72: 1346.

198. Riera, J., and F.A. Rodriguez. 1991. A comparison between two methods of measuring dynamic strength of the leg extensors: Isokinetic dynamometry and vertical jump testing [Abstract]. *Proceedings of the 2d World Congress on Sport Sciences*, 268–69. Barcelona: COOB '92.

199. Riezebos, M.L., D.H. Patterson, C.R. Hall, and M.S. Yuhasz. 1983. Relationship of selected variables to performance in women's basketball. *Canadian Journal of Applied Sport Science* 8(1): 34–40.

200. Rochcongar, P., R. Morvan, J. Jan, J. Dassonville, and J. Beillot. 1988. Isokinetic investigation of knee extensors and knee flexors in young French soccer players. *International Journal of Sports Medicine* 9: 448–50.

201. Roemmich, J.N., and W.E. Sinning. 1996. Sport-seasonal changes in body composition, growth, power, and strength of adolescent wrestlers. *International Journal of Sports Medicine* 17(2): 92–99.

202. Roetert, E.P., T.J. McCormick, S.W. Brown, and T.S. Ellenbecker. 1996. Relationship between isokinetic and functional trunk strength in elite junior tennis players. *Isokinetics and Exercise Science* 6: 15–20.

203. Rothstein, J.M. 1985. Measurement and clinical practice: Theory and application. In *Measurement in physical therapy*, ed. J.M. Rothstein, 1–46. New York: Churchill Livingstone.

204. Ryushi, T., and T. Fukanaga. 1986. Influence of sub-types of fast twitch fibers on isokinetic strength in untrained men. *International Journal of Sports Medicine* 7: 250–53.

205. Ryushi, T., T. Fukunaga, M. Kondo, K. Shiono, and T. Morimoto. 1982. Effects of muscle fiber composition and muscle cross-sectional area on isokinetic strength in

humans. *Japanese Journal of Physical Education* 27(2): 135–42 (in Japanese with English abstract).

206. Sale, D.G. 1991. Testing strength and power. In *Physiological testing of the high-performance athlete*, 2d ed. Ed. J.D. MacDougall, H.A. Wenger, and H.J. Green, 21–106. Champaign, IL: Human Kinetics.

207. Sale, D.G., J.D. MacDougall, S.E. Alway, and J.R. Sutton. 1987. Voluntary strength and muscle characteristics in untrained men and women and male bodybuilders. *Journal of Applied Physiology* 62(5):1786–1793.

208. Saltin, B., and Gollnick, P.D. 1983. Skeletal muscle adaptability: Significance for metabolism and performance. In *Skeletal muscle*. Handbook of Physiology, sec. 10. Ed. L.D. Peachey, 555–631. Bethesda, MD: American Physiological Society.

209. Sapega, A.A., J. Minkoff, J.A. Nicholas, and M. Valsamis. 1978. Sport-specific performance factor profiling: Fencing as a prototype. *American Journal of Sports Medicine* 6(5): 232–35.

210. Sapega, A.A., J. Minkoff, M. Valsamis, and J.A. Nicholas. 1984. Musculoskeletal performance testing and profiling of elite competitive fencers. *Clinics in Sports Medicine* 3(1): 231–44.

211. Schantz, P., E. Randall-Fox, W. Hutchison, A. Tyden, and P-O. Astrand. 1983. Muscle fiber type distribution, muscle cross-sectional area, and maximal voluntary strength in humans. *Acta Physiologica Scandinavica* 117: 219–26.

212. Schmidt, F.L., J.E. Hunter, and V.W. Urry. 1976. Statistical power in criterion-related validation studies. *Journal of Applied Psychology* 61(4): 473–85.

213. Schmidt-Nielsen, K. 1984. *Scaling: Why is animal size so important?* Cambridge: Cambridge University Press.

214. Secher, N.H., and O. Vaage. 1983. Rowing performance: A mathematical model based on analysis of body dimensions as exemplified by body weight. *European Journal of Applied Physiology* 52: 88–93.

215. Sharp, D.S., and P.M. Gahlinger. 1988. Regression analysis in biological research: sample size and statistical power. *Medicine and Science in Sports and Exercise* 20(6): 605–10.

216. Sharp, R.L. 1986. Muscle strength and power as related to competitive swimming. *Journal of Swimming Research* 2(2): 5–10.

217. Shields, C.L., F.E. Whitney, and V.D. Zomar. 1984. Exercise performance of professional football players. *American Journal of Sports Medicine* 12(6): 455–59.

218. Sjodin, B. 1982. The relationships among running economy, aerobic power, muscle power, and onset of blood lactate accumulation in young boys (11-15 years). In *Exercise and sport biology*, ed. P.V. Komi, 57–60. Champaign, IL: Human Kinetics.

219. Sleivert, G.G., R.D. Backus, and H.A. Wenger. 1995. Neuromuscular differences between volleyball players, middle distance runners and untrained controls. *International Journal of Sports Medicine* 16: 390–98.

220. Sleivert, G.G., and H.A. Wenger. 1993. Physiological predictors of short-course triathlon performance. *Medicine and Science in Sports and Exercise* 25(7): 871–76.

221. Smith, D.J. 1987. The relationship between anaerobic power and isokinetic torque outputs. *Canadian Journal of Sport Science* 12(1): 3–5.

222. Smith, D.J., H.A. Quinney, H.A. Wenger, R.D. Steadward, and J.R. Sexsmith. 1981. Isokinetic torque outputs of professional and elite amateur ice hockey players. *Journal of Orthopaedic and Sports Physical Therapy* 3(2): 42–47.

223. Smith, D.J., and D. Roberts. 1991. Aerobic, anaerobic, and isokinetic measures of elite Canadian male and female speed skaters. *Journal of Applied Sport Science Research* 5(3): 110–15.

224. So, C-H., T.O. Siu, K.M. Chan, M.K. Chin, and C.T. Li. 1994. Isokinetic profile of dorsiflexors and plantarflexors of the ankle: A comparative study of elite versus untrained subjects. *British Journal of Sports Medicine* 28(1): 25–30.

225. Suter, E., W. Herzog, J. Sokolosky, J.P. Wiley, and B.R. MacIntosh. 1993. Muscle fiber type distribution as estimated by Cybex testing and by muscle biopsy. *Medicine and Science in Sports and Exercise* 25(3): 363–70.

226. Svantesson, U., B. Ernstoff, P. Bergh, and G. Grimby. 1991. Use of Kin-Com dynamometer to study the stretch-shortening cycle during plantarflexion. *European Journal of Applied Physiology* 62: 415–19.

227. Svantesson, U., and G. Grimby. 1995. Stretch-shortening cycle during plantarflexion in young and elderly women and men. *European Journal of Applied Physiology* 71: 381–85.

228. Swain, D.P. 1994. The influence of body mass in endurance bicycling. *Medicine and Science in Sports and Exercise* 26(1): 58–63.

229. Tanaka, K., and Y. Matsuura. 1982. A multivariate analysis of the role of certain anthropometric and physiological attributes in distance running. *Annals of Human Biology* 9(5): 473–82.

230. Taylor, J., J. Brown, and W. Chaffin. 1992. Relationship between knee and ankle isokinetic peak torques and vertical jump performance in selected intercollegiate basketball players [Abstract]. *Journal of Athletic Training* 27(2):152.

231. Taylor, N.A.S., J.D. Cotter, S.N. Stanley, and R.N. Marshall. 1991. Functional torque-velocity and power-velocity characteristics of elite athletes. *European Journal of Applied Physiology* 62: 116–21.

232. Telford, R.D., A.G. Hahn, D.B. Pyne, and D.McA. Tumilty. 1990. Strength, anaerobic capacities, and aerobic power of Australian track and road cyclists. *Excel* 6(4): 20–22.

233. Telford, R.D., D.McA. Tumilty, and A.G. Hahn. 1985. Leg strength of athletes in 14 different sports. *Excel* 2(1): 6–9.

234. Tesch, P.A. 1980. Muscle fatigue in man. *Acta Physiologica Scandinavica* Suppl.: 480.

235. Tesch, P.A. 1980. Fatigue patterns in subtypes of human skeletal muscle fibers. *International Journal of Sports Medicine* 1(2): 79–81.

236. Tesch, P.A. 1983. Physiological characteristics of elite kayak paddlers. *Canadian Journal of Applied Sports Science* 8(2): 87–91.

237. Tesch, P.A. 1995. Aspects of muscle properties and use in competitive alpine skiing. *Medicine and Science in Sports and Exercise* 27(3): 310–14.

238. Tesch, P.A., G.A. Dudley, M.R. Duvoisin, B.M. Hather, and R.T. Harris. 1990. Force and EMG signal patterns during repeated bouts of concentric or eccentric muscle actions. *Acta Physiologica Scandinavica* 138: 263–71.

239. Tesch, P., B. Sjodin, A. Thorstensson, and J. Karlsson. 1978. Muscle fatigue and its relation to lactate accumulation and LDH activity in man. *Acta Physiologica Scandinavica* 103: 413–20.

240. Tesch, P.A., and J.E. Wright. 1983. Recovery from short-term intense exercise: Its relation to capillary supply and blood lactate accumulation. *European Journal of Applied Physiology* 52: 98–103.

241. Tesch, P.A., J.E. Wright, J.A. Vogel, W.L. Daniels, D.S. Sharp, and B. Sjodin. 1985. The influence of muscle metabolic characteristics on physical performance. *European Journal of Applied Physiology* 54: 237–43.

242. Thorland, W.G., G.O. Johnson, C.J. Cisar, T.J. Housh, and G.D. Tharp. 1987. Strength and anaerobic responses of elite young female sprint and distance runners. *Medicine and Science in Sports and Exercise* 19(1): 56–61.

243. Thorland, W., G. Johnson, T. Housh, G. Tharp, and C. Cisar. 1988. Generality of strength and power in young male runners [Abstract]. *Medicine and Science in Sports and Exercise* 20(2, Suppl.): S76.

244. Thorstensson, A. 1976. Muscle strength, fiber types, and enzyme activities in man. *Acta Physiologica Scandinavica* Suppl.: 443.

245. Thorstensson, A., G. Grimby, and J. Karlsson. 1976. Force-velocity relations and fiber composition in human knee extensor muscles. *Journal of Applied Physiology* 40: 12–16.

246. Thorstensson, A., and J. Karlsson. 1976. Fatigability and fiber composition of human skeletal muscle. *Acta Physiologica Scandinavica* 98: 318–22.

247. Thorstensson, A., L. Larsson, P. Tesch, and J. Karlsson. 1977. Muscle strength and fiber composition in athletes and sedentary men. *Medicine and Science in Sports and Exercise* 9: 26–30.

248. Tittel, K., and H. Wutscherk. 1992. Anatomical and anthropometric fundamentals of endurance. In *Endurance in sport*, ed. R.J. Shephard and P-O. Astrand, 35–45. Oxford: Blackwell Scientific.

249. Togari, H., J. Ohashi, and T. Ohgushi. 1988. Isokinetic muscle strength of soccer players. In *Science and football*, ed. T. Reilly, A. Lees, K. Davids, and W.J. Murphy, 181–85. London: Spon.

250. Trappe, S.W., D.L. Costill, T.A. Trappe, and G.A. Lee. 1995. Calf muscle strength in humans [Abstract]. *Medicine and Science in Sports and Exercise* 27(5, Suppl.): S40.

251. Triplett, T., S.J. Fleck, S.L. Smith, R.J. Bielen, and M. Smith. 1991. Isokinetic torque and throwing velocity in water polo [Abstract]. *Medicine and Science in Sports and Exercise* 23(4, Suppl.): S11.

252. Vandervoort, A.A., D.G. Sale, and J. Moroz. 1984. Comparison of motor unit activation during unilateral and bilateral leg extension. *Journal of Applied Physiology* 56: 46–51.

253. van Ingen Schenau, G.J., J.J. DeKoning, F.C. Bakker, and G. DeGroot. 1996. Performance-influencing factors in homogeneous groups of top athletes: A cross-sectional study. *Medicine and Science in Sports and Exercise* 28(1): 1305–10.

254. Webber, B.C., K.L. Kluckhuhn, J.F. Signorile, P.C. Miller, and M. Garcia. 1997. High speed isokinetics, anthropometrics, and pitching [Abstract]. *Medicine and Science in Sports and Exercise* 29(5, Suppl.): S223.

255. Weiss, L.W., G.E. Relyea, C.D. Ashley, and R.C. Propst. 1997. Using velocity spectrum squats and body composition to predict standing vertical jump ability. *Journal of Strength and Conditioning Research* 11(1): 14–20.

256. Westblad, P., J. Svedenhag, and C. Rolf. 1996. The validity of isokinetic knee extensor endurance measurements with reference to treadmill running capacities. *International Journal of Sports Medicine* 17: 134–39.

257. Westing, S.H., J.Y. Seger, and A. Thorstensson. 1991. Isoacceleration: A new concept of resistive exercise. *Medicine and Science in Sports and Exercise* 23(5): 631–35.

258. Wiklander, J., and J. Lysholm. 1987. Simple tests for surveying muscle strength and muscle stiffness in sportsmen. *International Journal of Sports Medicine* 8: 50–54.

259. Williams, C.A., and M. Singh. 1997. Dynamic trunk strength of Canadian football players, soccer players, and middle to long distance runners. *Journal of Orthopaedic and Sports Physical Therapy* 25(4): 271–76.

260. Wilmore, J.H., R.B. Parr, W.L. Haskell, D.L. Costill, L.J. Milburn, and R.K. Kerlan. 1976. Football pros' strength—and CV weaknesses—charted. *Physician and Sports Medicine* 4(10): 45–54.

261. Wilson, G.J., A.D. Walshe, and M.R. Fisher. 1997. The development of an isokinetic squat device: Reliability and relationship to functional performance. *European Journal of Applied Physiology* 75: 455–61.

262. Wrigley, T.V., and M. Grant. 1995. Isokinetic dynamometry. In *Sports physiotherapy: Applied science and practice*, ed. M. Zuluaga, C. Briggs, J. Carlisle, V. McDonald, J. McMeeken, W. Nickson, P. Oddy, and D. Wilson, 259–287. Edinburgh: Churchill Livingstone.

263. Yates, J.W., and E. Kamon. 1983. A comparison of peak and constant angle torque-velocity curves in fast and slow twitch populations. *European Journal of Applied Physiology* 51: 67–74.

264. Zakas, A., K. Mandroukas, E. Vamvakoudis, K. Christoulas, and N. Aggelopoulou. 1995. Peak torque of quadriceps and hamstring muscles in basketball and soccer players of different divisions. *Journal of Sports Medicine and Physical Fitness* 35(3): 199–205.

265. Zefrang, W. 1993. On the force moment of stretching or flexing the knee and the height of vertical jumping. In *Biomechanics of sport* XI, ed. J. Hamill, T.R. Derrick, and E.H. Elliott, 56–59. Amherst, MA: ISBS.

# Part II
---
# Limitations

$P$art II is intended to make the reader aware of what isokinetic technology *cannot* do. Chapter 4 discusses force-velocity characteristics of both the dynamometer and the human subject. Chapter 5 explores limitations of constant velocity settings within an acceleration and deceleration paradigm. Chapter 6 investigates the combination of force-velocity and length-tension curves utilizing a three-dimensional approach.

Without a thorough understanding of the limitations of this technology one might presume that isokinetic technology might be applied in any situation requiring muscular assessment. This is certainly not the case. An isokinetic dynamometer is but one tool available to the technician for testing and training. No matter what the cost or space requirements of the equipment, the technician should use isokinetics judiciously and not as a fill-in for other more appropriate equipment. In other words, isokinetics can perform many varied functions within a velocity spectrum across diverse human muscle actions. However, the end user must be acutely aware of biomechanical factors such as lever arm length and range of motion considerations as well as physical torque, force, work, and power components within the specialized velocity constraints of isokinetic dynamometry.

It should be stated up front that exercise on an isokinetic dynamometer is not isokinetic, or at least only a portion of the available range of motion occurs as such. All motion within a defined repetition transpires across some sort of accelerative and decelerative pattern. Any use of this technology, then, should be undertaken with these constraints in mind.

# Chapter 4

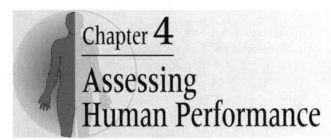

# Assessing Human Performance

Louis R. Osternig

Isokinetic exercise is not a modern concept for measuring muscle contractile characteristics. In 1922, Hill (18) used a flywheel, a series of pulleys, and a hand tachometer to control and record velocity in calculating work and the mechanical efficiency of human muscles (see figure 4.1). It was not until the late 1960s, however, that isokinetic dynamometers became popular tools to provide information about dynamic muscular actions. Because the changing mechanical advantage of the human limb-lever system alters the force applied

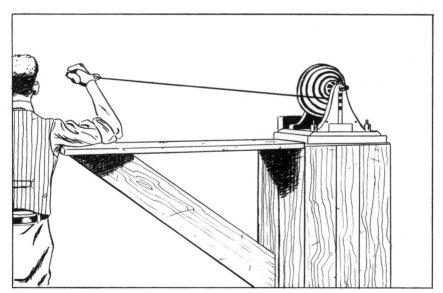

**Figure 4.1** Flywheel and pulley apparatus used to calculate work and mechanical muscle efficiency.

From *Journal of Physiology* 1922.

to the muscles through the range of motion in dynamic exercise, measurements of force, work, and power are not easily obtained where velocity is not
regulated (29).

This chapter focuses on the use of isokinetic dynamometry as a tool to measure human muscle force characteristics. As with many instruments designed
to assess human function, isokinetic dynamometers have constraints that limit
the types of information that can be obtained. These limitations, as well as the
purported advantages of this kind of exercise, are presented.

Since many principles of muscle training are based on the classic force-
velocity characteristics derived in the 1920s and 1930s, a considerable amount
of study has concentrated on evaluating the fit of isokinetic curves to those
derived with prepared muscle specimens. A synopsis of these studies is presented along with a discussion on the variables influencing force and power
production in isokinetic exercise. In recent years, considerable interest has
centered on the use of eccentric muscle loading. Isokinetic dynamometers have
the capacity to load lengthening as well as shortening muscle, thus concentric
as well as eccentric muscle actions are included in these discussions.

## Speed Control

An isokinetic dynamometer controls the velocity of an exercising limb by means
of a preset, integrated variable speed-governing mechanism. As more force is
exerted against the lever arm of the apparatus, the energy of the moving limb
is absorbed by the apparatus and converted to increased resistance encountered
by the limb (7, 50). Movement, therefore, occurs at a constant predetermined
speed.

## Accommodating Resistance in the Passive Mode

Most isokinetic dynamometers are passive devices in that they resist rather
than generate forces, and, unlike with weightlifting, no potential energy is
stored. Since the speed of movement is controlled, the resistance provided by
the dynamometer is considered to be proportionate to the amount of force
exerted by the muscle. Consequently, a maximal load can be applied at all
points throughout the arc of motion (21, 33). Other types of isokinetic dynamometers, however, in addition to having a passive mode, utilize a motor that
generates forces against which muscles can resist. This "active" mode permits
the measurement of force while the muscle is lengthening or undergoing "eccentric" loading.

Since passive isokinetic dynamometers apply no external load to the limb in
concentric exercise, any resistance encountered by the musculature is a function of the force applied to the apparatus. Conventional free weight training,
such as with a weighted boot, can generate relatively high joint forces at the
point of least mechanical advantage (see figure 4.2). It may be argued that

isokinetic exercise devices adjust resistance to varying anatomical or pathological deficiencies present at certain points in the joint range, whereas free weight systems are limited to the largest load that can be moved at the weakest point in the joint range. Researchers have suggested, however, that isokinetic exercise optimally loads muscles and joints through the joint range, thereby minimizing potential for injuries (see figure 4.3). Passive isokinetic dynamometers do not store potential energy, and eccentric muscular action does not follow

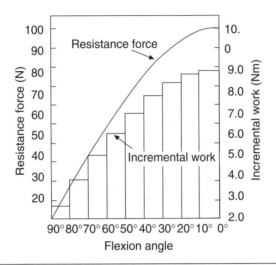

**Figure 4.2** Change in resistance force and incremental work for knee extensors from 90° to 0° of knee flexion.

From *Physical Therapy* 1979, with permission of the American Physical Therapy Association.

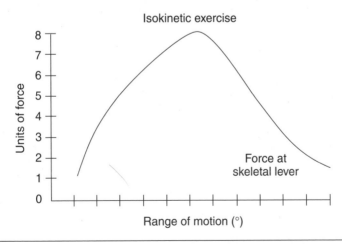

**Figure 4.3** Resistance encountered by skeletal lever during isokinetic exercise.

From *Physical Therapy* 1967, with permission of the American Physical Therapy Association.

a concentric action as occurs in gravity-loaded exercise. Hence, the development of muscle soreness due to training may be reduced. McCully and Faulkner (32) used a mouse model to support their hypothesis that lengthening (eccentric) actions resulted in greater injury to skeletal muscle fibers than isometric or shortening actions.

Another possible safety advantage of isokinetic exercise, compared to free weight exercise, relates to exercise skill requirements. Considerable skill and effort are needed to balance and stabilize free weights during exercises (13, 30). Because most types of isokinetic exercise are performed with a passive dynamometer, these requirements are reduced considerably. Thus, isokinetic exercise may minimize the risk of muscular and joint strain that can result from efforts to control the applied load.

## Accommodating Resistance in the Active Mode

Those isokinetic dynamometers, however, that have the capacity to apply a motor-driven external force to muscle (eccentric loading) introduce safety considerations not present with passive dynamometers. Eccentric exercise can generate much higher tension than concentric exercise and has been strongly implicated in delayed onset muscle soreness and frank muscle injury (12). Secondly, successful and safe training or testing using isokinetic eccentric exercise requires greater skill and experience on the part of the test administrator and subject than is required with passive dynamometers. Hence, while isokinetic dynamometers with passive and motor-driven "active" functions may offer enhanced training and testing capacities, users must prepare adequately, to reduce injury potential.

## Acceleration and Deceleration Components

The facility by which isokinetic dynamometers display muscle force information through a joint range has been viewed as a major advantage of this technique when compared to other forms of dynamic exercise in which measurement of muscle qualities is difficult to obtain. Since isokinetic dynamometers allow the operator to specify the desired angular velocity, torque at the rotating joint as a function of time and angle of displacement can be measured by computer. In spite of the advantages that isokinetic dynamometry provides, however, the user should consider a number of limitations for accurate interpretation of isokinetic dynamometer data.

Although isokinetic dynamometers permit a constant angular velocity to be designated by the user, the exercising limb must accelerate to the preset speed before isokinetic torque can be recorded (16, 30, 35, 38, 53, 54, 62). Consequently, a portion of the arc of motion is not isokinetic (see chapter 6 for full discussion). Similarly, the limb must decelerate at the end of the exercising range and a segment of the arc must be allocated for this to occur. Figure 4.4

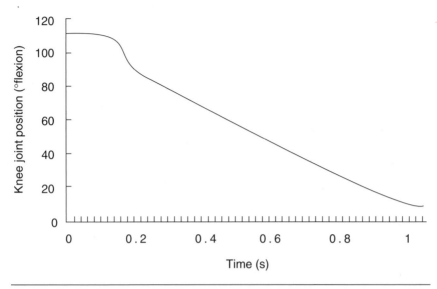

**Figure 4.4**    Change of knee joint position during isokinetic knee extension at 100°/s.

illustrates the change in knee joint position for knee extension generated on an isokinetic dynamometer set at 100°/s. Note that the rate of change in joint position is not constant throughout the range tested.

It has also been shown that the limb continues to accelerate well beyond the dynamometer speed before the subject makes adjustments to control angular velocity. Sapega and colleagues (53) measured lever arm displacement and time during exercise on an isokinetic dynamometer. They found that dynamic loading of hip abductors produced a 42 to 200% "overshoot" at speeds of 180°/s and 30°/s. They considered this to be due to normal limitations in internal and external mechanical couplings and dynamometer deformation under loading. Similarly, Osternig and associates (42) reported that subjects accelerated their limbs through an arc of movement that exceeded the preset dynamometer speed by up to 150% before constant velocity was attained (see figure 4.5).

As the speed of the dynamometer increases, peak torque occurs later in the range of motion (33, 38, 58; see figure 4.6). Thus, at fast speeds of motion, the limb can pass the position of peak torque prior to the muscle attaining full tension. Therefore, the peak torque recorded may not represent the muscle's fullest torque capacity. Since the position at which peak torque occurs may vary with speed of motion, it is important to analyze maximal values at specific joint angles across speeds in addition to the peak values generated throughout a joint range. Comparisons of peak torque across speeds irrespective of joint position may yield erroneous conclusions regarding the state of muscle function.

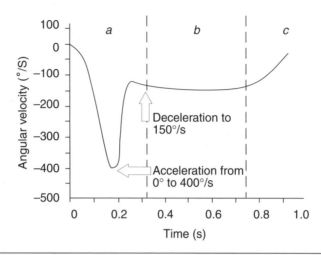

**Figure 4.5**   Angular velocity during isokinetic knee extension at 150°/s. A: Initial acceleration/deceleration phase. B: Isokinetic phase. C: Final deceleration phase.

From Osternig, Sawhill, Bates, and Hamill 1983.

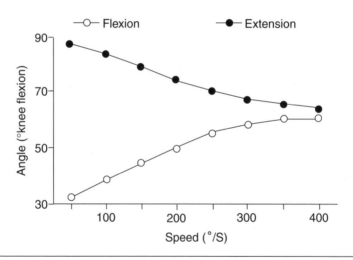

**Figure 4.6**   Peak torque knee angle relative to exercise speed.

Adapted from Osternig, Sawhill, Bates, and Hamill 1983.

# Influences on Force and Power Production

A number of variables may influence force and power production in isokinetic exercise. The amount of force generated in a musculotendinous unit is greatly influenced by interactions between the characteristics of the muscle action (concentric or eccentric), the position at which force is measured, and the speed of movement. Power produced or absorbed by the musculotendinous unit is similarly influenced by these variables.

## Concentric Force-Velocity Curves

The classic concentric force-velocity curve described by Hill in 1938 (19) was derived from prepared, in vitro specimens and revealed an inverse relationship between force and velocity of the muscle action (17; see figure 4.7). Osternig (45) summarized several in vivo studies on the isokinetic muscle force-velocity relationship and indicated that a drop in peak isokinetic torque with increasing speed was generally demonstrated. However, the shape of the isokinetic force-velocity curve differs from the curve derived from artificially stimulated muscle specimens. As speed approaches zero, the isokinetic muscular force tends to rise much less steeply than the force of the in vitro curve. Some studies (6, 31, 42, 44, 51) show a flattening or an actual decline in force production as the speed of movement slows (see figure 4.8). Because measurements of absolute maximal force or velocity are subject to constraints in human studies, the direct comparison of in vitro to in vivo force-velocity curves is not justified. Neural inhibition of force in the intact muscle as tension rises has been postulated as a possible mechanism retarding the force curve at slow speeds (6, 51).

## Eccentric Force-Velocity Curves

Eccentric muscle actions exhibit force-velocity relationships that are distinct from concentric actions. Figure 4.9 depicts the force-velocity curves for concentric and eccentric muscle actions measured in vitro; it shows that tension generated in the musculotendinous unit is greatest during eccentric actions compared to concentric or isometric actions. The steady rise in eccentric torque

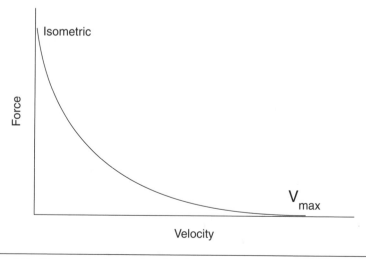

**Figure 4.7** Force-velocity relationship derived from prepared muscle specimens.

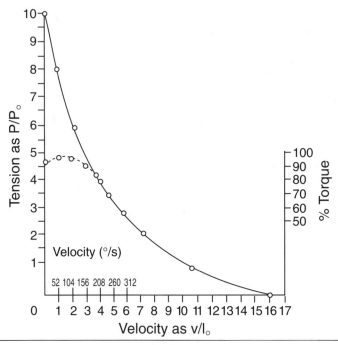

**Figure 4.8** Force-velocity relationships of artificially stimulated isolated animal muscle (solid line) and in vivo muscle under isokinetic loading (dotted line).

From *Medicine and S        cience in Sports* 1978.

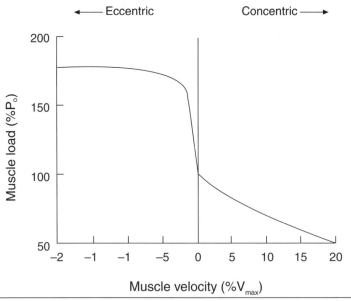

**Figure 4.9** Force-velocity relationships of eccentric and concentric muscle contractions.

Adapted from Garrett and Best 1994.

with speed was noted in the early work by Katz (26), who, using prepared specimens, calculated force-velocity relationships for lengthening muscle. Later work with human muscle (3, 5) demonstrated that eccentric actions produced greater force as lengthening velocity increased up to high velocities where force leveled off. Abbott and Aubert (3) reported that when stretch at constant speed is imposed on a muscle the rate of tension rise increases with the speed of stretch, but the tension has an upper limitation value independent of speed.

The eccentric curve suggests that muscles under active tension are highly resistive to forced lengthening. Friden and Lieber (12) and Garrett and Best (14) reported that a muscle lengthening at 1% of maximum velocity can increase tension by 50% over its maximum isometric contractile tension (see figure 4.9). In this case, tension rises about 10 times faster for lengthening than for an equivalent velocity of shortening as can be seen by the steepness of the slope at the beginning of the eccentric curve. Hence, muscles undergoing lengthening actions are well suited to resist opposing forces.

As indicated earlier, some isokinetic dynamometers are equipped with motors that generate forces, which can lengthen a resisting muscle and thus generate a measurable eccentric muscle action. Several studies have reported in vivo isokinetic eccentric force-velocity relationships (1, 2, 9, 22, 48, 59, 60).

Osternig and associates (48) tested uninjured controls and subjects after anterior cruciate ligament surgery and found that eccentric torque of the knee flexors rose steadily with speeds ranging from 15 to 60°/s in both groups (see figure 4.10). Hortobagyi and Katch (22) reported that arm flexion and extension eccentric torque rose with speed of stretch from 30 to 120°/s for subjects

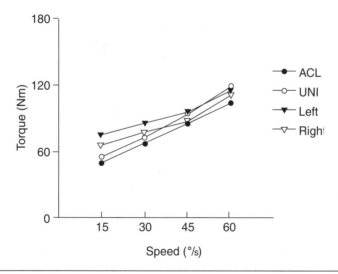

**Figure 4.10** Isokinetic eccentric torque-velocity relationships for contralateral limbs of post-ACL surgical and control subjects. For injured subjects: ACL = post-surgical side, UNI = uninjured side; for control subjects: Left = left side, Right = right side.

with "high strength" (HS) but not for those with "low strength" (LS). The researchers suggested that reduced neural inhibition in the HS subjects might have resulted in greater eccentric torque. Colliander and Tesch (9) found that eccentric peak torque of knee flexors increased with velocity (60–180°/s) in females but not in males. Since the female eccentric knee extensor torque appeared to drop between 120 and 180°/s, the researchers concluded that peak torque does not necessarily increase as a function of angular velocity.

The magnitude of the isokinetic eccentric torque appears to be influenced by the joint position at which torque is measured. Westing and colleagues (59) found that isokinetic eccentric knee extensor torque tended to increase from 30 to 70° of knee flexion while Osternig and associates (47) found that knee flexor eccentric torque decreased from 20 to 60° of knee flexion. These findings were not surprising since the knee flexor and extensor muscles exert maximum force at particular muscle lengths. According to the length-tension relationship (15), the maximum force, which corresponds to particular joint positions, occurs at about 30° of knee flexion for flexors and about 60° of knee flexion for extensors, when measured concentrically from the seated position (42, 60).

In summary, whether peak eccentric torque rises or remains stable across increasing speeds appears to be dependent upon subject gender (9), training condition (24), muscle group (9), and joint position (47, 59).

# Power-Velocity Relationships in Isokinetic Exercise

Power is considered to be a critical component in training and performance. Because isokinetic dynamometers provide information about the force of muscular action with respect to time and limb speed, they have been used to measure muscular power. Hill (19, 20) found that peak power occurred at approximately one third of the maximum speed of prepared and artificially stimulated shortening muscle. The mechanical constraints of isokinetic dynamometers, however, allow only a relatively narrow range of velocities that may be tested, and therefore, direct comparisons of power to studies of in vitro muscles are limited. As indicated earlier, as dynamometer speed increases, a decreasing portion of the arc of motion occurs in the isokinetic condition. Consequently, it is difficult to simulate the range of velocities generated in vitro. Studies on power production in isokinetic exercise suggest that power tends to rise as speed increases (38, 41), although there is evidence that power may level off at specific velocities of motion (10, 51; see figure 4.11). Force-velocity curves recorded with isokinetic dynamometers reveal a less dramatic drop in torque as speed is increased when compared to curves from in vivo measures. Since power is the product of force and velocity, this reduction in torque may be insufficient to offset the effect of speed in continuing to produce a rise in power as velocity increases.

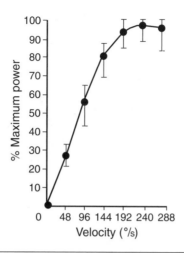

**Figure 4.11**   Power-velocity performance of 15 subjects during isokinetic knee extensions. Data are normalized with respect to maximum power attained. Dots represent means and vertical bars represent the range of values for all subjects.

From *Medicine and Science in Sports* 1978.

# Agonist/Antagonist Muscle Ratios

Practitioners have often used ipsilateral agonist/antagonist muscle ratios as standards by which to measure the progress of rehabilitation or to assess muscle imbalances (11, 55). Agonist/antagonist muscle groups, such as the quadriceps and hamstrings, function cooperatively to control the joints that they cross. Hence, the capacity of each muscle, forming the joint couple, to produce adequate force to balance its antagonist is considered important for joint stability.

## Concentric Muscle Function

Concentric hamstring-to-quadriceps torque ratios have been studied extensively (49) with reported averages ranging from about 0.5 to 0.75. However, a change in the angle of a joint alters the length-tension relationship of the antagonist muscles and the angle of pull in both muscle groups. This results in an increase in the physiological and mechanical advantage of one group and a decrease in the other. Therefore, ratios at changing angles throughout a joint arc will vary considerably (40). Comparisons of antagonist muscle ratios across isokinetic speeds are complicated further since the angle at which peak torque occurs varies with speed of movement. Thus, a ratio reported at 60°/s may be comparing the knee flexors at 35° of knee flexion and extensors at 75° of knee flexion, while at 180°/s, the comparison may be for the knee flexors at 50° and the extensors at 60° of knee flexion. The joint angular position and the isokinetic speed are important variables that influence the magnitude of the torque ratios between antagonist muscles. While agonist/antagonist muscle relationships are considered to be important factors in muscle performance screening (55), these relationships are not static and are affected by movement speed throughout the arc of motion (36, 37, 40).

## Eccentric Muscle Function

Although the knee flexors are activated eccentrically against the concentrically activated extensors, little has been reported on the eccentric knee flexor torque relative to concentric knee extensor torque. Eccentric knee flexor torque is believed to be a counter to anterior tibial shear produced by concentric knee extensors. In order to estimate the capacity of the knee flexors to eccentrically resist active knee extension, and potentially unload ligamentous structures, researchers have assessed the ratio of eccentric knee flexors to concentric knee extensors ( the E/C ratio) (1, 48). Theoretically, the higher the ratio, the greater the potential of the flexors to resist extensor-induced anterior tibial shear.

Aagaard and associates (1) found that the E/C ratio was close to 1.0 at fast speeds (240°/s) and dropped to 0.27 at 30°/s (1995). Osternig and coworkers (48) reported that the E/C ratio in post-ACL surgery subjects increased with speed of movement and approached 1.0 at 60°/s, nearly twice that of the controls (see figure 4.12). These studies suggest that as speed of motion increases the potential restraining action of the eccentric flexors may have an increasing capacity to counter the tibial anterior shear moment created by forceful knee extension or external loads.

As mentioned previously, the length of knee musculature changes with changes in joint position, and consequently, the agonist/antagonist forces may differ from one knee joint position to another. Therefore, the capacity of the

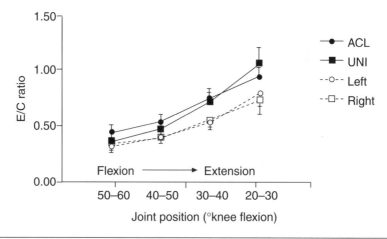

**Figure 4.12**   Isokinetic eccentric flexor/concentric extensor ratio (E/C ratio) for contralateral limbs of post-ACL surgical and control subjects at various joint position ranges. For injured subjects: ACL = postsurgical side, UNI = uninjured side; for control subjects: Left = left side, Right = right side.

knee flexors to counter knee extensor activity may vary throughout the joint range. Furthermore, since the knee flexors are activated eccentrically in this function, their exerted force may be greater at a given joint position than when activated concentrically (2, 47). The length-tension and force-velocity relationships of muscle, as well as the viscoelastic behavior of the musculotendinous unit, appear to contribute to these findings and should be considered in calculating knee flexor/extensor ratios.

# Coactivation

During forceful muscle actions, antagonist muscles such as the quadriceps and hamstrings often coactivate, with one group providing directional movement via concentric action while the opposing group provides control and joint support via simultaneous eccentric action.

The question of how active the antagonist knee muscles are during forceful agonist contractions has functional significance in that antagonist coactivation can influence the net force measured at the point of resistance in isokinetic or other forms of exercise. Since injuries can result from the rapid stretching of insufficiently relaxed muscles, the occurrence of antagonist coactivation may impose high resistance and possibly provoke antagonist muscle injury. In order to investigate the extent of coactivation in isokinetic exercise, researchers analyzed simultaneous recordings of joint position, torque, and (electromyographic) EMG activity from the quadriceps and hamstrings from untrained subjects (43) and trained intercollegiate sprinters and distance runners (44). Tests were conducted during maximal knee extension and flexion on an isokinetic dynamometer at slow (100–200°/s) and fast (300–400°/s) speeds. The results revealed that for all groups of subjects the hamstrings were quite active as an antagonist to knee extension, whereas the quadriceps generated little coactivation during flexion. This may be due to the more powerful quadriceps requiring greater antagonist coactivation for coordination and deceleration of extension than that required by the hamstrings during flexion. Figure 4.13 illustrates typical quadriceps and hamstring torque curves and agonist and antagonist EMG outputs during knee extension and flexion, in this case, for a sprinter at 100 and 400°/s. An examination of the athlete data revealed that the mean coactivation of the sprinters' hamstrings was four times greater than that of the distance runners. The researchers speculated that the explosive, high-intensity, short duration muscular efforts associated with sprinters' training may have induced residual hamstring tension that increased their sensitivity to stretch.

# Coactivation and ACL Dysfunction

From their work with animal models, Krauspe and colleagues suggested that stretching the ACL and PCL produced a change in the gamma motor neurons

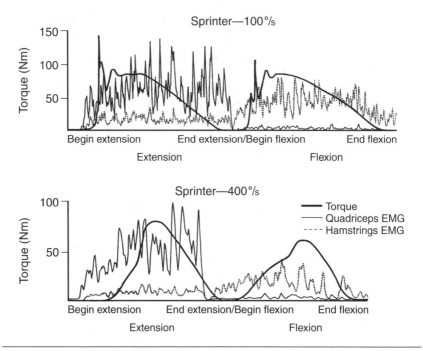

**Figure 4.13** Knee extension/flexion torque and electromyographic (EMG) output of quadriceps and hamstrings for a sprinter at 100 and 400°/s. Muscle coactivation is illustrated by hamstring activation during extension and quadriceps activation during flexion.

From *Medicine and Science in Sports and Exercise* 1986.

of the leg and thigh, indicating that cruciate sensory innervation may be important for control of movement and for protecting ligamentous tissue (28). Solomanow and associates (57) showed that direct stress to the ACL produces quadriceps inhibition and hamstring facilitation. These studies have functional significance in that knee ligament disruption and postinjury surgical reconstruction of the knee may disrupt ligamentous mechanoreceptors and consequently influence extremity function.

In an isokinetic study on hamstring coactivation in postsurgical ACL subjects and controls, researchers found that for the surgical group the injured limb generated significantly less knee flexor EMG activity during knee extension than did the uninjured contralateral limb (46). For the postsurgical subjects, mean coactivation of the uninjured contralateral limb averaged twice that of the postsurgical limb when data were collapsed across speeds. In contrast, no significant difference was observed for the same comparison between right and left limbs of the uninjured control group. The significant differences were more pronounced at the faster speed of movement. Explanation for this finding is speculative. It is possible that the ACL-injured knee may have suffered denervation of ligamentous tissue from trauma or operative repair, thus reducing afferent activity that triggers neuronal circuitry relevant for joint stability, as some researchers have suggested (27, 28).

In summary, these studies suggest that considerable antagonist coactivation of knee flexor musculature occurs during forceful knee extension in isokinetic exercise, and this can range from about 15 to 60% of maximum agonist activity (43, 44). The degree to which coactivation occurs appears to be related to type of training, speed of motion, the condition of the joint (postsurgical vs. uninjured), and the joint position tested (midrange vs. end range).

## Transfer of Training Across Speeds and Joint Positions

People often select isokinetic dynamometer speeds for conditioning purposes based on the extent to which a given exercise speed relates to some general strength concept. With varying results, several studies have addressed the question of transfer of force or power and training across speeds of movement in isokinetic exercise and other modalities (8, 23, 25, 31, 34, 39, 52). Kanehisa and Miyashita (25) investigated transfer of training for muscle power across isokinetic speeds. They used subjects who were trained under slow (60°/s), intermediate (180°/s), and fast (300°/s) velocity conditions and reported a specificity of isokinetic velocity effect: slow speed training resulted in power improvement primarily at slow speeds while fast speed training developed power only at fast speeds. However, they also reported that an intermediate training speed may exist that can enhance power output over a wide range of velocities. Coyle and associates (10) found that isokinetic training at slow speeds generated peak torque (PT) improvements only at the slow speed while fast speed training (300°/s) improved PT not only at the training velocity but also at a slower velocity of 180°/s. Since the fast group demonstrated a significant enlargement (+ 11%) of type II muscle fibers, the researchers suggested that type II fiber hypertrophy may be a plausible mechanism for the nonspecific improvement of the fast group. However, they noted that the existence of a neurological adaptation that enhances power at and below the training velocity could not be excluded.

Moffroid and Whipple (34) found that slow speed isokinetic training (36°/s) produced force gains only at slow speeds while fast speed training (108°/s) produced only nonsignificant force gains at any speed tested. Jenkins and colleagues (23) studied the effect of high speed (240°/s) and low speed (60°/s) isokinetic exercise on peak torque at 5 speeds (30–300°/s). The high speed group showed significant increases at all testing speeds while the low speed group produced increases only at 180 and 240°/s. Despite noting that transfer of training occurred for both groups, the researchers concluded that the range of transfer was insufficient to replace speed-specific training.

While several studies demonstrate that slow and fast speed training improves torque measures at slow and fast speeds, respectively, some researchers have reported notable exceptions to this tendency (8, 10, 23, 52). It seems reasonable to suggest that one cannot expect strength measures at a given speed to accurately reflect relative strength at a faster or slower speed. However, training at one speed may increase peak torque measures at other speeds of movement. The selection of appropriate speeds for testing and training using isokinetic dynamometers should be made with the understanding of a possible but limited transfer effect to other speeds of movement.

# Summary

Isokinetic human muscle assessment has been performed extensively over the past three decades. The facility by which isokinetic dynamometers provide information about muscle force and power throughout the range of motion has resulted in widespread use of these modalities in conditioning and research. Like other muscle assessment instruments, isokinetic dynamometers have constraints that limit the kind of data that can be generated. Due to the limb acceleration and deceleration that accompanies this form of exercise, the duration of "isokinetic" exercise decreases as the preset speed of the dynamometer increases. Hence, there is a velocity limit beyond which only relatively small amounts of constant velocity (load range) data can be obtained.

Concentric isokinetic force-velocity data partially simulate the classic inverse relationship curve derived from artificially stimulated, prepared muscle specimens in that they generally show a drop in peak force with increasing speed. However, as speed slows, isokinetic muscular force tends to rise much less steeply than that of the in vitro curve or may flatten or actually decline. Neural inhibition in the intact muscle may play a role in retarding the isokinetic force curve at slow speeds. Because measurements of absolute maximal force or velocity in human studies are subject to constraints, direct comparisons of in vivo to in vitro force-velocity curves are limited.

Some isokinetic instruments can lengthen resisting muscle and thereby generate measurable eccentric muscle actions. Muscle tension developed under the eccentric condition tends to increase with speed of muscle lengthening and can significantly surpass tension generated in voluntary maximum isometric actions. Whether eccentric torque rises or remains stable across increasing speeds appears to be dependent upon prior training, gender, muscle group, and joint position.

Eccentric knee flexor torque is believed to be a counter to anterior tibial shear produced by concentric knee extensors. Isokinetic studies have shown that the lengths of knee musculature change with changes in joint position and that the agonist/antagonist forces differ from one knee joint position to another. Therefore, the capacity of the knee flexors to counter knee extensor activity may vary throughout the joint range.

The results from studies on the transfer of isokinetic measures and training across speeds vary. The data suggest that measures of strength at a given speed do not accurately reflect relative strength at faster or slower speeds. However, training at one speed may increase measures of peak torque at other speeds of movement.

Despite the limitations of isokinetic dynamometers, these devices provide a reliable means of measuring force, power, and velocity in many types of human movement. An understanding of the capabilities and limitations of these tools will help to improve their usefulness in the assessment of muscle function.

# References

1. Aagaard, P., E.B. Simonsen, M. Trolle, J. Bangsbo, and K. Klausen. 1995. Isokinetic hamstring/quadriceps strength ratio: Influence from joint angular velocity, gravity correction, and contraction mode. *Acta Physiologica Scandinavica* 154: 421–27.

2. Aagaard, P., E.B. Simonsen, S. Magnusson, B. Larsson, and P. Dyhre-Poulsen. 1998. A new concept for isokinetic hamstring/quadriceps muscle strength ratio. *American Journal of Sports Medicine* 26: 231–37.

3. Abbott, B., and S. Aubert. 1951. Changes in energy in a muscle during very slow stretches. *Proceedings of the Royal Society* B139: 104–17.

4. Abbott, B., B. Bigland, and J. Ritchie. 1952. The physiological cost of negative work. *Journal of Physiology* 117: 380–90.

5. Asmussen, E. 1953. Positive and negative muscular work. *Acta Physiologica Scandinavica* 28: 364–82.

6. Barnes, W.S. 1975. The relationship of motor unit activation to isokinetic muscular contraction at different contractile velocities. *Physical Therapy* 55: 1152–57.

7. Barnes, W.S. 1980. The relationship between maximum isokinetic strength and isokinetic endurance. *Research Quarterly for Exercise and Sport* 51: 714–17.

8. Caiozzo, V.J., J.J. Perrine, and V.R. Edgerton. 1981. Training-induced alterations of the in vivo force-velocity relationship of human muscle. *Journal of Applied Physiology* 51: 750–54.

9. Colliander, E., and P. Tesch. 1989. Bilateral eccentric and concentric torque of quadriceps and hamstring muscles in females and males. *European Journal of Applied Physiology* 59: 227–32.

10. Coyle, E.F., D.C. Feiring, T.C. Rotkis, R.W. Cote, F.B. Roby, W. Lee, and J.H. Wilmore. 1981. *Journal of Applied Physiology* 51: 1437–42.

11. Davies, G.J. 1984. *A compendium of isokinetics in clinical usage,* 1–451. LaCrosse, WI: S & S.

12. Friden, J., and R.L. Lieber. 1992. Structural and mechanical basis of exercise-induced muscle injury. *Medicine and Science in Sports and Exercise* 24: 521–30.

13. Garhammer, J.J. 1979. Performance evaluation of Olympic weightlifters. *Medicine and Science in Sports* 11: 284–87.

14. Garrett, W.E., and T.M Best. 1994. Anatomy, physiology, and mechanics of skeletal muscle. In *Orthopaedic basic science,* ed. S.R. Simon, 89–125. Park Ridge, IL: American Academy of Orthopaedic Surgeons.

15. Gordon, A.M., A.F. Huxley, and F.J. Julian. 1966. The variation in isometric tension with sarcomere length in vertebrate muscle fibers. *Journal of Physiology* 184: 17–192.

16. Gransberg, L., and E. Knutsson. 1983. Determination of dynamic muscle strength in man with acceleration-controlled isokinetic movements. *Acta Physiologica Scandinavica* 119: 317–20.

17. Guyton, A.C. 1981. *Textbook of medical physiology.* 6th ed. Philadelphia: Saunders.

18. Hill, A.V. 1922. The maximum work and mechanical efficiency of human muscles and their most economical speed. *Journal of Physiology* 56: 19–41.

19. Hill, A.V. 1938. The heat of shortening and the dynamic constants of muscle. *Proceedings of the Royal Society* B126: 136–95.

20. Hill, A.V. 1940. The dynamic constants of human muscle. *Proceedings of the Royal Society* B128: 263–74.

21. Hislop, H.J., and J.J. Perrine. 1967. Isokinetic concept of exercise. *Physical Therapy* 47: 114–17.

22. Hortobagyi, T., and F. Katch. 1990. Eccentric and concentric torque-velocity relationships during arm flexion and extension. *European Journal of Applied Physiology* 60: 395–401.

23. Jenkins, W.L., M. Thackaberry, and C. Killian. 1984. Speed-specific isokinetic training. *Journal of Orthopaedic Sports Physical Therapy* 6: 181–83.

24. Johansson, H. 1991. Role of knee ligaments in proprioception and regulation of muscle stiffness. *Journal of Electromyography and Kinesiology* 1: 158–79.

25. Kanehisa, H., and M. Miyashita. 1983. Specificity of velocity in strength training. *European Journal of Applied Physiology* 52: 104–6.

26. Katz, B. 1939. The relation between force and speed in muscular contraction. *Journal of Physiology* 96: 45–64.

27. Kennedy, J.C., I.J. Alexander, and K.C. Hayes. 1982. Nerve supply of the human knee and its functional importance. *American Journal of Sports Medicine* 10: 329–35.

28. Krauspe, R., M. Schmidt, and H. Schable. 1992. Sensory innervation of the anterior cruciate ligament. *Journal of Bone and Joint Surgery* A74: 390–97.

29. Laird, C.E., and C.K. Rozier. 1979. Toward understanding the terminology of exercise mechanics. *Physical Therapy* 59: 287–92.

30. Lander, J.E., B.T. Bates, J.A. Sawhill, and J. Hamill. 1985. A comparison between free weight and isokinetic bench pressing. *Medicine and Science in Sports and Exercise* 17: 344–53.

31. Lesmes, G.R., D.L. Costill, E.F. Coyle, and W.J. Fink. 1978. Muscle strength and power changes during maximal isokinetic training. *Medicine and Science in Sports* 10: 266–69.

32. McCully, K.K., and J.A. Faulkner. 1985. Injury to skeletal muscle fibers of mice following lengthening contractions. *Journal of Applied Physiology* 59: 119–26.

33. Moffroid, M., R. Whipple, J. Hofkosh, E. Lowman, and H. Thistle. 1969. A study of isokinetic exercise. *Physical Therapy* 49: 735–46.

34. Moffroid, M.T., and R.H. Whipple. 1970. Specificity of speed of exercise. *Physical Therapy* 50: 1692–1700.

35. Murray, M.P., C.M. Gardner, L.A. Mollinger, and S.B. Sepic. 1980. Strength of isometric and isokinetic contractions. *Physical Therapy* 60: 412–19.

36. Murray, S.M., R.F. Warren, J.C. Otis, M. Kroll, and T.L. Wickiewicz. 1984. Torque-velocity relationships of the knee extensor and flexor muscles in individuals sustaining injuries of the anterior cruciate ligament. *American Journal of Sports Medicine* 12: 436–40.

37. Nosse, L.J. 1982. Assessment of selected reports on the strength relationship of the knee musculature. *Journal of Orthopaedic Sports Physical Therapy* 4: 78–85.

38. Osternig, L.R. 1975. Optimal isokinetic loads and velocities producing muscular power in human subjects. *Archives of Physical Medicine and Rehabilitation* 56: 152–55.

39. Osternig, L.R., B.T. Bates, and S.L. James. 1977. Isokinetic and isometric torque force relationships. *Archives of Physical Medicine and Rehabilitation* 58: 254–57.

40. Osternig, L.R., J.A. Sawhill, B.T. Bates, and J. Hamill. 1981. Function of limb speed on torque ratios of antagonist muscles and peak torque joint position [abstract]. *Medicine and Science in Sports and Exercise* 13: 107.

41. Osternig, L.R., J. Hamill, J.A. Sawhill, and B.T. Bates. 1983. Influence of torque and limb speed on power production in isokinetic exercise. *American Journal of Physical Medicine* 62: 163–71.

42. Osternig, L.R., J.A. Sawhill, B.T. Bates, and J. Hamill. 1983. Function of limb speed on torque patterns of antagonist muscles. In *Biomechanics* VIII-A, edited by H. Matsui and K. Kobayashi, 251–57. Champaign, IL: Human Kinetics.

43. Osternig, L., J. Hamill, D. Corcos, and J. Lander. 1984. Electromyographic patterns accompanying isokinetic exercise under varying speed and sequencing conditions. *American Journal of Physical Medicine* 63: 289–97.

44. Osternig, L.R., J. Hamill, J.E. Lander, and R. Robertson. 1986. Coactivation of sprinter and distance runner muscles in isokinetic exercise. *Medicine and Science in Sports and Exercise* 18: 431–35.

45. Osternig, L.R. 1986. Isokinetic dynamometry: Implications for muscle testing and rehabilitation. *Exercise and Sports Science Reviews* 14: 45–80.

46. Osternig, L., B. Caster, and C. James. 1995. Contralateral hamstring (biceps femoris) coactivation patterns and anterior cruciate ligament dysfunction. *Medicine and Science in Sports and Exercise* 27: 805–8.

47. Osternig, L.R., C.R. James, and D. Bercades. 1996. Effects of movement speed and joint position on knee flexor efficiency following anterior cruciate ligament surgery [abstract]. *Medicine and Science in Sports and Exercise* 28(Suppl.): S196.

48. Osternig, L.R., C.R. James, and D.T. Bercades. 1996. Eccentric knee flexor torque following anterior cruciate ligament surgery. *Medicine and Science in Sports and Exercise* 28: 1229–34.

49. Perrin, D. 1993. Isokinetic exercise and assessment, 153–58. Champaign, IL: Human Kinetics.

50. Perrine, J.J. 1968. Isokinetic exercise and mechanical energy potentials of muscle. *Journal of Health and Physical Education* 39: 40–44.

51. Perrine, J.J., and V.R. Edgerton. 1978. Muscle force-velocity relationships under isokinetic loading. *Medicine and Science in Sports* 10: 159–66.

52. Pipes, T.V., and J.H. Wilmore. 1975. Isokinetic vs. isotonic strength training in adult men. *Medicine and Science in Sports* 7: 262–74.

53. Sapega, A.A., J.A. Nicholas, D. Sokolow, and A. Saraniti. 1982. The nature of torque overshoot in Cybex isokinetic dynamometry. *Medicine and Science in Sports and Exercise* 14: 368–75.

54. Sawhill, J.A. 1981. Biomechanical characteristics of rotational velocity and movement complexity in isokinetic performance. PhD dissertation, University of Oregon, Eugene.

55. Schlinkman, B. 1984. Norms for high school football players derived from Cybex data reduction computer. *Journal of Orthopaedic Sports Physical Therapy* 5: 243–54.

56. Smith, M.J., and P. Melton. 1981. Isokinetic versus isotonic variable resistance training. *American Journal of Sports Medicine* 9: 275–79.

57. Solomonow, M., R. Baratta, and B.H. Zghou. 1987. The synergistic action of the anterior cruciate ligament and thigh muscles in maintaining joint stability. *American Journal of Sports Medicine* 15: 207–13.

58. Thorstensson, A., G. Grimby, and J. Karlsson. 1976. Force-velocity relations and fiber composition in human knee extensor muscles. *Journal of Applied Physiology* 40: 12–16.

59. Westing, S., J. Seger, E. Karlson, and E. Ekblom. 1988. Eccentric and concentric torque-velocity characteristics of the quadriceps femoris in man. *European Journal of Applied Physiology* 58: 100–4.

60. Westing, S.H., and J.Y. Seger. 1989. Eccentric and concentric torque-velocity characteristics, torque output comparisons, and gravity effect torque corrections for the quadriceps and hamstring muscles in females. *International Journal of Sports Medicine* 10: 175–80.

61. Westing, S., A. Cresswell, and A. Thorstensson. 1991. Muscle activation during maximal voluntary eccentric and concentric knee extension. *European Journal of Applied Physiology* 62: 104–8.

62. Winter, D.A., R.P. Wells, and G.W. Orr. 1981. Errors in the use of isokinetic dynamometers. *European Journal of Applied Physiology* 46: 397–408.

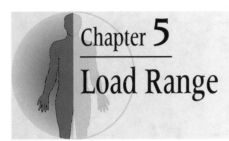

# Chapter 5
# Load Range

Lee E. Brown and Michael Whitehurst

Exercise on an isokinetic device involves three main phases of movement: acceleration, constant velocity, and deceleration. Inherent in these phases are unique occurrences that may confound test data and, thereby, test interpretation. Constant velocity is by definition isokinetic and represents a match between a mechanically imposed velocity and the subject's movement (e.g., knee extension). However, the acceleration phase, which is spent "catching" or matching the isokinetic velocity, is done without resistance or load. In other words, there is a portion of the available range of motion (ROM) during which there is no quantifiable external load. The ROM with external load or that ROM when there is a match between isokinetic velocity and limb movement is referred to as load range. Load range becomes increasingly smaller as velocity is increased. That is to say, there is an inverse relationship between velocity and load range (7, 8, 10, 28). Osternig and colleagues (29–31), in their pioneering work, were the first investigators to point out this inverse relationship. They detailed load range decreases from 92 to 16% at isokinetic speeds of 50 to 400°/s (see figure 5.1).

As a practical matter, this means that as the preselected velocity of an isokinetic device is increased, an exercising individual receives external overload through an ever decreasing portion of the full ROM. Couple this effect with the fact that torque is inversely related to velocity and the result is short arc, low-resistance exercise at high speeds, with the remaining ROM as acceleration or deceleration (see figure 5.2).

In other words, the exerciser on an isokinetic device set at high velocities is primarily attempting to reach the predetermined speed (accelerate and catch the lever arm) or slow down prior to contacting the end stop (decelerate). Acceleration and deceleration are performed without the benefit of externally imposed resistance. Thus, acceleration and deceleration should not be considered during test interpretation. However, data from these phases are often included in analyses and may result in spurious conclusions.

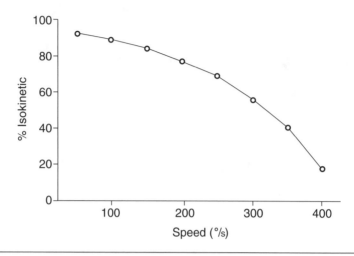

**Figure 5.1**　Percent of ROM spent in load range across velocities.
From Matsui and Kobayashi 1983.

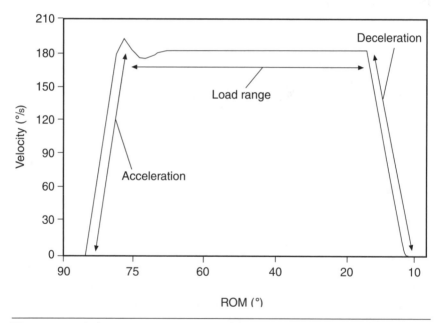

**Figure 5.2**　Velocity tracing at 180°/s showing the three major phases of an isokinetic repetition.

The reliability and validity of isokinetic dynamometers have been measured repeatedly (4, 36, 40) and found to be high when correlated over time. However, researchers have identified errors associated with artifacts inherent in the nonload range portions of the repetition. Taylor and coworkers (36) documented increased errors with increased velocity from 60 to 450°/s, and they caution against ascribing artifact torque to the exercising limb. Tis and Perrin (40) caution that using a data reduction technique that eliminates the first and last 10° of ROM may eliminate acceleration and deceleration areas but may also eliminate the peak torque range.

This book is designed to identify those circumstances where the dynamometer may be used to collect valid reliable data pertaining to muscle strength and apply that to human performance. In this chapter we point out various drawbacks and pitfalls in the use of the dynamometer as well as remedies available to the isokinetic practitioner.

# Standardized Test Measures

Prior to discussing load range in full it is necessary to explore basic test measures that help to insure proper subject setup in the dynamometer. In the ensuing pages we delineate confounding elements that may impact velocity-specific tests, and we focus on standardized testing procedures that should be considered when utilizing an isokinetic device. Following the consideration of these factors, we present a detailed discussion of investigations focusing on load range.

## Preliminary Considerations

An examiner must determine why he is using the dynamometer prior to its use, not after. The isokinetic machine is a specialized tool that returns specialized information based on specific anatomical configurations, muscle length-tension relationships, and velocities of muscle action. The dynamometer has been criticized for any number of reasons; critics say that it is not functional in movement pattern or speed. However, the fact of the matter may be that the dynamometer was never designed to be a functional tool but rather was designed for the specific circumstances stated previously, and it should be used judiciously in that manner. Before using any dynamometer the examiner should have a thorough plan as to what type of strength data is required. This data may include peak strength, peak or average power, work performed, or endurance capabilities of a specific muscle group at a specific length and speed.

An isokinetic evaluation is designed to determine muscle strength at a constant velocity. In addition, practitioners may use the dynamometer to strength-train muscle groups at constant velocities. We have stated that, when using the dynamometer, only a portion of the ROM is spent in load range. This being the case, the practitioner must be aware of data reduction techniques, which are designed to eliminate extraneous information. We discuss these techniques in detail later in this chapter. If a clear understanding of the limitations of this technology is established during test interpretation, there will be little chance for erroneous conclusions.

Researchers have identified known faults associated with isokinetic dynamometry; these include artifacts that are manifested during overspeeding of the limb at the onset of movement (35), decelerative torque spikes (44), mechanical work errors due to gravitational forces, and angle of torque changes due to deceleration (46), axis alignment (34), and lever arm oscillation (3).

## Isolation and Stabilization

With few exceptions, an isokinetic device is designed to test and exercise muscles using the open kinetic chain. Since only the muscles of one joint are being examined, isolation of those muscles is of paramount importance. The information gathered from testing will lead the examiner to specific conclusions regarding the physiological assessment of a joint. Without proper isolation this information may contain errors that could lead to spurious conclusions.

Isolation of one muscle group merely excludes any other group from adding to the test outcome. The practitioner may best achieve isolation of the desired group through proper positioning and strapping (i.e., stabilization) of the subject in the dynamometer. For example, if the examiner wants to isolate the muscles used for knee extension, he will stabilize the waist and thigh. The objective is to restrict motion to knee extension and flexion without extraneous joint movement about the hip. This will insure that only the quadriceps and hamstring muscle groups are producing measured torque through the dynamometer. Without stabilization the lower leg is left to flex at the hip joint, which may artificially inflate muscle performance.

This potential for error is present at all joints if the practitioner does not take care to control for extraneous movement. Shoulder internal/external rotation muscle torque may be inflated through the addition of trunk rotation torque if proper stabilization of the torso is not achieved. While one may argue that trunk rotation is a functional counterpart of shoulder rotation and is performed simultaneously, it is not the intent of isolated open kinetic chain testing to include trunk rotation in the measurement scheme. Weir and colleagues (41), measuring knee extension torque at 60, 180, and 300°/s with stabilized and nonstabilized conditions, have shown that extraneous movements may reduce torque output and change the angle of peak torque production secondary to changes in muscle length.

## Axis of Motion

Each dynamometer on the market consists of a lever arm attached to a dynamometer head. Resultant muscle torque is recorded at this juncture through rotation of the lever. Since torque is the product of force and lever arm length ($T = F \times L_A$), it is of vital importance that the axes of motion of the machine and the joint being tested are congruent. If the lever axis and the joint axis are not in alignment, torque measurements will be invalid.

Using the shoulder as an example, the axis of rotation is located at the center of the humeral head. Assuming a distal lever attachment from this point of testing, muscle torque output is the product of force generated and lever length. In other words, varying the attachment at the distal end may alter shoulder rotation torque. Each different testing position may be reliable and valid (and therefore repeatable) so long as the axis of rotation is held constant, yet torque values will vary greatly. Deviation of the axis of rotation will render the test invalid secondary to the introduction of an artificial lever arm.

Rothstein and colleagues (34) make a cogent argument for the use of aligned axes of rotation by stating that errors associated with misalignment may be amplified in torque measurements in joints where the axis changes with movement. The knee and shoulder are such joints. They further state that since the axis of the machine is stable, measurement in any joint with uncontrolled movement will result in error.

## Gravity Compensation

Since exercise on an isokinetic device is most often performed under a gravitational force, the practitioner must account for its effects. Considering, for example, seated knee extension/flexion, one can see that performing a knee extension movement requires an individual to lift the weight of the limb and the dynamometer lever arm against gravity. However, during seated knee flexion, gravity assists the motion by pulling down on the limb and lever. In this scenario, flexion torque may be artificially inflated due to gravity while the opposite is true for extension.

Without compensation for the effects of gravity the test results are subject to large errors. Winter and colleagues (46) documented mechanical work errors ranging from 26% to over 500% during knee extension and flexion exercise at 60 and 150°/s. These errors also caused early peaks in the torque curves, making test interpretation inaccurate.

## Range of Motion

Two types of ROM, physiological and total, need to be considered when performing exercise on a dynamometer. The physiological ROM is the anatomical beginning and end of the movement as measured by a goniometer. Total ROM is the arc traveled between the two physiological measurements. In other words, a shoulder motion from 0 to 90° or from 90 to 180° of flexion has the same total ROM (90°) but a very different physiological ROM. Since most joint torque curves resemble an inverted U shape, it follows that a valid measure of torque production must account for where in the ROM the torque was produced. The length-tension relationship of the muscle (by ROM determination) must be considered, to accurately assess true muscle performance capabilities. Physiological ROM will determine what portion of the inverted U is being evaluated (i.e., upslope or downslope).

Errors associated with ROM measurements may be magnified when interpreting work and power variables. Since work is the product of torque and distance ($W = T \times D$) and power is a function of work and time ($P = W/T$), distance traveled must be precise for comparative purposes. In other words, if total ROM is 50° on pretest and subsequently is compared with total ROM of 70° on a posttest, work and power may be artificially inflated.

## Verbal Instructions

Any instructions given to a subject should be consistent from one test to the next and from one subject to another. Not all individuals respond to the same form of verbal encouragement. Instructions, therefore, should be concise and parsimonious. Furthermore, since the dynamometer is a unique piece of equipment, most subjects may not be familiar with it. This unfamiliarity may cause anxiety in some subjects and lead to misunderstandings regarding test procedures. Therefore, verbal commands should be explicit as to every facet of the procedure. This includes, but is not limited to, where to grasp the attachment, how to breath, what to do with the contralateral limb, how to push in both directions, how to give a maximal effort, what constitutes one full repetition (e.g., extension and flexion), and how many repetitions to perform.

Sufficient practice repetitions are analogous to verbal commands for proper instruction. Since the dynamometer is novel to most subjects, they may require several practice trials in order to achieve reliable torque tracings. We recommend that each subject perform as many repetitions as needed to completely understand what is required during the testing or training process. This may be as few as 3 for experienced resistance-trained individuals or as many as 15 for naive subjects.

## Repetitions

A repetition is defined as completing a ROM movement for both the agonist and antagonist muscle groups. The practitioner chooses the number of repetitions to include in a test or exercise session based on what information is desired from the test or what outcome from the exercise session. For strength testing there is no need to perform more than 5 repetitions, but one may choose to perform as many as 50 repetitions when endurance is a factor. The total distance traveled within the predetermined ROM will have a significant effect on some physiological variables. Total work and power primarily are affected by ROM and therefore by repetitions. By setting hard stops at each end of the ROM, the practitioner can insure that all subjects traverse the same total distance. This is especially important for retest purposes, as some test variables (i.e., work and power) may be artificially inflated by increasing ROM.

## Velocity Order

Many dynamometers on the market today have a velocity range between 0 and 500°/s. The practitioner must decide which speed to use for testing or training depending on the desired result. When testing at multiple speeds it may be beneficial to randomize the sequence in order to control for order effects. However, conflicting evidence exists that velocity order does not significantly affect strength variables such as peak torque, work, and power.

Timm and Fyke (39) have shown no significant difference in torque measurements of knee extension at 60, 180, and 300°/s when varying test speed sequence. However, Kovaleski and Heitman (24, 25) and Kovaleski and others

(26) have shown that velocity progression order plays a role in torque, work, and power production during knee extension at 30 through 210°/s. The major difference between these studies appears to be number of repetitions performed. While Timm and Fyke (39) performed only 5, the Kovaleski group (24–26) performed 10. Therefore, fatigue may have been a factor in the latter studies and rest intervals may need to be adjusted accordingly.

## Static Preload

Placing a limb in a preactivated state has been shown to significantly affect strength variables. Neural preactivation of muscle units in the exercising limb places that limb in a ready state, which in turn leads to greater torque production. Kovaleski and colleagues (27), using knee extension at 120 through 210°/s, have documented that preloading the limb produces results superior to isokinetic training and may afford individuals full ROM strength development based on a reduced acceleration range.

## Bilateral Deficit

In our lab we have adapted our dynamometers to accept both limbs simultaneously (5, 6, 9). When testing or training is performed in this manner the practitioner should be aware of the bilateral deficit phenomenon; that is, when two limbs are performing maximal muscle actions simultaneously the resultant torque will be less than the sum of the individual limbs tested in isolation. Studies we have performed conclude that females may show a decrease in the bilateral deficit with increasing velocity from 60 through 360°/s, which may be explained through decreased activation of primarily slow twitch muscle fibers (5, 9). We have also shown significant unilateral torque improvements following bilateral training of the knee extensors and flexors at 60 and 180°/s (5) along with a decrease in the bilateral deficit with increasing velocity. There also appears to be significant correlation between isokinetic bilateral knee extension at 180°/s and a cycle ergometry test of power (6). This last investigation may shed some light on the use of open kinetic chain isokinetics as a laboratory measurement device that may be used as a picture into closed kinetic chain assessments.

## Coefficient of Variation

A repetition may be measured for reproducibility by means of the coefficient of variation (CV). In its simplest form the CV is the standard deviation of the torque divided by the mean of the torque. In this way a group of repetitions may be quantifiably evaluated for reproducibility. The CV values used in testing are generally less than 15% for clinical use and less than 10% for research purposes (4). The CV value is not a reliable measure during endurance testing because it will be inflated as a function of increasing repetitions, since torque and work will decline over time. Furthermore, artifacts associated with constant velocity and ROM may affect CV values at high speeds. Those artifacts are covered in the following sections.

## Velocity Overshoot and Torque Overshoot

The limb must pass through a free acceleration phase prior to receiving machine resistance (35), and torque tracings of the movement manifest artifacts upon engagement of resistance (load range) by the limb. Immediately following the acceleration phase of motion the lever arm and attached limb exhibit speed that is greater than the preselected velocity by as much as 200% (32, 35, 36, 45; see figure 5.3). A braking mechanism inside the power head of the dynamometer then attempts to slow the limb. Velocity overshoot occurs as a function of the limb accelerating past the desired speed. The subsequent braking results in an obvious torque spike as the limb slows to the preselected velocity. The effect of this braking is mild at slow speeds such as 60°/s (see figure 5.4) but increases in magnitude with increased velocity. Figure 5.5 shows that velocity and torque overshoot are coincident at the beginning of the flat load range.

This resultant torque overshoot is caused by the preceding velocity overshoot. As mentioned earlier, this spike will grow with increasing velocity (see figure 5.6) as the braking mechanism of the dynamometer must account for ever-increasing amounts of velocity overshoot. As shown in figure 5.7, the torque spike (flexion in this case) may dwarf actual peak torque produced by the human muscle.

It is important to remove this artifact prior to test interpretation. At present no dynamometer on the market will automatically remove torque overshoot, so it is incumbent on the practitioner to recognize the artifact and not consider

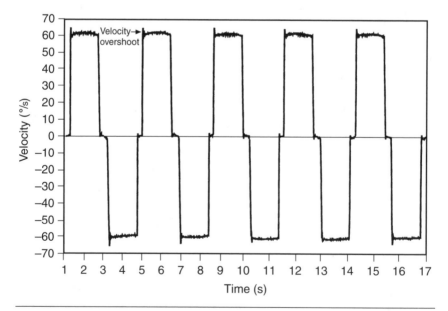

**Figure 5.3**   Velocity tracing of knee extension (positive) and flexion (negative) at 60°/s. Notice the small velocity overshoot at the beginning of the load range.

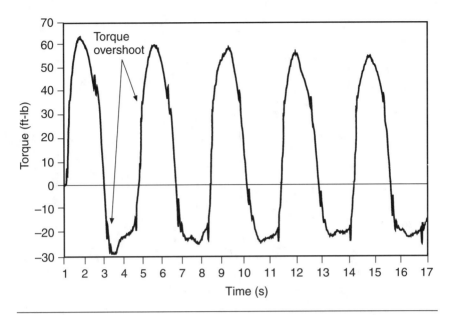

**Figure 5.4** Torque tracing of knee extension (positive) and flexion (negative) at 60°/s. Notice the small torque overshoot and impact artifacts at each end of the ROM.

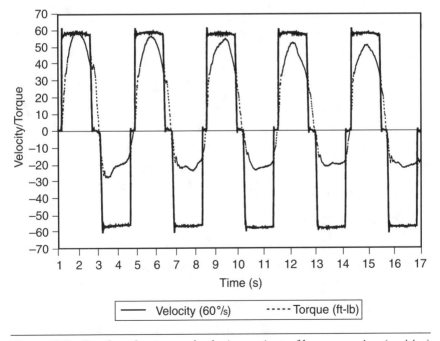

**Figure 5.5** Overlay of torque and velocity tracings of knee extension (positive) and flexion (negative) at 60°/s.

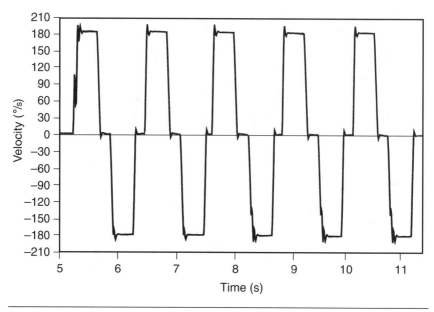

**Figure 5.6** Velocity tracing of knee extension (positive) and flexion (negative) at 180°/s. Notice the large velocity overshoot at the beginning of the load range.

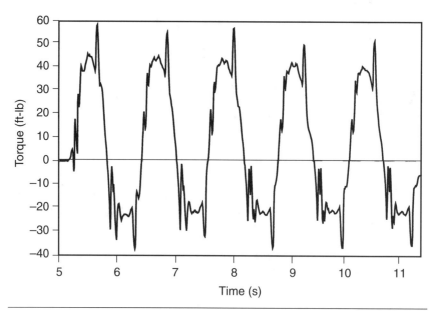

**Figure 5.7** Torque tracing of knee extension (positive) and flexion (negative) at 180°/s. Notice the large torque overshoot and impact artifacts at each end of the ROM.

it during analysis. In addition, some computer software (e.g., Biodex) attempts to control these effects by using a data reduction technique called windowing (43). During windowed analysis the acceleration and deceleration phases of the repetition are eliminated and only the load range data is preserved (see figure 5.8). This technique has been shown to increase the reliability of testing via the control of aberrant torque production (44).

It is interesting to note that figures 5.7 and 5.8 depict the same torque tracings at 180°/s. Notice the absence of torque overshoot during the positive extension curve but maintenance of this variable during flexion.

## Lever Arm Oscillation

The classic velocity tracing will look similar to figure 5.9 (180°/s). It contains an acceleration phase at the beginning of the ROM followed by velocity overshoot, then a load range phase, and finally a deceleration phase at the end of the ROM.

Another artifact inherent in the torque tracing is oscillation. Figure 5.10 depicts oscillation immediately following torque overshoot (11, 35). Notice also in figure 5.10 how windowing the data would remove some of the extraneous data.

Immediately after the acceleration phase there is a period of lever arm oscillation, which is caused by the length of the lever and the braking procedure

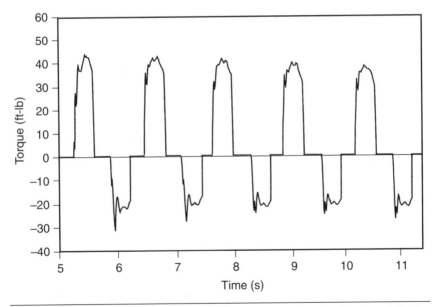

**Figure 5.8** Windowed torque tracing of knee extension (positive) and flexion (negative) at 180°/s. Notice the absence of large torque overshoot and impact artifacts during extension. However, a large torque overshoot remains during knee flexion.

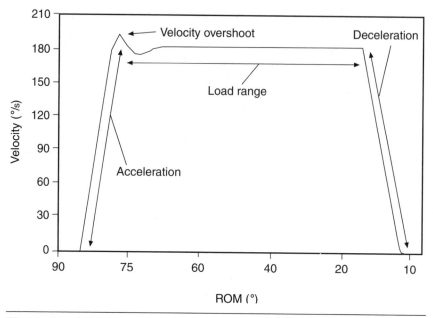

**Figure 5.9** Velocity tracing at 180°/s showing the three major phases of an isokinetic repetition plus velocity overshoot.

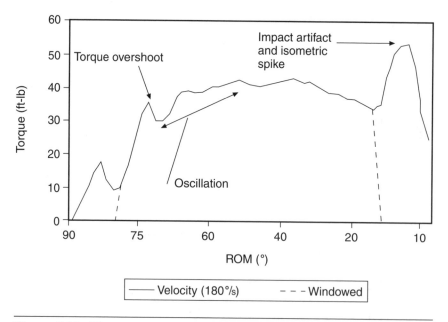

**Figure 5.10** Torque tracing at 180°/s demonstrating how windowed data reduces the effects of confounding elements.

that counteracts velocity overshoot. The exercising limb is attached to the dynamometer lever arm shaft distally but produces torque proximally; it may therefore be thought of as analogous to a long fishing pole. If one grasps a fishing pole at one end and applies a quick whipping motion, the distal end will oscillate back and forth for a short period of time until it stabilizes. Greater oscillation occurs with greater lever arm length and greater velocities as the distal end attempts to "catch up" and then decelerate to the speed of the proximal end (11, 35). Figure 5.10 shows oscillation in a close-up view. The probability of error is increased with the inclusion of lever arm artifacts such as these because it may be impossible to determine actual torque measurements apart from extraneous data.

## Impact Artifact and Isometric Spikes

From acceleration to deceleration, the repetition culminates in the eventual stopping of the lever arm. Many of the confounding elements already mentioned during the acceleration phase occur in reverse order during deceleration. First the dynamometer begins to slow the lever arm in preparation for stopping at the turnaround point. This causes the lever arm to oscillate somewhat and ultimately results in a large isometric spike at the end of the repetition due to the lever arm impacting the mechanical end stop (see figure 5.10). The spike is greater with increasing velocity as the limb and lever are moving faster upon impact. These spikes can be as much as twice as great as the torque seen during load range and should not be confused with actual muscle torque production.

Figure 5.11 demonstrates knee extension at 250°/s and the subsequent isometric spike at the end stop during the deceleration phase. As can be seen in figure 5.12, the velocity tracing at 250°/s exhibits no load range at all (absence of the flat portion of the curve), which is the result of knee extension exercise without machine resistance. Isometric spikes that are greater than peak torque and are coincident with deceleration are depicted in figures 5.13 and 5.14.

# Constant Velocity

It is somewhat paradoxical that one major criticism of isokinetic dynamometry is that functional movements in real life do not occur at a constant velocity (34). However, these same detractors point out that movements on an isokinetic device include only a small constant velocity phase. The classic early work of Fitts (13) demonstrated that limb motion occurs within an acceleration and deceleration paradigm. It has been shown many times (2, 7, 8, 10, 14, 16–18, 21, 22, 28–31, 46) that isokinetic devices, despite their claims of isokinetic movement, repeatedly fail to demonstrate isokinetic movement. Previous studies have advocated increasing the ROM at speeds from 60 through 300°/s to compensate for acceleration (18), have cautioned that peak torque may occur later in the ROM subsequent to acceleration at speeds greater than 180°/s, and have cautioned that maximum muscle tension may occur during the acceleration

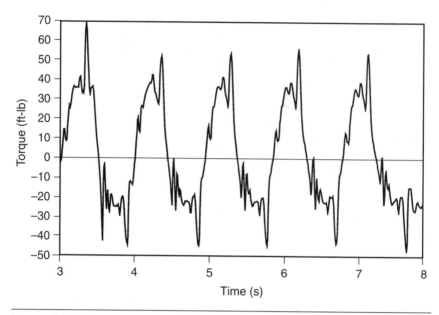

**Figure 5.11**    Torque tracing of knee extension (positive) and flexion (negative) at 250°/s. Notice the very large torque overshoot and impact artifacts at each end of the ROM.

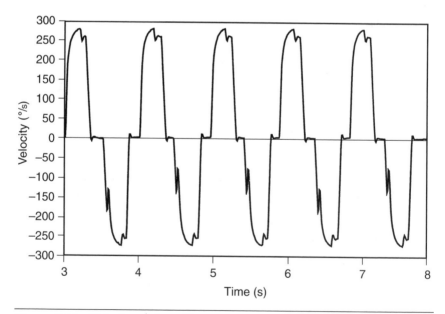

**Figure 5.12**    Velocity tracing of knee extension (positive) and flexion (negative) at 250°/s. Notice the absence of load range.

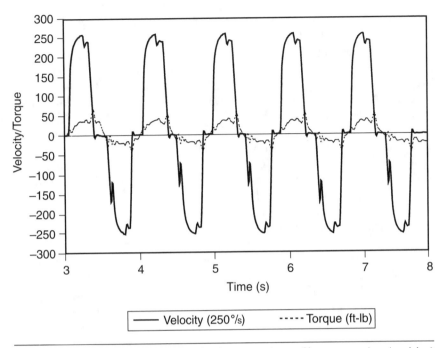

**Figure 5.13**  Overlay of torque and velocity tracings of knee extension (positive) and flexion (negative) at 250°/s.

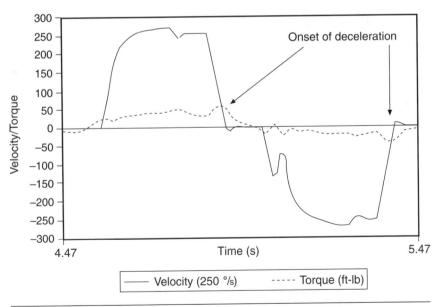

**Figure 5.14**  One repetition overlay of torque and velocity tracings of knee extension (positive) and flexion (negative) at 250°/s. Notice the artifact at the onset of deceleration.

phase (14). Further studies have documented quasi-isokinetic devices showing a load range of only 80% at moderate speeds (16) and closed kinetic chain devices with the same 80% load range (46). Other studies have shown acceleration and deceleration movements to be consistent with real-life activity (2) and that these phases are distinguished through individual difference (22). In addition, Abernethy and Jurimae (1) have shown that strength-training timing and magnitude adaptations vary greatly across modality. Collectively, this evidence points to a technology that may be functional within a penurious definition but does not rely on function as justification for existence.

It is apparent that while periods of constant velocity do occur in the context of isokinetic performance, they do so within boundaries determined by the speed of exercise performance. The acceleration and deceleration phases limit the range in which limb motion occurs at load range. The percentage of load range has been reported to decrease with increased dynamometer speed (7, 8, 10, 28–31). Figure 5.15 shows that when speed is increased during knee extension exercise, from 60 to 450°/s, load range decreases significantly as a portion of the total ROM. Figure 5.16 shows the same negative relationship between velocity and load range using shoulder internal/external rotation.

Since isokinetic dynamometers require an acceleration period prior to applying resistance to the exercising muscle, limitations exist in the extent to which

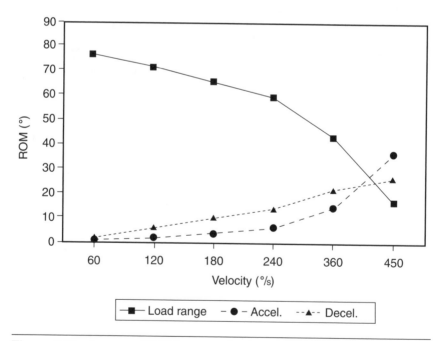

**Figure 5.15** Amount of ROM spent in load range, acceleration, and deceleration across velocities during knee extension.

From Brown et al. (8).

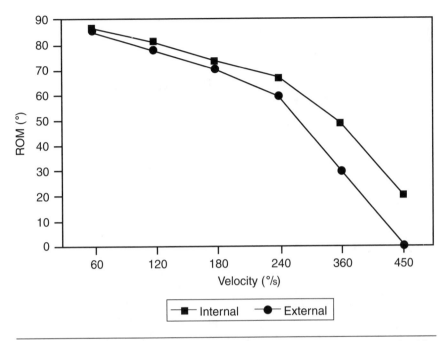

**Figure 5.16**  Amount of ROM spent in load range across velocities during shoulder internal/external rotation.

From Brown et al. (7).

dynamometers may be effective for either strength gains or strength evaluation in the total ROM. Sufficient time is needed for the muscle to develop its fullest contractile capacity (15, 19, 20, 23); thus, isokinetic exercise within a small joint range requires rapid acceleration of the limb to produce resistance within the desired range or muscle loading may not occur (7, 8, 28, 31). Hence, short arc isokinetic exercises may be limited to relatively slow dynamometer speeds if overload is a concern. However, if overload is not a concern then short arc isokinetics may prove advantageous for other reasons (i.e., neural and limb velocity training).

The dynamometers on the market today generally control deceleration, thus making load range a function of acceleration only. This means that the dynamometer will begin mechanical deceleration of the exercising limb at a predetermined position in the ROM in order to reduce collision with the end stop. Therefore, quick limb acceleration will result in reaching load range sooner, thereby enhancing the overload phase of the repetition. Conversely, slow acceleration will result in less load range or, in some cases, none at all (7, 9).

Initial investigations into acceleration focused on acceleration time. Chen and colleagues (11) tested knee extension and flexion at speeds from 30 to 300°/s. Their table 9 represents almost no change in acceleration time across speeds, which may mean that this variable is not sensitive enough to acceleration motion. Furthermore, errors due to oscillation and velocity overshoot have caused researchers to accept movement that varies around the preset speed from 2% to 10% (8, 12, 33, 36). This further illustrates the extent to which load range may be compromised during isokinetic exercise.

# The Major Phases of a Repetition

Initial investigations in our laboratory have focused on direct quantification of the three major phases of an isokinetic repetition. We have investigated knee extension/flexion (8, 10) and shoulder internal/external rotation (7) as well as the influence of repetition type and number (10). Each of these studies, and its conclusions, is summarized below.

## Knee Testing Methods

Nine male and nine female subjects with no history of orthopedic knee pathology volunteered to participate. Testing was performed on the Biodex System 2 isokinetic dynamometer (Biodex Corp., Shirley, NY), which has been shown to be a reliable instrument for collecting data (4) and a valid measurement tool of human torque, joint position, and limb velocity (36). The dynamometer shaft was aligned with the assumed axis of rotation (lateral femoral condyle) of the dominant knee with the subject in a seated position and the back reclined at approximately 110°. Both thighs were secured with straps as were the waist and thoracic torso. Arms were placed across the chest with hands grasping the straps. Range of motion mechanical stops were set at 90 and 10° of knee flexion (0° at full extension). The lever arm pad was positioned to place the inferior aspect immediately superior to the medial malleolus. Warm-up on the isokinetic device consisted of 3 submaximal reciprocal concentric extension and flexion repetitions with increasing intensity (i.e., first repetition at 25% perceived effort, second repetition at 50% perceived effort, etc.) at 60 through 450°/s (4, 39). In addition the subject completed two maximal intensity repetitions at each speed, then rested for 1 min prior to testing. Testing began from a dead stop with the subject's leg at 90° of flexion and consisted of 3 maximal concentric reciprocal knee extension and flexion gravity-corrected repetitions in a fixed order at 60, 120, 180, 240, 360, and 450°/s with 30 s rest between velocities (39). Each subject was encouraged to contact the mechanical end stops during both extension and flexion motions. Consistent and identical verbal encouragement was provided during the test, but no visual feedback of torque generation was provided.

## Test Results

Multivariate analysis of variance with repeated measures was used to determine the difference in load range and acceleration and deceleration ROM between velocities. Load range significantly ($p < .05$) decreased and acceleration and deceleration ROM significantly increased with each increase in velocity for knee extension (see figure 5.15). Analysis of variance results revealed that females exhibited significantly greater acceleration ROM and significantly less load range than males at 240, 360, and 450°/s during extension while deceleration ROM was not gender dependent. Extension load range, as a percentage of the total test ROM, decreased from 96.1% to 21.1% for males and from 95.9% to 0.0% for females at 60 through 450°/s. Additionally, no females were able to attain velocity during knee extension at 450°/s.

These results are not surprising with consideration given to the fact that deceleration is controlled by the dynamometer and therefore should not be different across subjects. In light of this study we concluded that acceleration is the determining factor in load range. The faster one accelerates the limb, the greater the load range that will be experienced. This led Wilk and colleagues (44) to measure the relationship between acceleration and functional testing in the knee. The Wilk group demonstrated significant correlation between knee acceleration at 180 and 300°/s with the timed hop test and triple crossover hop tests in ACL-reconstructed patients. Gender differences have been demonstrated prior to this study by other researchers, including the documentation of different concentric/eccentric ratios (17) and different maximal velocities of limb movement (20). These may be explained by the different force-time relationships exhibited across gender (23).

## Shoulder Testing Methods

In this study 12 elite male junior tennis players with no history of orthopedic shoulder pathology who were actively involved in a tennis training program volunteered to participate. Testing was performed on the Biodex System 2. The dynamometer shaft was aligned with the olecranon process of the dominant arm at approximately 45° of abduction. The subject was seated with his back reclined at approximately 110°. Straps secured his waist and thoracic torso. Total ROM was 90°, from +45° to –45° of internal and external rotation. Testing began from a dead stop and consisted of 3 maximal concentric reciprocal shoulder internal and external gravity-corrected repetitions in a fixed order at 60, 120, 180, 240, 360, and 450°/s with 30 s rest between velocities (39). Each subject was encouraged to contact the mechanical end stops during both internal and external motions. Consistent and identical verbal encouragement was provided during the test, but no visual feedback of torque generation was provided.

## Test Results

Multivariate analysis of variance with repeated measures was used to determine the difference in load range and acceleration and deceleration ROM between velocities. Load range significantly ($p < .05$) decreased with each increase in velocity for shoulder internal and external rotation (see figure 5.16). Results further revealed that external rotation load range, as a percentage of the total test ROM, decreased from 95.4% to 0.0%, while internal rotation decreased from 96.3% to 21.8% at 60 through 450°/s. No subject was able to attain velocity during external rotation at 450°/s.

Muscle architecture and fiber type may account for the variation in acceleration rate differences between subjects. Previous investigations have shown that muscle length and cross-sectional area (42) as well as a greater percentage of fast twitch fibers (19, 38) may alter the force-velocity curve.

# Reciprocal Versus Single and Multiple Repetitions

The previous two studies are similar in that they document that acceleration is a determining factor in load range. The following study (10) looked at acceleration ROM with the knowledge of its effect on load range. Multiple repetitions performed on an isokinetic device may take one of two forms: reciprocal, defined as a repetition that is immediately preceded by another repetition, or single, a repetition that begins from a dead stop. The following study examined the difference in acceleration ROM as a function of these two repetition types.

## Testing Methods

Fifteen male and 20 female subjects completed a practice session on the isokinetic dynamometer prior to participation. Testing was performed on the Biodex System 2 isokinetic dynamometer. Range of motion mechanical stops were set at 90 and 0° of knee flexion (0° at full extension). Two different test sessions (multiple speed and multiple repetition) were performed on two different days separated by one week with test session order randomized.

Multiple speed testing began from a dead stop with the subject's leg at 90° of flexion and consisted of 3 maximal concentric reciprocal knee extension and flexion gravity-corrected repetitions. Velocities were presented in a fixed order at 60, 120, 180, 240, 300, 360, 400, and 450°/s with 30 s rest between velocities (39). The first repetition was identified as single while repetitions two and three were reciprocal. The acceleration ROM mean of repetitions two and three was used for data analysis.

Multiple repetition testing was performed at 180°/s with 50 extension motions only and a passive return to flexion as described by Thorstensson (37). The mean value of every tenth repetition was recorded for trend analysis. Methods were the same as described earlier for knee testing and each subject was encouraged to contact the mechanical end stop during the extension motion. Consistent and identical verbal encouragement was provided during each test session, but no visual feedback of any kind was provided.

## Test Results

Data were divided into three phases by the Biodex software based on velocity and position curves. Total ROM prior to velocity attainment was termed acceleration, ROM during sustained velocity was termed load range, and ROM after load range was termed deceleration. Only the acceleration phase during knee extension was recorded and used for data analysis. The Biodex dynamometer controls deceleration, therefore only the subject's individual rate of acceleration determines the load range. Multivariate analysis of variance with repeated measures was used to determine the difference in acceleration between repetitions, repetition type, and gender. During the multiple repetition test at 180°/s, acceleration significantly ($p < .05$) increased every 10 repetitions between 20 and 50 yet was not gender dependent (see figure 5.17). During multiple speed testing, reciprocal repetitions exhibited significantly less acceleration than single repetitions at all speeds for both genders (see figure 5.18). Males demonstrated significantly less acceleration than females during reciprocal repetitions at 120 through 450°/s and significantly less acceleration than females during single repetitions at 240 through 450°/s (see figure 5.18).

There is a direct positive correlation between acceleration ROM and velocity during knee extension exercise. There is also a positive correlation between acceleration ROM and number of repetitions when the number exceeds 20. The ability of reciprocal repetitions to produce a greater acceleration rate than single repetitions may be explained as a function of the antagonist muscle action that serves to influence the agonist muscle unit activation (15). As a result the extensors may be preactivated and therefore are able to react more quickly, which results in greater acceleration rates.

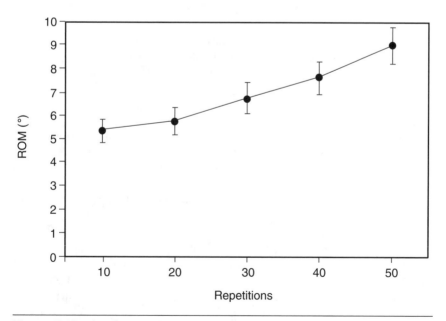

**Figure 5.17**  Acceleration ROM at 180°/s across 50 repetitions.

From Brown et al. (10).

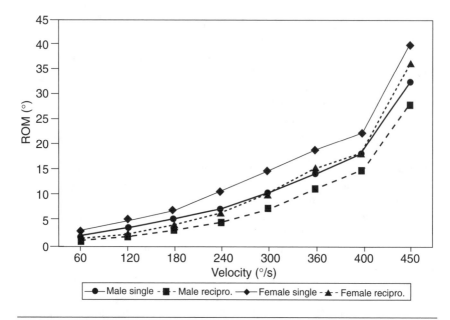

**Figure 5.18** Acceleration ROM between single and reciprocal repetitions by speed and gender.

From Brown et al. (10).

# Summary

The practitioner must use the isokinetic dynamometer properly and interpret the isokinetic data carefully. He or she should be aware of standardized testing procedures such as determining the desired information prior to testing, knowing how to isolate and stabilize a subject and the muscle group being tested, and properly aligning the limb and machine axes of rotation. Gravity compensation should be used when exercising against gravity; total and physiological ROM must be equal for proper comparative reasons. Verbal instructions should be clear and identical across subjects; repetition number and type should be chosen based on the desired outcome of testing. Velocity order should be chosen on the basis of whether one is testing or training, static preload may be used to reduce acceleration effects, bilateral deficit concerns will impact testing limbs alone or together, and the coefficient of variation will shed light on the reproducibility of a set of repetitions.

Confounding factors such as velocity and torque overshoot may be reduced through data reduction techniques as may lever arm oscillation, impact artifacts, and isometric spikes. Failure to interpret isokinetic tests in light of the foregoing discussion may result in erroneous information and spurious conclusions. Furthermore, the data should be separated into phases of acceleration, load range, and deceleration, and inherent artifacts should be eliminated where possible prior to interpretation. Additionally, gender and muscle fiber effects on acceleration and load range should be taken into account prior to testing as should velocity variation between individuals.

With the exception of the X-ray machine, no other tool designed to interpret the human condition has been more abused by uninformed and ill-informed practitioners. We hope the preceding chapter will assist those engaged in training and research designed to evaluate athletic and human performance.

# References

1. Abernethy, P.J., and J. Jurimae. 1996. Cross-sectional and longitudinal uses of isoinertial, isometric, and isokinetic dynamometry. *Med. Sci. Sports Exer.* 28(9): 1180–87.

2. Aagaard, P., E.B. Simonsen, M. Trolle, J. Bangsbo, and K. Klausen. 1994. Moment and power generation during maximal knee extensions performed at low and high speeds. *Eur. J. Appl. Physiol.* 69: 376–81.

3. Baltzopoulos, V., J.G. Williams, and D.A. Brodie. 1989. Isokinetic dynamometry: Applications and limitations. *Sports Med.* 8: 101–16.

4. Brown, L.E., M. Whitehurst, J.R. Bryant, and D.N. Buchalter. 1993. Reliability of the Biodex System 2 isokinetic dynamometer concentric mode. *Isokinetics Exer. Sci.* 3(3): 160–63.

5. Brown, L.E., M. Whitehurst, and D.N. Buchalter. 1993. Bilateral isokinetic knee rehabilitation following bilateral total knee replacement surgery. *J. Sport Rehab.* 2: 274–80.

6. Brown, L.E., M. Whitehurst, and D.N. Buchalter. 1994. Comparison of bilateral isokinetic knee extension/flexion and cycle ergometry tests of power. *J. Strength Cond. Res.* 8(3): 139–43.

7. Brown, L.E., M. Whitehurst, B.F. Findley, R. Gilbert, and D.N. Buchalter. 1995. Isokinetic load range during shoulder rotation exercise in elite male junior tennis players. *J. Strength Cond. Res.* 9(3): 160–64.

8. Brown, L.E., M. Whitehurst, R. Gilbert, and D.N. Buchalter. 1995. The effect of velocity and gender on load range during knee extension and flexion exercise on an isokinetic device. *J. Ortho. Sports Phys. Ther.* 21(2): 107–12.

9. Brown, L.E., M. Whitehurst, R. Gilbert, B.W. Findley, and D. Buchalter. 1994. Effect of velocity on the bilateral deficit during dynamic knee extension and flexion exercise in females. *Isokinetics Exer. Sci.* 4(4): 153–56.

10. Brown, L., M. Whitehurst, B. Findley, P. Gilbert, D. Groo, and J. Jimenez. 1998. The effect of repetitions and gender on acceleration range of motion during knee extension on an isokinetic device. *J. Strength Cond. Res.* 12(4): 222–25.

11. Chen, W.L., F.C. Su, and Y.L. Chou. 1994. Significance of acceleration period in a dynamic strength testing study. *J. Ortho. Sports Phys. Ther.* 19(6): 324–30.

12. Chow, J.W., W.G. Darling, and J.G. Hay. 1997. Mechanical characteristics of knee extension exercises performed on an isokinetic dynamometer. *Med. Sci. Sports Exer.* 29(6): 794–803.

13. Fitts, P.M. 1954. The information capacity of the human motor system in controlling the amplitude of movement. *J. Exper. Psych.* 47: 381–91.

14. Gransberg, L., and E. Knutsson. 1983. Determination of dynamic muscle strength in man with acceleration controlled isokinetic movements. *Acta Physiol. Scand.* 119: 317–20.

15. Grabiner, M.D. 1994. Maximum rate of force development is increased by antagonist conditioning contraction. *J. Appl. Physiol.* 77(2): 807–11.

16. Greenblatt, D., W. Diesel, and T.D. Noakes. 1997. Clinical assessment of the low-cost VariCom isokinetic knee exerciser. *Med. Eng. Phys.* 19(3): 273–78.

17. Griffin, J.W., R.E. Tooms, R. Vander Zwaag, T.E. Bertorini, and M.L. O'Toole. 1993. Eccentric muscle performance of elbow and knee muscle groups in untrained men and women. *Med. Sci. Sports Exer.* 25(8): 936–44.

18. Handel, M., H.H. Dickhuth, F. Mayer, and R.W. Gulch. 1996. Prerequisites and limitations to isokinetic measurements in humans: Investigations on a servomotor-controlled dynamometer. *Eur. J. Appl. Physiol.* 73: 225–30.

19. Houston, M.E., R. W. Norman, and E.A. Froese. 1988. Mechanical measures during maximal velocity knee extension exercise and their relation to fiber composition of the human vastus lateralis muscle. *Eur. J. Appl. Physiol.* 58: 1–7.

20. Ives, J.C., W.P. Kroll, and L.L. Bultman. 1993. Rapid movement kinematic and electromyographic control characteristics in males and females. *Res. Quart.* 64(3): 274–83.

21. Kannus, P., and B. Beynnon. 1993. Peak torque occurrence in the range of motion during isokinetic extension and flexion of the knee. *Int. J. Sports Med.* 14(8): 422–26.

22. Kaufman, K.R., K.N. An, and E.Y.S. Chao. 1995. A comparison of intersegmental joint dynamics to isokinetic dynamometer measurements. *J. Biomechanics* 28(10): 1243–56.

23. Komi, P.V., and J. Karlsson. 1978. Skeletal muscle fiber types, enzyme activities, and physical performance in young males and females. *Acta Physiol. Scand.* 103: 210–18.

24. Kovaleski, J.E., and R.J. Heitman. 1993. Interaction of velocity and progression order during isokinetic velocity spectrum exercise. *Isokinetics Exer. Sci.* 3: 118–22.

25. Kovaleski, J.E., and R.J. Heitman. 1993. Effects of isokinetic velocity spectrum exercise on torque production. *Sports Med. Training Rehab.* 4: 67–71.

26. Kovaleski, J.E., R.J. Heitman, F.M. Scaffidi, and F.B. Fondren. 1992. Effects of isokinetic velocity spectrum exercise on average power and total work. *J. Athletic Training* 27: 54–56.

27. Kovaleski, J.E., R.J. Heitman, T.L. Trundle, and W.F. Gilley. 1995. Isotonic preload versus isokinetic knee extension resistance training. *Med. Sci. Sports Exer.* 27(6): 895–99.

28. Lander, J.E., B.T. Bates, J.A. Sawhill, and J.A. Hamill. 1985. Comparison between free weight and isokinetic bench pressing. *Med. Sci. Sports Exer.* 17(3): 344–53.

29. Osternig, L.R. 1986. Isokinetic dynamometry: Implications for muscle testing and rehabilitation. In *Exercise and sport sciences reviews.* Vol. 14, ed. K.B. Pandolf, 45–80. New York: Macmillan.

30. Osternig, L.R. 1975. Optimal isokinetic loads and velocities producing muscular power in human subjects. *Arch. Phys. Med. Rehab.* 56: 152–55.

31. Osternig, L.R., J.A. Sawhill, B.T. Bates, and J. Hamill. 1983. Function of limb speed on torque patterns of antagonist muscles. In: *Biomechanics* VIII-A. Vol. 4A, ed. H. Matsui and K. Kobayashi, 251–57. Champaign, IL: Human Kinetics.

32. Perrine, J.J., and V.R. Edgerton. 1978. Muscle force-velocity and power-velocity relationships under isokinetic loading. *Med. Sci. Sports Exer.* 10(3): 159–66.

33. Rathfon, J.A., K.M. Matthews, A.N. Yang, P.K. Levangie, and M.C. Morrissey. 1991. Effects of different acceleration and deceleration rates on isokinetic performance of the knee extensors. *J. Ortho. Sports Phys. Ther.* 14(4): 161–68.

34. Rothstein, J.M., R.L. Lamb, and T.P. Mayhew. 1987. Clinical uses of isokinetic measurements. *Phys. Ther.* 67(12): 1840–44.

35. Sapega, A.A., J.A. Nicholas, D. Sokolow, and A. Saranti. 1982. The nature of torque "overshoot" in Cybex isokinetic dynamometry. *Med. Sci. Sports Exer.* 14(5): 368–75.

36. Taylor, N.A.S., R.H. Sanders, E.I. Howick, and S.N. Stanley. 1991. Static and dynamic assessment of the Biodex dynamometer. *Eur. J. Appl. Physiol.* 62: 180–88.

37. Thorstensson, A., and J. Karlsson. 1976. Fatigability and fiber composition of human skeletal muscle. *Acta Physiol. Scand.* 98: 318–22.

38. Thorstensson, A. 1976. Muscle strength, fiber types, and enzyme actions in man. *Acta Physiol. Scand.* 443(Suppl.): 1–45.

39. Timm, K.E., and D. Fyke. 1993. The effect of test speed sequence on the concentric isokinetic performance of the knee extensor muscle group. *Isokinetics Exer. Sci.* 3(2): 123–28.

40. Tis, L.L., and D.H. Perrin. 1993. Validity of data extraction techniques on the kinetic communicator (KinCom) isokinetic device. *Isokinetics Exer. Sci.* 3(2): 96–100.

41. Weir, J.P., S.A. Evans, and M.L. Housh. 1996. The effect of extraneous movements on peak torque and constant joint angle torque-velocity curves. *J. Ortho. Sports Phys. Ther.* 23: 302–8.

42. Wickiewicz T.L., R.R. Roy, P.L. Powell, J.J. Perrine, and V.R. Edgerton. 1984. Muscle architecture and force-velocity relationships in humans. *J. Appl. Physiol.* 57(2): 435–43.

43. Wilk, K.E., C.A. Arrigo, and J.R. Andrews. 1992. Isokinetic testing of the shoulder abductors and adductors: Windowed vs. nonwindowed data collection. *J. Ortho. Sports Phys. Ther.* 15(2): 107–12.

44. Wilk, K.E., W.T. Romaniello, S.M. Soscia, C.A. Arrigo, and J.R. Andrews. 1994. The relationship between subjective knee scores, isokinetic testing, and functional testing in the ACL-reconstructed knee. *J. Ortho. Sports Phys. Ther.* 20(2): 60–73.

45. Wilson, G.J., A.D. Walshe, and M.R. Fisher. 1997. The development of an isokinetic squat device: Reliability and relationship to functional performance. *Eur. J. Appl. Physiol.* 75: 455–61.

46. Winter, D.A., R.P. Wells, and G.W. Orr. 1981. Errors in the use of isokinetic dynamometers. *Eur. J. Appl. Physiol.* 46: 397–408.

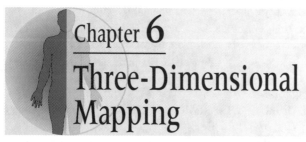

# Chapter 6
# Three-Dimensional Mapping

Joseph F. Signorile and Brooks Applegate

**T**wo inherent properties of isolated skeletal muscle are the bases for the three-dimensional maps described in this chapter. These properties, which must be considered part of the history of muscle physiology, are the length-tension and force-velocity relationships. Each can be visualized as a curve with its respective components defining their axes. Before examining the three-dimensional maps developed at our laboratory, it may be helpful to look at each curve separately to understand the basis of its shape and its applicability to the isokinetic analysis we describe in this chapter.

## The Length-Tension Curve

The length-tension relationship in isolated skeletal muscle was recognized in the late 1800s, but the characteristic shape (see figure 6.1*a*) with which we are currently familiar was the result of the independent experiments by Gordon, Huxley, and Julian (13) and Edman (10) in the mid-1960s.

The curve is a combination of two components, a contractile component (the sarcomere) and an elastic component (the costamere and connective tissue). These components are represented, respectively, as the dashed and dotted lines in figure 6.1*a*. As can also be seen from figure 6.1, *a* through *c*, individual muscles may produce differently shaped curves due to the variations in either component or the relationship between the two.

The active or contractile portion of the curve was developed using isolated muscle preparations, which enabled the researcher to test their maximal isometric tensions at predetermined lengths. Figure 6.2 illustrates the tension of the contractile portion of a muscle and its relationship to sarcomere length.

The shape of the length-tension curve of an isolated muscle preparation is often very different from that of an intact muscle due to a number of factors. First, a muscle fiber will produce its maximal tension at approximately 120%

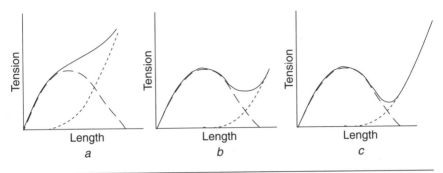

**Figure 6.1**   Length-tension curves from three isolated muscle preparations containing progressively lower connective tissue contents. The solid line represents the additive tension of the contractile (dashed line) and connective tissue (dotted line) components.

From Carlson and Wilke 1974.

of its equilibrium length, and the fiber lengths for intact skeletal muscles range from 70% to 140% of their equilibrium length depending on the range of motion of the joints over which they cross (1). Second, each intact muscle will have its own inherent length-tension curve, which is dependent on its connective tissue content, its equilibrium length, and its mechanical relationship to the joint on which it acts. Finally, the bones of the body are levers, and maximal force is applied to any lever at an angle of 90°. Therefore, any limb position causing the muscle to pull at an angle other than 90° would dictate less than maximal force production.

# The Force-Velocity Curve

Initial descriptions of the force-velocity relationship in skeletal muscle were presented by A.V. Hill (20) and Bernard Katz (24) in the late 1930s. As was the case with the length-tension curve, the force-velocity curve was developed using isolated muscle preparations. The characteristic curve produced during such experiments is shown in figure 6.3.

A review of the curve reveals the relationship between force and velocity, that is, as force increases, velocity decreases. Examining the points where the curve touches the ordinate (y axis) and abscissa (x axis), it can also be seen that maximal force ($F_{max}$) is exerted at a velocity of zero ($V_{min}$) and that maximal velocity ($V_{max}$) is produced at the point of minimal force application ($F_{min}$). It should be recognized that in intact skeletal muscle a condition of complete unloading ($F_{min}$ or $V_{max}$) can not exist due to the attachment of the muscle to the bony levers of the skeletal system.

The second curve appearing in figure 6.3, the power curve (dashed line), is the product of force and velocity:

$$\text{Power} = \text{force} \times \text{velocity}.$$

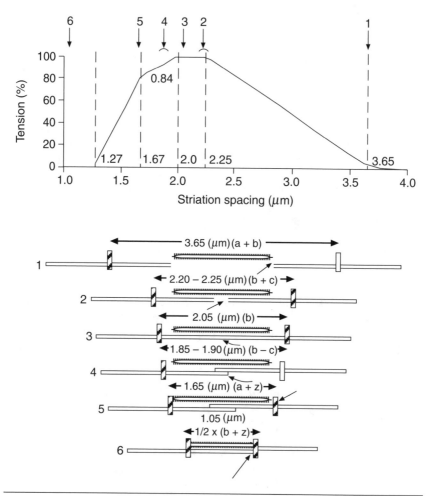

**Figure 6.2**    Contractile component of the length-tension curve showing the overall curve and related sarcomere lengths as well as filament overlap.

From *Journal of Physiology* 1966.

The point at which peak power ($P_{peak}$) is produced in this relationship has been estimated at approximately 30% of $F_{max}$ and $V_{max}$ (11). Given this relationship, specific shifts in the force-velocity curve would dictate shifts in $P_{peak}$. In figure 6.4, the dotted lines represent the pretraining curves and the solid lines show increased values for both force and velocity with training and the related shift in $P_{peak}$.

As was the case with the length-tension curve, applying the force-velocity curve, which was constructed in vitro, to in vivo applications is complicated by a number of factors. These factors include neuromuscular influences (37), distribution of fiber types (21), differences in velocity within fiber types (43), coactivation of agonists and antagonists (2, 29, 44, 47), and the nature of the testing device (17, 36).

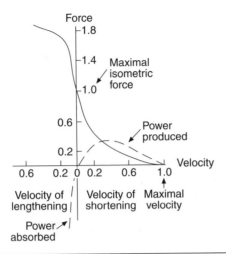

**Figure 6.3**   Classic force-velocity curve obtained from isolated skeletal muscle preparations. Note that force and velocity are presented on normalized axes. The power curve (Power = force × velocity) is shown as a dashed line.

From Astrand and Rodahl 1986.

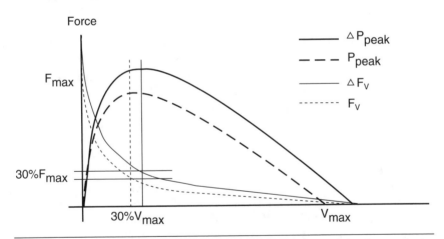

**Figure 6.4**   An example of a shift upward and to the right of the force-velocity curve, due to the effects of training the muscle, and the increase in peak power.

# Hypothetical Models for Length-Force-Velocity Surfaces

A number of authors have presented models of length-force-velocity surfaces. For example, Richard L. Lieber, in his text *Skeletal muscle structure and function*, provides a three-dimensional surface map that includes both the overall surface and individual "slices" at specific velocities and lengths (30). These slices illustrate the individual length-tension and force-velocity components that frame the surface. A model more closely associated with the surfaces presented in this chapter was offered by Everett Harmon in his chapter on "The Biomechanics of Resistance Training" contained in the National Strength and Conditioning Association text, *Essentials of strength training and conditioning* (16). The axes in Harmon's model are joint angle, torque, and angular velocity rather than length, force, and velocity. Harmon's variables are more appropriate when describing intact muscle function, since all forces and movement patterns are applied through the bony levers of the body and are therefore angular in nature.

Although these models are available, to our knowledge, no studies to this point have provided maps that show relationships between the contours of these surfaces and the specific training patterns employed by individual athletes.

# Modifications in the Length-Tension Curve Due to Training

The ability of the length-tension relationship to change with respect to specific training protocols has been hypothesized by a number of researchers (35, 45). While there are few studies that have examined this question explicitly, a number of studies confirm the feasibility of this hypothesis (3, 12, 18, 19, 25–27, 31, 42, 45, 46).

Studies of isometric training have shown that strength improvements are specific to the joint angle at which the training occurs (3, 12, 25, 26, 42). However, conflicting data do exist (38). The degree of carryover from the joint angle used in training to other angles of force application is dependent on a number of factors including the muscle groups involved (25, 26, 42), the joint angle and related length of the muscle (12, 25, 26, 42), and the duration of the action (32). However, the fact that joint angle-specific increases in strength do occur with isometric training demonstrates that the length-tension curve can be modified at particular points along its length by training.

In two separate experiments, Williams and Goldspink (45, 46) showed that immobilized cat soleus muscle either added (20%) or reduced (40%) sarcomere number when held in full dorsiflexion or full plantarflexion, respectively. They determined that these changes reset the length-tension relationship to optimize force production at the immobilization length.

Lynn and Morgan (31) showed that sarcomere number, and thus the length-tension relationship, could be increased in the vastus intermedius muscles of rats using downhill running, due to the large eccentric component of the exercise.

Herzog and his colleagues (18, 27) have shown that the torque-angle curve is highly dependent on the mechanical dictates of the synergistic muscles, especially the additive effects of their force-length relationships. Herzog and coworkers (19) provided convincing proof of the modification of the moment-length relationship for the rectus femoris muscle with training by comparing the moment-length relationships of one speedskater and three cyclists to those of four runners. They showed that cyclists produced greater force at shorter rectus femoris lengths since cycling is performed at a small hip angle, while the runners exhibited the opposite relationship since running requires a greater hip angle.

These studies help to support the hypothesis that the torque-angle relationship of our three-dimensional maps should assume a specific shape dictated by the individual training protocols of the athletes studied.

# Modifications in the Force-Velocity Curve Due to Training

The force-velocity relationship in skeletal muscle is also quite plastic. A number of cross-sectional population studies and longitudinal training studies confirm specific adaptations to different training protocols.

## Population Studies

A study by de Koning and coworkers (9) compared the differences in the force-velocity curve within samples of 123 untrained males, 110 untrained females, and 48 arm-trained competitive athletes. Although they reported no significant differences among the groups in the shapes of the force-velocity curves, the curves for untrained males and untrained females showed a smaller moment at any velocity than those of the athletes. The athletes also produced greater maximal static moments, maximal angular velocity, and maximal power values. The authors suggested that the similar shapes of the curves among groups might have been due to the lack of training specificity (9).

These results confirmed those reported earlier by de Koning and colleagues (8) indicating no changes in the shape of the force-velocity curves among rowers, tug-of-war athletes, or runners across a season of training. However, significant differences in maximal static moment and maximal power values were found among the groups due to exercise specificity.

Labrecque and coworkers (28) produced force-velocity curves using a Nautilus knee extension machine and reported that the curve that was produced by a sprinter (100 m in 11.2 s) was positioned furthest up and to the right and that produced by a marathoner (42.2 km in 2 h 35 min) was furthest down and to the left.

## Training Studies

Coyle and coworkers (6) examined the effect of low speed (1.05 rad/s), high speed (5.24 rad/s), and mixed speed (1.05 and 5.24 rad/s) training protocols on isokinetic mean torque at 0, 1.05, 3.14, and 5.24 rad/s. Results confirmed the theory of speed-specific training. The low speed training group produced their greatest increases in torque (31.8%) at 1.05 rad/s, the high speed group improved significantly at both 3.14 rad/s (16.8%) and 5.24 rad/s (18.5%), and mixed speed training proved the second most effective technique at 1.05 rad/s (23.6%) and 5.24 rad/s (16.1%). It is interesting to note that the mixed speed group showed the least improvement at 3.14 rad/s, the speed at which they did no training.

A study by Caiozzo and colleagues (4) also demonstrated that speed-specific training regimens could elicit changes in specific portions of the force-velocity curve. Individuals trained at either 1.68 or 4.19 rad/s. When increases in torque were plotted against velocity, the regression lines for each group showed slopes going in opposite directions. The group training at 1.68 rad/s made greatest improvements at the low velocities (downward slope) and the group that trained at 4.19 rad/s improved most at the highest velocities (upward slope).

Kanehisa and Miyashita (23) examined knee extension power at 1.05, 2.09, 3.14, 4.19, and 5.24 rad/s in 21 male volunteers before and after isokinetic training. Training was performed at 1.05 rad/s (slow speed), 3.14 rad/s (intermediate speed), or 5.24 rad/s (high speed). The results of their study were similar to those of Caiozzo and his coworkers. Kanehisa and Miyashita reported significant gains in power at all isokinetic speeds tested for the slow speed training group. However, as testing speed was increased, these gains declined from 24.8% at 1.05 rad/s to 8.6% at 5.24 rad/s. The intermediate speed group showed consistent increases in power across all testing speeds (18.5–22.4%) except 2.09 rad/s (15.4%). The high speed training group, however, showed increases in power only at the faster speeds of testing (23.9% at 4.19 rad/s and 22.8% at 5.24 rad/s).

In a study examining the effects of slow resistance training on jump performance, Hakkinen and Komi (14) noted that a significant shift occurred in the high force (low velocity) portion of the force-velocity curve; however, these changes became consistently smaller at higher leg extension velocities. These same investigators examined the effect of explosive, low resistance exercise on the force-velocity curve and found that the greatest improvements were in the high velocity portion of the curve (15).

As was the case with the studies showing changes in the length-tension curve due to training, the studies examining changes in the force-velocity relationship also supported our hypothesis that the three-dimensional maps presented in this chapter would be unique to the training distances and events of the athletes tested.

# Discrimination of Runners Using Three-Dimensional Mapping

This section presents the results of our study designed to determine if isokinetic torque-angle-velocity surfaces could be used to identify track athletes according to their specific training regimens.

## Test Subjects

Fifteen competitive runners participated in our study. Subject characteristics are presented in table 6.1. Subjects were assigned to one of four groups ac-

## Table 6.1    Subject Characteristics

| Subject | Age (yr) | Weight (kg) | Gender | Event |
|---------|----------|-------------|--------|-------|
| 1 | 20 | 48.92 | F | 10 km |
| 2 | 43 | 54.81 | F | 10 km |
| 3 | 55 | 81.54 | M | 10 km |
| 4 | 32 | 71.57 | M | 10 km |
| 5 | 17 | 81.54 | M | 100 m, 400 m, hurdles |
| 6 | 19 | 78.37 | M | 100 m, 200 m |
| 7 | 21 | 67.95 | M | 100 m, 200 m |
| 8 | 19 | 73.39 | M | 100 m, 400 m |
| 9 | 20 | 60.70 | F | 400 m |
| 10 | 21 | 57.98 | F | 400 m, long jump |
| 11 | 22 | 67.04 | M | 400 m, 800 m |
| 12 | 19 | 59.80 | F | 400 m, 800 m |
| 13 | 18 | 63.42 | M | 800 m, 1500 m |
| 14 | 19 | 59.80 | F | 800 m |
| 15 | 19 | 75.65 | M | 800 m, 1500 m |
| Mean | 24.25 | 68.32 | M = 9, F = 6 | |
| SE | 2.62 | 11.35 | | |

cording to their predominant competitive event. The groups included sprinters (SP, 100–200 m, n = 4); short middle distance runners (SMD, 400–800 m, n = 3); long middle distance runners (LMD, 800–1500 m, n = 4); and long distance runners (LD, 10 km, n = 4).

## Test Procedure

Knee extension torques were measured for each participant on a Biodex isokinetic dynamometer (Biodex Medical Systems, Inc., Shirley, NY) at 14 different speeds (0.52 rad/s, 1.05 rad/s, 1.57 rad/s, 2.09 rad/s, 2.62 rad/s, 3.14 rad/s, 3.67 rad/s, 4.19 rad/s, 4.71 rad/s, 5.24 rad/s, 5.76 rad/s, 6.28 rad/s, 6.98 rad/s, and 7.85 rad/s) through his or her full range of motion. The calibration of the Biodex was confirmed before each testing session. The seat depth, seat angle, and height of the powerhead were adjusted to ensure that each subject had his or her hip flexed at 90°, and the lateral femoral epicondyle of the knee was aligned with the axis of the powerhead. In addition, the length of the lever arm was adjusted so that the contact pads were positioned between the ankle and the inferior edge of the lateral head of the gastrocnemius. Velcro stabilization straps were used to maintain this position throughout all testing conditions.

Five warm-up trials, each followed by a 30 s rest, were allowed before each speed to increase blood flow and decrease tissue viscosity and to familiarize the subject with the resistance provided by the new speed setting. Subjects performed three perceived maximal muscle actions at each speed. The order of the speeds was fully randomized among subjects. At each speed the repetition that yielded the highest peak torque was used to construct the component curve.

The raw data from the Biodex dynamometer for each speed was then exported to a spreadsheet program (PSIPlot 2.9, Poly Software International, Salt Lake City, UT). Due to the restrictions imposed by the graphing program in the three-dimensional mode, all speeds were required to have the same number of data points throughout the range of motion. Since the Biodex dynamometer collects data at a constant sampling rate, it collected a progressively fewer number of points per test session as the speed of the test increased. Therefore it was necessary to interpolate the missing data. This was done by considering the changes in at least three points preceding and following the specific missing angle.

If successive torque-angle slices at increasing velocities (0.52 rad/s through 7.85 rad/s) are examined, an increasingly larger impulse artifact due to the need to decelerate the leg will be noted (40). Although the application of a damping force would have reduced this artifact, it also would have distorted the shape of the curve earlier in the range of motion (39). Sinacore and coworkers (41) have encouraged the use of zero damping when accurate determination of angle-specific torque is desired. Therefore, we chose to employ a "hard stop" during our testing procedure, thereby increasing the impulse artifact at the end of the range of motion, especially at higher isokinetic speeds. The data was then truncated at 179° to reduce the impact this artifact might have on the statistical analysis.

## Statistical Analysis

Discriminant function analysis is a statistical technique that allows researchers to study differences between two or more known groups with respect to several variables simultaneously. Parallel discriminant function analyses were examined separately for raw torque, normalized torque, and data adjusted by body weight. Normalized torque was derived by dividing a torque value at a specific angle and speed by the maximum torque value measured over the entire surface map. Similarly, torque values were adjusted for body weight by dividing the measured torque by the individual's body weight.

Predictor variables for each of the three separate discriminant function analyses were torque (raw torque, normalized torque, or torque adjusted by body weight), angle torque, velocity torque, and angle × velocity × torque. Together these three interaction variables allow the three-dimensional surface defined by torque-angle-velocity to flex into any shape, thus accounting for subtle differences in the torque-velocity-angle surfaces among the four groups.

## Test Results

Representative surface graphs for the raw torque data are presented in figure 6.5, *a* through *d*. Surfaces representing the average raw torque data for each group are presented in figure 6.6, *a* through *d*. Discriminant function analysis findings for this model indicated that the first two discriminant functions were statistically significant ($p < .0001$), accounting for nearly 26% of the variance among the groups. The first canonical function accounted for 98.9% of the variance among the four groups, while the second canonical function accounted for only 1.1% of the between groups variance. Although the second canonical function was statistically significant it is of no practical value since virtually all of the explainable between groups variance is explained by the first canonical function. Table 6.2 presents summary data for the discriminant function analysis. The square of the total structure coefficients presented in this table can be used to identify the relative contribution of the different predictor variables in explaining the canonical function. Structural coefficients greater than .3 are considered meaningful. In a similar manner, the between structure coefficients represent the relative contribution of each predictor variable in explaining the differences among the four groups and the within structure

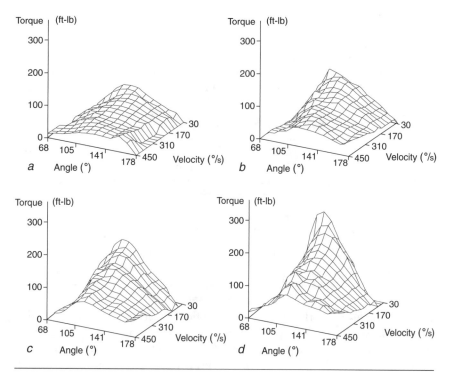

**Figure 6.5** Representative response surfaces for selected individual from each group using the raw torque data: (*a*) long distance, (*b*) long middle distance, (*c*) short middle distance, and (*d*) sprinters.

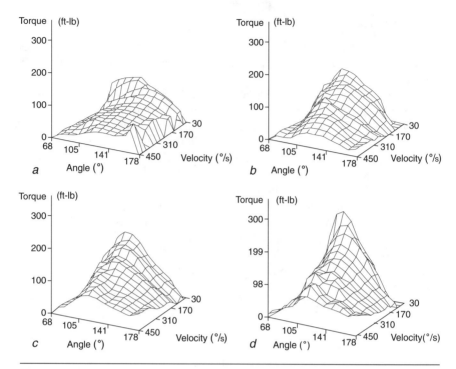

**Figure 6.6**   Response surfaces from each group using average of the raw data: (a) LD, (b) LMD, (c) SMD, and (d) SP. Note the variations in both the shapes of the curve and the level of torque production.

**Table 6.2   Raw Data: Structure of Canonical Function 1**

| Variable | Total structure | Between structure | Pooled within structure | Standardized canonical coefficients |
|---|---|---|---|---|
| Torque | 0.821 | 0.999 | 0.778 | 0.409 |
| Torque × angle | 0.762 | 0.997 | 0.712 | 0.259 |
| Torque × speed | 0.813 | 0.999 | 0.769 | 2.149 |
| Torque × angle × speed | 0.719 | 0.997 | 0.666 | −1.555 |

coefficients represent the relative contribution of each variable in explaining similarities within the group. Figure 6.7 provides a graph of the four group means showing the clear and significant differences between the SP and LD groups ($p < .0001$). Additionally, the middle distance runners (SMD and LMD) were also distinguishable from the SP and LD groups ($p < .0001$). However, the canonical function for the raw torque data did not differentiate the SMD from the LMD.

## Class means (raw)

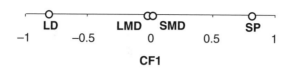

CF1

**Figure 6.7** Graph of class means of raw data for canonical function 1 (CF1). Note that the sprinters, middle distance runners, and long distance runners are clearly distinguished from each other by this analysis. However, the long middle distance runners (LMD) and short middle distance runners (SMD) could not be distinguished from each other by CF1.

Representative surface graphs for the normalized torque data are presented in figure 6.8, *a* through *d*. Surfaces representing the average normalized torque data for each group are presented in figure 6.9, *a* through *d*. Recall that the normalization procedure adjusts for the large individual variability in torque that would be expected due to the specific differences in body size and structure evident among the athletes tested. The discriminant function analysis for

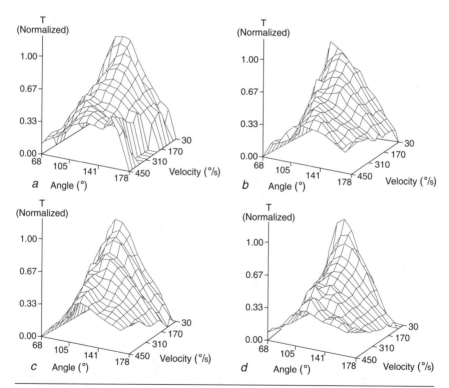

**Figure 6.8** Response surfaces for selected individuals from each group using the normalized data: (*a*) LD, (*b*) LMD, (*c*) SMD, and (*d*) SP.

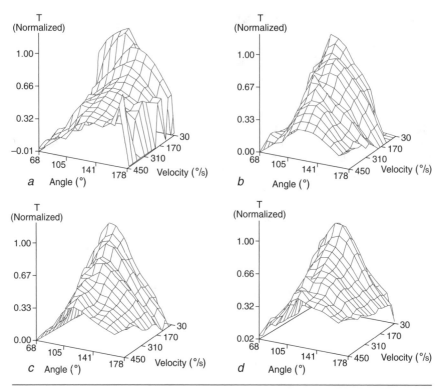

**Figure 6.9** Response surface from each group using average of normalized data: (a) LD, (b) LMD, (c) SMD, and (d) SP.

the normalized data yielded a slightly different picture than that produced by the raw torque data. Although the overall power of the analysis was drastically reduced, accounting for only 4% of the variance among the groups, the first two canonical functions were both significant ($p < .0001$). The first canonical function accounted for over 86% of the explained variance. Because the second canonical function accounted for over 13% of the variance and was statistically significant, we chose to include it in describing the differences among the groups. Table 6.3 presents the structure coefficients for the normalized analysis. Figure 6.10 presents the means for each group, which are all significantly different from each other ($p < .0001$). Note that two axes are included, one for each canonical function.

The final analysis presented is for the torque values adjusted by body weight. Surface graphs for selected individuals of the torque data adjusted for body weight are presented in figure 6.11, $a$ through $d$. Surfaces representing the average torque data corrected for body weight for each group are presented in figure 6.12, $a$ through $d$. Just as was the case for the raw data, discriminant function analysis findings for this model indicated that the first two discriminant functions were statistically significant ($p < .0001$). In this case they explained

## Table 6.3 Normalized Data

**Structure of Canonical Function 1**

| Variable | Total structure | Between structure | Pooled within structure | Standardized canonical coefficients |
|---|---|---|---|---|
| Norm. torque | 0.582 | 0.949 | 0.575 | 1.015 |
| Norm. torque × angle | 0.434 | 0.837 | 0.428 | –0.66 |
| Norm. torque × speed | 0.731 | 0.97 | 0.725 | 2.204 |
| Norm. torque × angle × speed | 0.562 | 0.909 | 0.555 | –1.594 |

**Structure of Canonical Function 2**

| Variable | Total structure | Between structure | Pooled within structure | Standardized canonical coefficients |
|---|---|---|---|---|
| Norm. torque | 0.477 | 0.309 | 0.479 | –0.993 |
| Norm. torque × angle | 0.71 | 0.544 | 0.712 | 1.463 |
| Norm. torque × speed | 0.458 | 0.242 | 0.462 | –1.328 |
| Norm. torque × angle × speed | 0.644 | 0.414 | 0.646 | 1.625 |

nearly 20% of the variance among the groups. The first canonical function now accounted for 99.0% of the variance among the four groups, while the second canonical function accounted for less than 1% of the between group variance. The second canonical function, though statistically significant, was once again of no practical value since over 99% of the explainable between group variance was explained by the first canonical function. The summary data for the discriminant function analysis is presented in table 6.4. Figure 6.13 provides a graph of the four group means showing the clear and significant differences among all groups ($p < .0001$). Unlike the canonical function 1 for the raw torque data, this single canonical function did allow us to differentiate all groups including the SMD from the LMD.

## Test Conclusions

The results of this study indicate that the isokinetic torque-angle-velocity surfaces produced during knee extension can be used to discriminate runners according to their individual events. However, the reader should recognize that these surfaces are presented as potential diagnostic templates for training and

**Class means (normalized)**

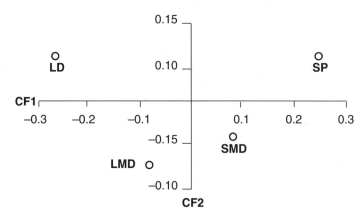

**Figure 6.10** Graph of class means of normalized data for canonical functions 1 (CF1) and 2 (CF2). Note that the sprinters (SP), distance runners (LD), long middle distance runners (LMD) and short middle distance runners (SMD) are all distinguishable from one another.

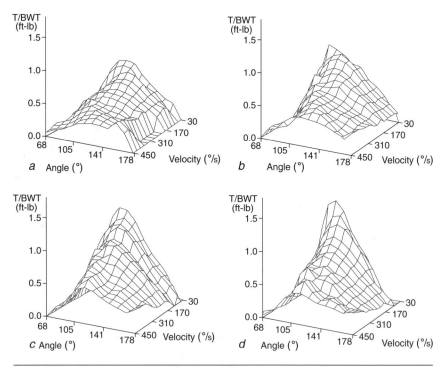

**Figure 6.11** Response surfaces for a representative individual from each group using the data adjusted for body weight: *(a)* LD, *(b)* LMD, *(c)* SMD, and *(d)* SP.

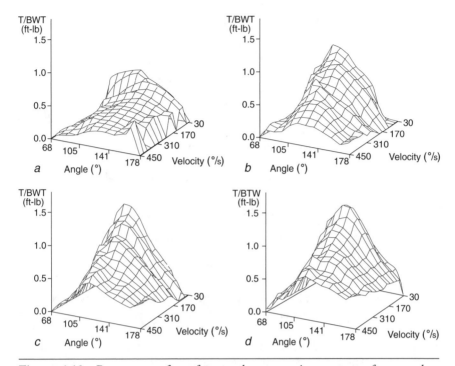

**Figure 6.12** Response surfaces from each group using average of torque data adjusted for body weight: *(a)* LD, *(b)* LMD, *(c)* SMD, and *(d)* SP.

**Table 6.4 Data for Torque Adjusted for Body Weight: Structure of Canonical Function 1**

| Variable | Total structure | Between structure | Pooled within structure | Standardized canonical coefficients |
|---|---|---|---|---|
| Torque/BW | 0.793 | 0.999 | 0.760 | 0.440 |
| Torque/BW × angle | 0.722 | 0.998 | 0.684 | 0.196 |
| Torque/BW × speed | 0.793 | 0.999 | 0.761 | 2.130 |
| Torque/BW × angle × speed | 0.689 | 0.996 | 0.649 | −1.550 |

not as representative force-length-velocity maps. The sections that follow partially dissect the surfaces into their component planes, present the relative importance of these planes and their relationship to previous research, and discuss the difference between our isokinetic results and those that might be expected from in vitro length-tension and force-velocity curves.

**Class means (body weight adjusted)**

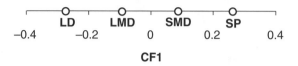

CF1

**Figure 6.13**  Graph of class means of torque adjusted by body weight data for canonical functions 1 (CF1). Note that the sprinters (SP), distance runners (LD), long middle distance runners (LMD), and short middle distance runners (SMD) are all distinguishable from one another using a single canonical function.

# Consideration of the Isokinetic Map Torque-Angle Plane

It may be tempting to compare the torque-angle plane of our isokinetically derived surfaces with the length-tension curve prepared from isolated skeletal muscle; however, it should be recognized that this comparison is inaccurate, especially in terms of isokinetics. Perhaps the simplest explanation for the disparity between these two sets of curves is the fact that the classic curve was produced from isolated muscle and, therefore, is not subject to the anatomical restrictions or neural mechanisms affecting muscle in vivo. However, the difference between the torque-angle curves produced in this study and the length-tension curves produced from isolated muscle goes beyond simple anatomical considerations to the basis of isokinetic testing itself. By definition, isokinetic devices measure torque only when the subject meets or exceeds the constant velocity (load range) set by the machine (36). Therefore, the shape of the torque-angle curve is not dictated simply by the length of the sarcomere (and related actin-myosin overlap) or the angle of pull of the muscle on the bony levers; it is also dependent on the subject's ability to meet or exceed the testing speed. For example, if representative 7.85 rad/s slices are compared for each of the four groups tested (see figure 6.14, *a-d*), it can be seen that the shapes of these curves vary considerably, and they do not resemble the typical parabolic curve that is produced using in vitro muscle preparations. The two-dimensional slices depicted in these views emphasize the plateauing effect that results when the speedier athletes attain the target speed and maintain it throughout the repetition. The initial portion of the sprinters curve (SP, see figure 6.14*d*) shows a sharp upward slope at the beginning of the repetition as the subject accelerated the lever arm to meet the testing speed dictated by the dynamometer, followed by a prolonged plateau as speed was maintained. In comparison, the curves for the middle distance runners (LMD and SMD, see figure 6.14, *b* and *c*, respectively) show a less extreme positive slope at the beginning of the curve (indicative of a slower acceleration), a peak, and an immediate drop in torque as the subjects failed to maintain the contractile speed required to meet the dictated angular velocity. Finally, the curves for the long distance runners (LD,

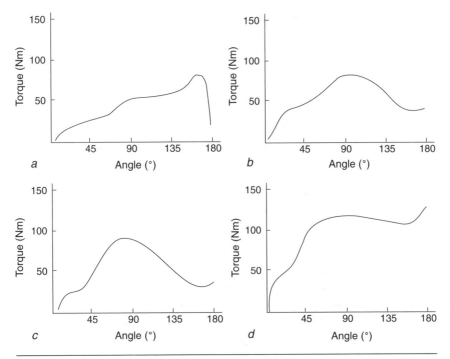

**Figure 6.14**   Two-dimensional torque by angle slices at a velocity of 7.85 rad/s for each group: (*a*) LD, (*b*) LMD, (*c*) SMD, and (*d*) SP. Note the difference between these isokinetic torque-angle curves and the typical length-tension curves in figures 6.1 and 6.2, which were produced using isometric contractions of isolated skeletal muscle.

see figure 6.14*a*) show only a gradual upward slope; this was likely due to the subjects' inability to meet the speed of the dynamometer until the deceleration point was reached.

In fact, these differences allow discrimination between groups. As can be seen, these differences are dependent on at least two performance variables, strength (raw data analysis only) and limb velocity. Researchers have attributed these differences to a number of possible factors including differences in motor unit firing frequency (7), motor unit activation and synchronization (33, 34), cross-sectional muscle area (22), fiber type distribution and cross-sectional area (6, 22), and the related differences in myosin ATPase activity and $Ca^{++}$ kinetics.

# Consideration of the Isokinetic Map Torque-Velocity Plane

Given the close relationship between isokinetics and limb velocity, it can be seen that the torque-velocity relationship illustrated by the other axis of our isokinetic surface maps is an important defining factor. Examining previous studies that have addressed the impact of training on the force-velocity relationship in humans is especially meaningful.

These studies support our current findings showing significant differences among runners due to their event-specific training (see section entitled Modifications in the Force-Velocity Curve Due to Training). Coincidentally, using measured torques at 30°/s (0.52 rad/s) to 180°/s (3.14 rad/s), Johansson and coworkers (22) projected that the highest mean power for sprinters would occur at an isokinetic speed of 450°/s (7.85 rad/s) and for marathon runners at 270°/s (4.71 rad/s). In fact, these researchers calculated a nearly linear decline in power output for the marathoners at speeds above 270°/s (4.71 rad/s). These results are substantiated by plots of the average peak power measured for each group during the tests used to construct the surface plots presented in the present study. Graphs encompassing the entire range of velocities from 0.52 to 7.85 rad/s show that the actual peak power outputs for the SP and LD groups occurred at 6.98 rad/s and 4.71 rad/s, respectively. The SMD group produced its greatest power at 5.24 rad/s, while the LMD group peaked at 4.71 rad/s (see figure 6.15). When our three-dimensional maps are examined, it is this high speed portion of the graph that most clearly shows distinctions among the groups. It is also of interest that one subject in the SP group pro-

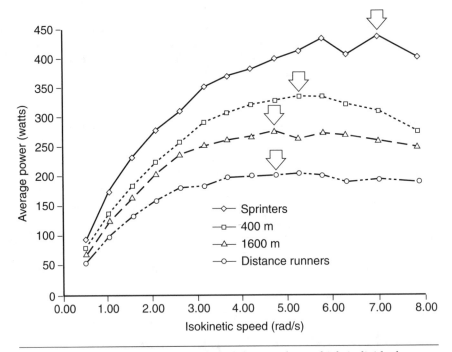

**Figure 6.15**  Graphic representation of the speeds at which individual groups attained their highest power outputs. The open arrows denote the point of highest average power among all speeds tested.

duced values at 7.85 rad/s and 6.28 rad/s, which were more than two standard deviations below the mean. If the values for this athlete were not used in the analysis the peak power would have occurred at 7.85 rad/s, since the other three athletes in the group all produced their highest power values at that speed.

## Conclusions

Given the uniqueness of the surfaces produced from data generated by the different groups of runners in our study, a number of uses for these three-dimensional maps can be postulated. First of all, they may provide templates that can identify deficiencies among athletes training for an event and allow specific training prescriptions to target these weaknesses. Thus, if world-class athletes generate data from which the templates are created, the surfaces produced from data provided by athletes in training could be superimposed on these "world-class templates" to identify specific deficits in one variable (torque, velocity, or angle) in relation to the other two. This, for example, could allow the coach or trainer to target specific needs for velocity training at angles showing the greatest deficits from the "ideal" surface.

The surfaces could also serve as a diagnostic tool, providing feedback concerning the success or shortcomings of training programs, so that specific modifications could be made to increase the rate of improvement. Since all training for performance enhancement is dependent on the response of the individual, and individuals respond uniquely due to their inherent physiological and biomechanical differences, these surfaces could be used to map the training responses and provide feedback for the modification of the program as it progresses.

The use of these surfaces may not be limited to the athletic community. For example, if population-specific surfaces are developed, they have the potential to be used in the analysis of speed- and angle-specific strength deficits resulting from muscle atrophy related to age, illness, or job-related injury.

We find the analysis of the weight-adjusted torque curves especially promising since they allow comparisons of individuals relative to their individual body masses. This may be seen as analogous to reporting maximum oxygen uptake in absolute terms (L/min) compared to its body weight-adjusted or relative form (ml/kg/min). The predictive strength of the weight-adjusted model, combined with its dependence on a single canonical function and its potential to compare athletes relative to their individual body weights, makes it a powerful tool for comparative analysis.

Having said this it must also be recognized that both raw torque curves and normalized curves have their own potential applications. For example, in sports or activities where absolute strength rather than strength-to-weight ratio is the important controlling factor, surfaces constructed from the raw data may be preferable. In addition, normalized curves may be used as generalized templates for diagnosis of specific injuries or illnesses, as well as coaching tools to point out specific areas requiring strength or speed training.

# Summary

The data used to produce these surfaces reflect the isokinetic performances of a limited number of highly motivated competitive athletes. All of the athletes tested were runners, and only a single movement, knee extension, was used. If these surfaces are to be used for diagnosis, prescription, and monitoring during training, the database will need to be expanded in at least three ways. First, a greater number of runners, trained at different distances and performing at different skill levels, will need to be recruited, to examine differences in the topography of their surface plots. This will not only allow the assessment of differences between events, it will also provide information concerning potential differences between the elite runners and those at other performance levels.

Second, the database should also be expanded to examine knee function in other competitive athletes who may use the same muscle group but in a different biomechanical pattern. For example, the angles of peak force or the speeds at which they are produced may be very different for a rower, a tennis player, an American football lineman, or a long jumper, even though all of these athletes rely heavily on their quadriceps for success in their specific sport. This was evidenced in the study of cyclists and runners cited earlier in this chapter (19).

Finally, the database needs to be expanded to other movements and other joints that may be performance-specific for different sports. For example, it would be interesting to compare differences in shoulder extension and flexion between and within groups of pitchers, tennis players, shot-putters, and swimmers, to evaluate differences among athletes competing in different sports and among athletes of different skill levels within a sport.

Given the development of such a database, and the systematic testing of athletes during their training and competitive season, these surfaces may serve as an excellent tool to target specific weaknesses, give the appropriate exercise prescription, and evaluate the progress of the athlete.

# References

1. Astrand, P.-O., and Rodahl, K. 1986. *Textbook of work physiology.* New York: McGraw-Hill.

2. Behm, D.G., and Sale, D.G. 1996. Influence of velocity on agonist and antagonist activation in concentric dorsiflexion muscle actions. *Can. J. Appl. Physiol.* 21(5): 403–16.

3. Bender, J., and Kaplan, H. 1963. The multiple angle testing method for evaluation of muscle strength. *J. Bone Joint Surgery* 45A: 135–40.

4. Caiozzo, V.J., Perrine, J.J., and Edgerton, V.R. 1981. Training-induced alterations of the in vivo force-velocity relationship of human muscle. *J. Appl. Physiol.: Respirat. Environ. Exerc. Physiol.* 51(3): 750–54.

5. Carlson, F.D., and Wilke, D.R. 1974. *Muscle physiology.* Englewood Cliffs, NJ: Prentice Hall.

6. Coyle, E.F., Feiring, D.C., Rotkis, T.C., Cote III, R.W., Roby, F.B., Lee, W., and Wilmore, J.H. 1981. Specificity of power improvements through slow and fast isokinetic training. *J. Appl. Physiol.: Respirat. Environ. Exerc. Physiol.* 51(6): 1437–42.

7. Cracroft, J.D., and Petajan J.H. 1977. Effect of muscle training on the pattern of firing of single motor units. *Am. J. Phys. Med.* 56: 183–94.

8. de Koning, F.L., Vos, J.A., Binkhorst, R.A., and Vissers, A.C.A. 1984. Influence of training on the force-velocity relationship of the arm flexors of active sportsmen. *Int. J. Sports Med.* 5: 43–46.

9. de Koning, F.L., Binkhorst, R.A., Vos, J.A., and vant Hof, M.A. 1985. The force-velocity relationship of arm flexion in untrained males and females and arm-trained athletes. *Eur. J. Appl. Physiol.* 54: 89–94.

10. Edman, K.A. 1966. The relation between sarcomere length and active tension in isolated semitendinosus fibers of the frog. *J. Physiol. (Lond.)* 183: 407–17.

11. Faulkner, J.A., Chaflin, D.R., and McCully, K.K. 1986. Power output of fast and slow fibers from human skeletal muscles. In *Human muscle power,* ed. N.L. Jones, N. McCartney, and A.J. McComas. Champaign, IL: Human Kinetics.

12. Gardner, G. 1963. Specificity of strength changes of the exercised and nonexercised limb following isometric training. *Res. Quart.* 34: 98–101.

13. Gordon, A.M., Huxley, A.F., and Julian, F.J. 1966. The variation in isometric tension with sarcomere length in vertebrate muscle fibers. *J. Physiol.* 184: 170–92.

14. Hakkinen, K., and Komi, P.V. 1985. Changes in electrical and mechanical behavior of leg extensor muscles during heavy resistance strength training. *Scand. J. Sports Sci.* 7: 55–64.

15. Hakkinen, K., and Komi, P.V. 1985. The effect of explosive-type strength training on electromyographical and force production characteristics of leg extensor muscles during concentric and various stretch-shortening cycle exercises. *Scand. J. Sports Sci.* 7: 65–76.

16. Harmon, E. 1994. The biomechanics of resistance training. In *Essentials of strength training and conditioning,* ed. T.R. Baechle, 19–50. Champaign, IL: Human Kinetics.

17. Herzog, W. 1988. The relation between the resultant moments at a point and the moments measured by an isokinetic dynamometer. *J. Biomech.* 21: 5–12.

18. Herzog, W., Hasler, E., and Abrahamse, S.K. 1991. A comparison of knee extensor strength curves obtained theoretically and experimentally. *Med. Sci. Sports Exerc.* 23(1): 108–14.

19. Herzog, W., Guimaraes, A.C., Anton, M.G., and Carter-Erdman, K.A. 1991. Moment-length relations of rectus femoris muscles of speed skaters/cyclists and runners. *Med. Sci. Sports Exerc.* 23(11): 1289–96.

20. Hill, A.V. 1938. The heat of shortening and the dynamic constraints of muscle. *Proc. R. Soc. Lond. (Biol.)* 126: 136–95.

21. Ivy, J.L., Withers, R.T., Brose, G., Maxwell, B.D., and Costill, D.L. 1981. Isokinetic contractile properties of the quadriceps with respect to fiber type. *Eur. J. Appl. Physiol. Occup. Physiol.* 47: 247–55.

22. Johansson, C., Lorentzon, R., Sjostrom, M., Fagerlund, M., and Fugl-Meyer, A.R. 1987. Sprinters and marathon runners: Does isokinetic knee extensor performance reflect muscle size and structure? *Physiol. Scand.* 130: 663–69.

23. Kanehisa, H., and Miyashita, M. 1983. Specificity of velocity in strength training. *Eur. J. Appl. Physiol.* 52: 104–6.

24. Katz, B. 1939. The relation between force and speed in muscular contraction. *J. Physiol.* 96: 45–64.

25. Kitai, T.A., and Sale, D.G. 1989. Specificity of joint angle in isometric training. *Eur. J. Appl. Physiol.* 58: 744–48.

26. Knapik, J.J., Mawdsley, R.H., and Ramos, M.U. 1983. Angular specificity of isometric and isokinetic strength training. *J. Ortho. Sports Phys. Ther.* 5: 58–65.

27. Koh, T.J., and Herzog, W. 1995. Evaluation of voluntary and elicited dorsiflexor torque-angle relationships. *J. Appl. Physiol.* 79(6): 2007–13.

28. Labrecque, S., Grondin, S., and Nadeau, M. 1983. The force-velocity curve on a Nautilus machine. *Am. Correct. Ther. J.* 37(2): 53–55.

29. Latash, M.L. 1998. *Neurophysiological basis of movement.* Champaign, IL: Human Kinetics.

30. Lieber, R.L. 1992. *Skeletal muscle structure and function.* Baltimore: Williams & Wilkins.

31. Lynn, R., and Morgan, D.L. 1994. Decline running produces more sarcomeres in rat vastus intermedius muscle than does incline running. *J. Appl. Physiol.* 77(3): 1439–44.

32. Meyers, C.R. 1967. Effects of two isometric routines on strength, size, and endurance in exercised and non-exercised arms. *Res. Quart.* 38: 430–40.

33. Milner-Brown, H.S., Stein, R.B., and Lee, R.G. 1975. Synchronization of human motor units: Possible roles of exercise and supraspinal reflexes. *Electroencephal. Clin. Neurophysiol.* 38: 245–54.

34. Moritani, T., Muro, M., Ishida K., and Taguchi, S. 1987. Electrophysiological analysis of the effects of muscle power training. *Res. J. Phys. Ed.* 1: 23–32.

35. Muller, W. 1975. Isometric training of young rats—effects upon hind limb muscles: Histological, morphometric, and electron microscopic studies. *Cell Tissue Res.* 161(2): 225–37.

36. Perrin, D.H. 1993. *Isokinetic exercise and assessment.* Champaign, IL: Human Kinetics.

37. Perrine, J.J., and Edgerton, V.R. 1978. Muscle force-velocity and power-velocity relationships under isokinetic loading. *Med. Sci. Sports* 10: 159–66.

38. Rasch, P.J., and Pierson, W.R. 1964. One position versus multiple positions in isometric exercise. *Am. J. Phys. Med.* 43: 10–12.

39. Rothstein, J.M., Lamb, R.L., and Mayhew, T.P. 1987. Clinical use of isokinetic measurements. *Phys. Ther.* 67: 1840–44.

40. Spega, A.A., Nicholas, J.A., Sokolow, D., and Saraniti, A. 1982. The nature of torque "overshoot" in Cybex isokinetic dynamometry. *Med. Sci. Sports Exerc.* 14(5): 368–75.

41. Sinacore, D.R., Rothstein, J.M., Delitto, A., and Rose, S.J. 1983. Effect of damp on isokinetic measurements. *Phys. Ther.* 63: 1248–50.

42. Therpaut-Mathieu, C., Van Hoecke, J., and Martin, B. 1988. Myoelectrical and mechanical changes linked to length specificity during isometric training. *J. Appl. Physiol.* 64: 1500–5.

43. Widrick, J.J., Trappe, S.W., Costill, D.L., and Fitts, R.H. 1996. Force-velocity and force-power properties of single muscle fibers from elite master runners and sedentary men. *Am. J. Physiol.* 271 (*Cell Physiol.* 40): C676–83.

44. Wilke, D.R. 1950. The relation between force and velocity in human muscle. *J. Physiol. Lond.* 110: 249–80.

45. Williams, P., and Goldspink, G. 1973. The effect of immobilization on the longitudinal growth of striated muscle fibers. *J. Anat.* 116: 45–55.

46. Williams, P., and Goldspink, G. 1978. Changes in sarcomere length and physiological properties in immobilized muscle. *J. Anat.* 127: 459–68.

47. Zehr, E.P., and Sale, D.G. 1994. Ballistic movement: Muscle activation and neuromuscular adaptation. *Can. J. Appl. Physiol.* 19(4): 363–78.

# Part III
# Functional Applications

This section attempts to cover, in a broad manner, the collective concepts underlying isokinetics usage and specifically, what this technology *can* do. Chapters 7 and 8 cover upper extremities and lower extremities, respectively, forming the base of practically all open kinetic chain testing and training principles. Chapter 9 discusses the seldom-used closed kinetic chain capabilities of isokinetics while focusing on multijoint movement. Chapter 10 examines muscular control as viewed through submaximal voluntary torque production. Chapter 11 investigates how modern dynamometers incorporate eccentrics into a testing and training protocol. Chapter 12 considers the use of isokinetics in evaluating the functional capacity of working individuals in strength-dependent occupations. Chapter 13 presents data relative to one of the sites in our bodies subject to the most debilitating injury—the spine. Finally, chapter 14 probes the cardiovascular adaptations and effects of isokinetic intervention.

The chapters mentioned above provide a comprehensive view into how the present-day dynamometer may be utilized across an expansive spectrum of subjects. This information may be applied to a diverse population covering a wide range of both laboratory and on-site settings.

The review of literature in this section should provide the reader with a basis for forming protocols suitable to serve the needs of his or her particular population. Furthermore, specific information is furnished regarding testing and training standards as well as normative data that may serve as a starting point for the reader to more critically examine his or her own procedures presently in use.

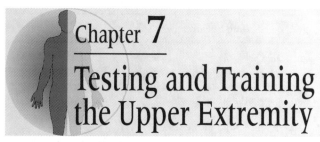

## Chapter 7

# Testing and Training the Upper Extremity

T. Jeff Chandler

This chapter focuses on the rationale of isokinetic testing and training for upper body sports and athletic movements. The main concept of isokinetic exercise is to control the speed of muscular actions by preventing acceleration beyond a set speed. In theory, isokinetic training for the upper extremity develops maximal speed and power at each angle through the range of motion. Researchers have suggested that, by loading the muscle to capacity throughout the range of motion, isokinetic exercise develops greater muscular endurance and power than isometric or isoinertial training (29).

Limitations of isokinetic devices have been reviewed in this text and in the scientific literature (62, 49). This chapter discusses the advantages and disadvantages of isokinetic testing and training specifically related to upper body activities relative to improving muscular performance (see table 7.1).

Many factors affect the results of isokinetic measurement of strength and power, including age, gender, weight, history of athletic performance, disability, and limb dominance (34). In practical use, isokinetic dynamometers do not produce truly isokinetic muscle actions due to oscillations between acceleration and deceleration (49), so some of the limitations of isokinetic devices are related to the device itself. The methods chosen to interpret the data may also affect the results of the measurements (62).

Most of the reported research on isokinetics deals with rehabilitation rather than performance. Thus, to discuss the effect of isokinetic training on performance, in many cases we must interpret research performed in the rehabilitative realm. So another limitation in discussing the topic of isokinetics and performance is the lack of research dealing specifically with the topic.

## Characteristics of Upper Extremity Movement

Despite their limitations, isokinetic devices are being used for testing and training athletes who participate in upper body sporting activities. Upper body

## Table 7.1  Advantages and Disadvantages of Isokinetic Testing and Training

### Testing advantages

- Testing is reproducible
- Makes use of set protocols for specific isokinetic devices
- Isolates joints
- Generates data that can be stored and used later
- Some units allow isoinertial and isometric testing
- Some units allow for active (eccentric) mode testing

### Testing disadvantages

- Lack of specificity
- Devices are expensive
- Calibration required at regular intervals, and calibration is more difficult than with free weights
- Limited number movement patterns possible for testing
- Maximal effort is assumed, but can not be measured
- Muscle actions not specific to sports activities
- Eccentric strength measurements not specific to dynamic activities
- Difficult to isolate some joints, such as the shoulder joint, in many movement patterns
- Some question the safety of active (eccentric) mode
- Spikes in torque may be related to other factors besides strength or power in the athlete being tested

### Training advantages

- Visual feedback to the athlete may be motivational
- Exerts maximal resistance at each angle during a range of motion
- Allows training specifically of eccentric strength
- Can isolate specific muscle groups for training
- Active eccentric training is possible

### Training disadvantages

- Lack of specificity with dynamic movements
- Difficulty in simulating sport-specific movement patterns
- Joints are isolated and generally not specific to sports performance
- Limited movement patterns
- Maximal effort is assumed for training, but can not be measured
- Muscle actions, eccentric and concentric, not specific to most sports activities
- Difficult to isolate the shoulder for specific movement patterns
- Active eccentric training may not be safe for all participants
- Spikes in torque should be adequately dampened

sports include a wide variety of movements and activities that place unique and varied demands on the upper torso and upper extremity. This section discusses these movements relative to the speed of movement, the specific movement pattern, and the specific muscle action involved.

## Speed of Movement

An important consideration in testing and training the upper extremity, speed of movement determines the type of muscle fiber recruited and imposes specific demands on both the accelerator and decelerator muscles. One limitation of many isokinetic devices is their inability to test and train at the highest movement speeds.

To improve performance, we tend to focus on muscles that accelerate a body part. Deceleration is most often viewed as a factor in injury risk. However, deceleration is also important in positioning the upper extremity, which strongly relates to accuracy. Shoulder strength depends on cocontractions of specific musculature, particularly at the end ranges of motion (56). In high-performance athletes who are involved in activities like pitching in baseball and serving in tennis, this is an important consideration that directly relates to functional performance.

Sport-specific movements require constant acceleration and deceleration of specific body parts. This does not occur with isokinetic exercise, which limits the applicability of isokinetic training in sport-specific musculoskeletal training.

## Movement Patterns

Movement patterns of the upper extremity vary from sport to sport, from one player to another, and even within an individual athlete. Using baseball as an example, different pitchers' movement patterns may range from overhead to sidearm or below. It is likely that there are differences between specific pitches in the same pitcher. As a pitcher fatigues, one possible result is the arm may drop, changing the mechanics of the movement and likely the accuracy of the athlete.

In most upper body sports, the arm is used as an open kinetic chain either to throw or strike an object. The determination of open vs. closed kinetic chain is an important distinction, particularly in upper body activities (15). In an open kinetic chain, the arm is free to move in any direction. In a closed kinetic chain, the upper extremity meets significant resistance. Thus heavy sets of bench press are a closed chain upper body activity. In open kinetic chain upper body activities precision and accuracy are often required, as in pitching a baseball. This means that slight perturbations or a diskinesis in the movement patterns could lead to failure to perform at the desired level.

Upper body isokinetic testing and training is joint specific. More research has been performed on the elbow than other joints of the upper extremity. However, sporting movements of the upper extremity often involve a combination of the shoulder, the elbow, and the wrist. The shoulder is a complex joint with a wide variety of possible movement patterns. The ball-and-socket design of the shoulder allows freedom of movement but is inherently unstable. Function of the shoulder also depends, to some extent, on the ability of the athlete to control and stabilize the scapula (37), which serves as an anchor for muscles around the shoulder. Because we can not measure scapular function with isokinetic testing, this is just one of the variables that must be considered in addition to isokinetic test results.

## Specific Muscle Actions

The actions of the specific muscles of the upper extremity are also an important consideration. Concentric action causes shortening of the muscles and subsequent movement. In many instances, the forces in the upper extremity result from ground reaction forces transferred from the legs through the torso to the arm. At the shoulder some muscles must act isometrically, cocontracting to stabilize the humeral head (56).

Upper extremity muscles also work eccentrically to decelerate the arm in the throwing motion. Therefore, it is important to know the action of the muscles involved in a specific activity, concentric, isometric, or eccentric. Concentric and eccentric actions can be isoinertial or isokinetic. Isometric actions are also present to stabilize the shoulder during dynamic activities. Dynamic activities may cause muscle damage, which occurs primarily from eccentric actions. Repeated eccentric muscle damage may cause changes in the properties of the muscle tissue, translating into decreased range of motion in specific muscle groups. Range of motion measurements have demonstrated that ROM decreases on the dominant side (9), that ROM decreases are positively correlated with both years of intense participation in a sport and age (36), and that these ROM changes can be modified with standard flexibility exercises (38).

Currently, the relationship between eccentric isokinetic strength and decreased range of motion has not been studied. It is possible that resistance training, isokinetic or isoinertial, or isometric training might have an effect on modifying the changes in range of motion or the process of regaining normal range of motion once the changes have occurred.

In one study looking at the muscles that decelerate the shoulder, baseball players were placed on a free weight dumbbell program or the same program plus an eccentric elastic tubing strengthening program. Tested isokinetically, significant improvement was seen in the elastic tubing group at 60°/s but not at 180°/s (51). For training, one should consider that deceleration generally occurs at relatively high rotational velocities that can not be simulated with isokinetic equipment. However, injury risk factors such as eccentric strength, muscle strength balance, and range of motion do affect performance. It should be noted that subjects in this study trained dynamically but tested isokinetically. This lack of adherence to the specificity principle is an important consideration, and the results of this and other similar studies should be interpreted with that in mind.

# Interaction of Speed, Patterns, and Muscle Actions

Most sports can be characterized in terms of movement patterns common to that sport. Across a variety of sports, the upper extremity is required to move in a variety of patterns and speeds, with the actual movement speed being a result of the effort and the resistance met. For example, an implement such as a baseball bat or a tennis racket can slow movement speed. The most common example of a high speed upper extremity is the throwing arm of a pitcher in baseball. The velocity of internal rotation of an arm throwing a baseball has been estimated at over 6000°/s (52). A tennis stroke might serve as an example of a moderately high speed movement. The internal rotation of the arm has been reported ranging from approximately 1100 to 1700°/s (35). A limitation of isokinetic devices is they do not approach these movement speeds.

Swimming and sports related to movement of an object through water (rowing, canoeing, etc) are unique because the resistance met by the upper extremity increases as the effort and intensity increases, which is also a characteristic of isokinetic exercise. Some authors refer to muscle actions performed during activities such as rowing as isokinetic (11). It may be that swimming, rowing, canoeing, and the like, are sports in which the athlete is more likely to benefit by speed-specific isokinetic training.

The possible movement patterns of the upper extremity, as previously discussed, are almost unlimited. It is difficult with typical isokinetic equipment to train isokinetically using a wide variety of movement patterns. Thus another limitation of isokinetics for the upper extremity is the difficulty in simulating sport-specific upper extremity movement patterns.

For example, the tennis athlete is required to hit a first serve, second serve, overhead, forehand, backhand, high, low, and normal forehand volley, high, low, and normal backhand volley, running forehand, and running backhand, to name a few of the possibilities. It would be very difficult to simulate all of these specific movement patterns with a typical isokinetic device.

The interaction of movement speed and movement patterns is sport specific. The athlete must not only accelerate the body part, but he or she also must efficiently decelerate the body part, both to perform well and to minimize injury risk. The muscle action in deceleration is eccentric, so eccentric testing and training is related to the ability of an athlete to decelerate a part of the body efficiently. As we discuss why isokinetics may be useful to athletes, we must include the role of deceleration in both performance and injury risk.

Eccentric muscle actions are also more likely to cause microtraumatic changes in the muscle. Musculoskeletal adaptations that occur with intense sport participation—decreased range of motion adaptations and muscle strength imbalances—affect both performance and injury risk (10, 35, 36, 38). With isokinetic eccentric testing and training, microtraumatic damage to muscle should be further evaluated. This damage may be the stimulus for protein synthesis and subsequent increases in strength. If so, does eccentric isokinetic exercise cause the same microtraumatic changes as functional eccentric exercise?

The basic question to consider in this chapter is why isokinetic training would produce greater performance improvement than other forms of exercise training. The rationale of isokinetic exercise is that maximal work is performed at each angle during the full range of motion. But it is important to note that no studies comparing isokinetic and isoinertial exercise conclude that isokinetic training is superior to improve performance.

Training to improve performance is usually discussed in terms of skill sports such as baseball and tennis. But performance can also be evaluated in high-power sports. To train to improve performance in an activity such as the bench press, you can choose isokinetic or isoinertial resistance, or isometric resistance at a variety of angles. Isokinetic resistance, if the effort is maximal, provides maximal resistance at each angle, causing the speed of movement to be constant. Isoinertial resistance provides a fixed amount of resistance such that, with maximal effort, the speed of movement is maximal at each angle. While isokinetic training provides variety in a nonspecific phase of training, the specificity of training principle suggests that isoinertial resistance is superior, particularly in a competitive phase of training.

Wilson and Murphy (66) used isometric tests of muscular function to assess athletes. The authors question the external validity of isometric testing of athletes. Since athletic activities are dynamic, dynamic testing was deemed more appropriate than isometric testing. A similar argument can be made in favor of dynamic testing over isokinetic testing in athletes.

# Rationale for Isokinetic Testing of the Upper Body in Sports

Isokinetic testing of the upper body includes testing the shoulder in internal/external rotation, flexion/extension, abduction/adduction, the elbow in flexion/extension, the forearm in pronation/supination, and the wrist in flexion/extension. Many of these tests are performed with the body in a variety of positions. Shoulder internal/external rotation, for instance, is performed on a person who is in a supine position, seated, or standing. The supine position is best if isolation of the joint is the goal, because the other positions, particularly standing, likely allow some substitution of lower body muscles. The "modified neutral" test position in shoulder internal/external rotation may be more specific to some sports, but it also allows some substitution of other muscle groups. So the choice of test positions depends on the goals of testing. If the goal of testing is to evaluate a specific muscle group, the test position should allow for a valid and reliable test by isolating the joint being tested.

## Stabilization

Stabilization of the athlete during upper extremity testing is important if the test values are to be accurate. One study (58) estimated that for shoulder flexion/

extension on a Cybex II isokinetic dynamometer, the glenohumeral joint elevated an average of 8 cm. The author estimated this to be 12.5% of the distance from the shoulder to the handle, meaning the strength and power values should be reduced by that amount to be accurate.

## Plane of the Scapula

At the shoulder, testing in the plane of the scapula is currently a popular concept. However, Whitcomb, Kelley, and Leiper (60) demonstrated no differences in peak and mean torque produced at 90 and 210°/s in shoulder abduction testing in the coronal and scapular plane. They concluded that although there are anatomical, functional, and clinical reasons cited for testing shoulder abductors in the scapular plane, no differences in torque production were found between the coronal and scapular planes. Greenfield and coworkers (24) reported rotational shoulder strength in 20 subjects with 45° abduction at 60°/s in the frontal and scapular planes. The results indicated no significant differences between the two positions for internal rotation. External rotation strength was significantly higher in the frontal plane. Hartsell and Forwell (27) evaluated isokinetic concentric and eccentric torque production of the shoulder in internal/external rotation in the scapular and neutral planes. The scapular plane produced significantly higher peak torques concentrically. These authors concluded that while both planes produced acceptable results, the scapular plane was preferred because it was more functional and less injurious to the rotator cuff.

Isolating a joint is rarely specific to sport performance. While isokinetic testing isolates the joint being tested, sports require joint movements that take place in a synchronized pattern to produce the desired movement. Therefore, joints are generally not isolated in sport performance, although there are exceptions.

## Test Positions

The most common isokinetic test of the shoulder is internal/external rotation. Most often, this test is performed on a supine subject with 90° of humeral abduction allowing up to 90° for external rotation and 90° for internal rotation. Other testing positions, such as the modified neutral test position can be utilized. When interpreting research results, test position is an important consideration.

## Calibration

One distinct advantage of isokinetic dynamometry in testing is the reproducibility of the results. Because the test position isolates specific muscles, and because the test position is reproducible, then the reliability of the tests is relatively high. Isometric reliability coefficients have been reported for the upper body ranging from .88 to .96 for test-retest reliability (16). In that study, interrater reliability differences were apparently related to the way the examiners provided verbal encouragement, which would also be a variable in isokinetic testing.

## Reliability

For isokinetic test results to be accurate, regular calibration of the testing device is a must. In the analysis of torque curves, Williamson and coworkers (61) discuss the importance of calibrating the instrument, dampening to insure that peak torque is not movement artifact, and correcting for gravity when appropriate. Backman (5) reported that a simple handheld dynamometer produced the most accurate measures of muscle function in children. In the study, three of six age groups demonstrated greater isometric force in elbow flexion on the dominant side. Isokinetic tests required more time and more experienced evaluators, caused difficulty at high speeds where children could not overcome gravity, and were regarded as complementary to isometric testing. In the same group of children, Duchenne muscular dystrophy was followed in 16 boys. Isokinetic measurements proved unreliable in tracking these individuals, possibly due to the difficulty in activating muscles at a variety of speeds.

The reliability of three isometric shoulder strength testing dynamometers was evaluated by Leggin and coworkers (40). Strength testing was measured in internal rotation, external rotation, and abduction. Interclass correlation coefficients ranged from .84 to .99. Measurements taken on the same day by the same examiner appeared to be highly reliable with all three devices. Therefore, the reliability of isokinetic dynamometry appears to be generally high, even when compared to isometric strength measurements.

Wilk, Arrigo, and Andrews (62) discussed several problems with isokinetic data collection, including the use of windowed vs. nonwindowed data. They tested shoulder abduction/adduction in 50 healthy baseball pitchers and obtained statistical differences using windowed and nonwindowed data. They concluded that the use of windowed data might help to identify spikes in peak torque and control aberrant torque production during testing.

The results of isokinetic testing of the upper body are reported under a variety of conditions. Often correlations are reported to compare the dominant to the nondominant side. In some instances, correlations to a specific performance variable are reported. In all instances, it is important to evaluate the methods of data collection before comparing the results of different studies.

## Isokinetic Shoulder Testing

The results of isokinetic testing in skill sports such as tennis and baseball are widely reported in the literature. These sports are discussed elsewhere in this text in detail and are mentioned here in terms of general isokinetic testing of the upper body in athletes. Sport-specific training data from isokinetic profiling studies of the shoulder in internal/external rotation have been reported in baseball (19) and tennis (9, 18).

# Tennis

Chandler and coworkers (9) demonstrated a decrease in concentric external rotation strength in the dominant arm of college tennis players. Ellenbecker (18) reported increased isokinetic strength in the dominant over the nondominant arms in highly skilled tennis players; he found no correlation between service velocity and isokinetic strength. Ellenbecker and Mattalino (19) reported a significant difference in isokinetic peak torque in internal but not external rotation in professional baseball pitchers.

Codine and coworkers (12) reported isokinetic rotator cuff strength of 12 nonathletes, 12 runners, 15 tennis players, and 12 baseball players. The comparison between dominant and nondominant extremities demonstrated no significant differences in tennis players, it showed higher peak torque and power values in the dominant extremities of nonathletes at 180°/s and of runners at 300°/s, and it showed higher peak torque and power values in the dominant extremities at both speeds for baseball players.

Wilk and coworkers (63) established a database on isokinetic muscular performance characteristics of internal/external rotation musculature in professional baseball pitchers. They evaluated 150 healthy professional baseball pitchers with concentric isokinetic testing at 180 and 300°/s in both the throwing and nonthrowing shoulders. There were no statistically significant differences between the dominant and nondominant arms in internal rotation at either speed or in external rotation at 300°/s. There was a statistically significant difference in external rotation between the dominant and nondominant arms at 180°/s. Wilk, Andrews, and Arrigo (65) reported the isokinetic abductor/adductor strength in 83 professional baseball players. The adductor muscle group was significantly stronger in the throwing shoulder. There were no side-to-side differences for the abductor muscle group.

Cohen and coworkers (13) reported a significant relationship between service velocity and isokinetic strength and between service velocity and flexibility. Elbow extension strength and both concentric and eccentric internal rotation/external rotation ratios correlated positively to service velocity. This only suggests the possibility that eccentric and concentric training may improve performance. Well-controlled studies must be performed and compared to typical dynamic training programs to determine that isokinetic training improves performance and is superior to other forms of training.

# Baseball

Bartlett, Storey, and Simons (4) reported a positive correlation between isokinetic torque production of the shoulder adductors and throwing speed in professional baseball players. In comparing the dominant to the nondominant arm, all values measured except shoulder adduction were significantly correlated. Measurements included elbow flexion/extension, forearm pronation/supination, shoulder abduction/adduction, shoulder internal/external rotation, shoulder flexion/extension, and shoulder horizontal abduction/adduction.

Mikesky and associates (44) reported on the isokinetic eccentric and concentric strength of shoulder and arm musculature in college baseball pitchers. Eccentric strength of shoulder rotators averaged 114% of concentric strength. These authors found no differences between the dominant and nondominant extremities for any strength measure or ratio. Brown and coworkers (7) tested the shoulder in internal/external rotation of 41 professional baseball players. Pitchers produced significantly greater torque in the dominant arm. In both pitchers and position players, the dominant arm did produce significantly more torque than the nondominant arm at all speeds tested. There were no significant differences in strength ratios in the dominant and nondominant arms.

Isokinetic torque patterns have been used to identify injury and injury risk patterns. Timm (57) identified a specific isokinetic torque curve for baseball pitchers with impingement syndrome. By developing characteristic torque curves for specific injuries, isokinetic testing becomes useful as a diagnostic tool.

## Swimming

Magnusson and coworkers (42) reported an isokinetic profile of masters level swimmers and related the profile to performance. Upper extremity isokinetic measurements included shoulder abduction and internal/external rotation. Neither shoulder isokinetic variables, range of motion variables, nor supraspinatus muscle strength correlated with swim performance. The only variable that did correlate with swim performance was isokinetic trunk flexion.

## Postsurgery

Rokito and coworkers (53) reported isokinetic strength after surgical repair of the rotator cuff. Isokinetic testing was performed in flexion/extension, abduction/adduction, and internal/external rotation at 60°/s. The strength of the injured extremity increased in all three movements with the greatest improvement in mean peak torque occurring during the first six months postsurgery. Significant increases in mean power and mean total work also occurred. By 12 months, mean work had increased to 70% of the uninvolved extremity in flexion and abduction and to 90% of the uninvolved extremity in external rotation. The degree of recovery of strength correlated primarily with the size of the tear, with recovery of the larger tears progressing much slower and with less consistency.

## Other Studies

Scoville and others (56) evaluated the isokinetic strength of the shoulder musculature in end range (60–90°) concentric/eccentric strength ratios. Because shoulder function in athletes participating in overhead sports is an interaction of eccentric and concentric muscle actions, this may be a more functional method of evaluating shoulder strength in these athletes. It is at the end range of movement that this concentric/eccentric muscle balance becomes most important. The end range ratios for the medial rotators functioning eccentrically and the lateral rotators functioning concentrically were 2.39:1 and 2.15:1, respectively, for the dominant and nondominant shoulders.

Ivey and others (32) reported normal isokinetic strength in 31 volunteers in shoulder flexion/extension, abduction/adduction, and internal/external rotation. No significant differences were found between the dominant and nondominant extremities, although the dominant shoulders were consistently stronger. Male shoulder strength was greater than female, although the difference was less when the measurements were normalized for lean body mass and exercise habit.

# Isokinetic Elbow Testing

Isokinetic elbow flexion/extension is a relatively common test in general training studies and is often used to compare upper body flexion/extension ratios with lower body flexion/extension ratios at the knee.

## General Studies

Otis and Godbold (48) measured the relationship between maximal isokinetic and maximal isometric torque at angular velocities of 24, 48, 96, and 192°/s for elbow flexion/extension. They tested 24 subjects bilaterally with torque values recorded at 60 and 90° of flexion compared in the isometric and isokinetic conditions. Confidence intervals were determined to predict isokinetic torque by measuring isometric torque.

Isokinetic torque measurements correlate highly to measurements at a similar speed. Knapik and Ramos (39) studied relationships between elbow flexion and extension in 16 healthy young men. Isokinetic torque values were obtained at 36, 108, and 180°/s. The study demonstrated that isokinetic torque declined with increasing velocity of muscle action. Correlations between isokinetic and isometric actions were moderate to high. The higher correlations were found at the lower velocities and between isokinetic velocities that were adjacent on the velocity spectrum.

One study attempted to correlate muscle fiber type with isokinetic torque production at specific speeds of muscle action (11). Muscle fiber type and isokinetic strength and fatigue were measured in nine elite rowers in canoeing and kayaking, and the results were compared to needle muscle biopsies. Elbow flexion/extension peak torques and fatigue were not related to fiber type.

## Males Versus Females

Most studies report that females produce less concentric torque in upper body testing than males. Frontera and associates (21) measured the isokinetic strength of the elbow flexors and extensors in 200 healthy 45- to 78-year-old men and women. Peak torque, measured at 60 and 180°/s, was significantly higher in 45- to 54-year-olds than in 65- to 78-year-olds. When strength was adjusted for fat free mass or muscle mass, the age-related differences were not significant in elbow flexion or extension. Absolute strength of women ranged from 42.2 to 62.8% of males.

One study reported that women generate greater eccentric torque than males in the elbow flexors (25). Both the eccentric and concentric isokinetic performance of the elbow flexor muscle group in 90 males and females ages 21 to 67 years were examined. Eccentric average torque did not change as a function of velocity, and concentric torque decreased as angular velocity increased. Women generated greater eccentric torque relative to concentric torque than men did.

## Bodybuilders

Alway and associates (2) compared male and female bodybuilders to male and female control groups on maximal elbow flexion on an isokinetic dynamometer. Velocities tested ranged between 1.02 and 5.24 rad/s. Elbow flexor cross-sectional area was measured by computed tomographic scanning. Lean body mass ratios were greater in the male bodybuilders. Correlations of peak torque were positively related to muscle cross-sectional area but negatively related to cross-sectional area lean body mass and peak torque/cross-sectional area ratios. Velocity-associated declines in peak torque from 1.02 to 5.24 rad/s averaged 28.4%, and were identical in men and women and among the bodybuilders and controls. In this study, neither gender nor training affected the decrease in peak torque at increasing velocities.

Sale, MacDougall, and Alway (55) compared elbow flexion in male bodybuilders and untrained men and women. Velocities of 30, 120, 180, 240, and 300°/s were used to collect impact torque, peak torque, and work. They used CT scans to determine muscle fiber area, fiber composition, and collagen volume density. Peak torque and work decreased at higher velocities in male controls and bodybuilders but not in females. Female controls had greater work/cross-sectional area ratios than male controls and bodybuilders at all velocities. Muscle fiber composition failed to correlate with any measure of strength. Sale and MacDougall (54) measured elbow extension strength in 6 power lifters, 7 bodybuilders, and 25 male controls. The weight trainers exceeded the controls by 73% in isokinetic strength of the elbow extensors.

## Endurance

Isokinetic endurance of the elbow flexor/extensor musculature was reported by Motzkin and associates (46). The study compared a healthy population of 32 male subjects, ages 21 to 39 years, on the isometric and isokinetic endurance with maximum effort in flexion and extension of the dominant and nondominant elbows. Isometric endurance was not related to isokinetic endurance. Dominant and nondominant elbow endurance were related, meaning the opposite extremity can adequately serve as a comparison for an injured or diseased extremity. Also, endurance was greater in flexion than in extension.

## Nonathletes

Gallagher and coworkers (23) reported on the isokinetic strength of the elbow in flexion/extension and pronation/supination in 60 nonathletic men. The men were subdivided into an older group, ages 50 to 60 years, and a younger group, ages 20 to 30 years. Peak torque, work, power, and angle of peak torque were measured at 90°/s and 180°/s. Highly significant differences were found between age groups in flexion/extension, but no significant differences were evident in pronation/supination. The dominant wrist had significantly higher levels of peak torque, work, and power in flexion but not in extension, pronation, or supination. Peak torque and work were greater at the slow speed, and power was significantly greater at the high speed with the exception of pronation. Age was suggested as a factor in determining the angle of peak torque.

# Wrist Testing

Hartsell, Hubbard, and Van Os (26) reported isokinetic testing of the wrist in pronation and supination. Testing was performed at 60, 120, and 180°/s. Interclass correlation coefficients calculated over one or two testing periods indicated greater consistency when the correlations were averaged over at least two test occasions. The dominant wrist was significantly stronger than the nondominant wrist at all velocities for pronation but only at the slowest velocity, 60°/s, for supination.

A similar study was reported on patients with a biceps brachii tendon rupture (14). Isokinetic strength testing indicated strength and total work levels returned to expected normal levels in elbow flexion. Six of eight patients continued to have less strength in supination of the injured arm than the uninjured arm. All eight patients performed less total work with repetitive supination of the injured arm compared to the uninjured arm.

Because wrist flexion/extension is a relatively simple movement in a single plane, reliability measurements should be high if the methods are well outlined and if the joint is well stabilized. Reliability measurements of isometric wrist extension using the Lido WorkSET demonstrated an intraobserver coefficient of .96, interobserver coefficient of .94, and an overall reliability of .92 (31).

# Rationale for Isokinetic Training of the Upper Extremity

The rational for using isokinetic training for specific sports should be critically evaluated. Maximal effort results in maximal speed at each angle throughout a range of motion. One problem is reliably measuring effort. Also, at the present time, there is a lack of studies to show that isokinetic training is superior to traditional isoinertial training. More research needs to be done comparing the effects of isokinetic training to other training modalities relative to the concentric or force-generating aspects of upper body athletic movements as well as eccentric actions of muscles in the upper body.

Wilk and Arrigo (64) state that the overhead-sport athlete must demonstrate functional stability in the overhead position. A balance of static (passive) and dynamic (active) stabilizers accomplish this stability. In the rehabilitation process, they recommended that athletes utilize the concepts of neuromuscular control, proprioception, force couples, plyometrics, eccentrics, and scapular stability. These rehabilitative concepts can be applied to training the noninjured overhead-sport athlete.

Since isokinetic training is by nature not specific to most sports, it is most likely to be effective as an adjunct form of exercise in the general phases of training as opposed to the sport-specific phases of training. When isokinetic training is performed, it should begin with a variety of movement speeds, then focus on the muscle action speeds specific to the sport. Following the specificity principle, baseball pitchers would be most likely to benefit from training at high movement speeds, tennis players at moderate to high movement speeds, and swimmers and power lifters at moderate to slow movement speeds.

## Isokinetic Shoulder Training

Researchers compared isokinetic vs. eccentric training of the shoulder internal and external rotators in elite tennis players (45). Groups consisted of an isokinetic concentric training group, an isokinetic eccentric training group, and a control group with no training. Service velocity increased by over 11% in both training groups, which was a significant increase over the control group. The success of isokinetic training is encouraging, but it was not compared with a group trained with fixed resistance equipment. Ellenbecker, Davies, and Rowinski (17) compared concentric and eccentric isokinetic internal rotation strengthening in college tennis players. Only the concentrically trained group significantly increased in service velocity.

Amiridis and coworkers (3) evaluated the effects of isokinetic concentric and eccentric training on muscular strength. For 12 weeks, subjects performed training including concentric and eccentric actions. After that, they were divided into three groups performing different combinations of eccentric and concentric training. All three groups increased in performance. The findings only partially supported the specificity of training for concentric/eccentric mode, but the velocity of training principle was strongly supported.

Heiderscheit, McLean, and Davies (28) studied the effects of isokinetic and plyometric training on the shoulder internal rotators. Since plyometric exercises are often used as a performance-enhancing exercise, the study may have application to performance as well. Female subjects were assigned to a control, isokinetic, or plyometric group. Tests included eccentric and concentric isokinetic tests for the internal rotators at 60, 280, and 240°/s and a softball throw for distance. There were no pre- to posttest differences in the softball throw. The isokinetic group did improve measures of concentric and eccentric power measured isokinetically. These results indicate the adaptations to isokinetic training were specific to the mode of testing. The softball throw is a specific skill and, at least at the performance level of these subjects, does not improve with either dynamic or isokinetic training.

Bronstrom and associates (6) reported on the effects of isokinetic training in patients with recurrent shoulder dislocations. Patients trained using an isokinetic pulley-weight apparatus 3 times a week for 8 weeks. After 1 year, 28 out of 33 shoulders had improved in stability. Of the shoulders that were not stabilized with training, subjects had either a multidirectional instability or a generalized overall joint laxity. Since no group used free weight exercises, it is not possible to determine the superiority of either mode of exercise over the other.

# Isokinetic Elbow Training

There are a number of studies that evaluate training the elbow flexors isokinetically, just as with the studies testing the elbow flexors. Some studies also evaluate elbow extension.

## General Studies

Kanehisa and Miyashiti (33) studied the effect of isometric and isokinetic muscle training on static strength and dynamic power. During the first 8 weeks, 12 males trained the elbow flexors in 4 different positions on an isometric dynamometer. Gains in isometric strength ranged from 27 to 36% and in isometric power from 34 to 46%. Afterward, subjects were divided equally into a fast group who trained at 157°/s and a slow group who trained at 73°/s. After 6 weeks of the second phase of training, the fast group produced significant gains in power with light equivalent masses. Neither group produced a significant increase in isokinetic strength.

Housh and Housh (30) examined the effects of unilateral velocity-specific concentric isokinetic training of the extensor and flexor muscles of the elbow. Twelve adult men volunteered to train their nondominant extremities 3 times per week for 6 sets of 10 maximal repetitions for 8 weeks using a velocity of 120°/s. Subjects were tested at the end of 8 weeks for increases in peak torque at 60, 120, 180, 240, and 300°/s. Training resulted in significant increases in peak torque on the trained side of the body for elbow flexion and extension. Increases in peak torque were found at torque velocities that were both greater than and less than the training velocity. In addition, there was a cross-training effect, with significant increases in peak torque on the contralateral side of the body for elbow extension at all velocities except 300°/s. The researchers concluded that unilateral single-velocity training in midrange was sufficient to elicit strength gains at a wide range of velocities in both the trained and contralateral limbs.

Martin, Martin, and Morlon (43) studied the effects of short-term eccentric isokinetic training on the force-velocity relationships of the elbow flexor muscles. On an isokinetic dynamometer, subjects performed 2 maximal concentric elbow flexions at 60, 120, 180, 240, 300 and 360°/s and held maximal and submaximal isometric actions at an elbow flexion angle of 90°. Training was conducted three times a week for four weeks. After training, the subjects' maximal shortening velocity increased significantly along with significant increases in EMG amplitude of the maximal isometric action. The researchers interpreted this as a change toward improving the fast characteristics of the elbow flexor muscles.

O'Hagen and others (47) compared an accommodating resistance device to coupled eccentric/concentric actions on a resistance device. Six women and 6 men trained the elbow flexors 3 days per week for 20 weeks, with one arm performing accommodating resistance and one arm performing concentric/eccentric actions. With the results collapsed across the two conditions, the women made significantly greater increases in elbow flexion strength as measured on both devices.

Young men and women respond similarly to training of elbow flexion using accommodating resistance. In response to the same short-term resistance training program, men and women make similar gains in muscle size, but women make greater relative changes in strength.

## Prepubescents

Ozmun, Mikesky, and Surburg (50) investigated the mechanisms responsible for strength increases in prepubescent children. Eight male and 8 female subjects, mean age 10.3 years, were randomly assigned to a training or a control group. Strength, IEMG, and arm anthropometrics were measured. Isoinertial and isokinetic strength gains occurred in the trained group without corresponding changes in arm circumference or skinfolds. Early gains in muscular strength in prepubescent youth were attributed to a neural effect causing increased muscular activation.

Training the elbow in isometric flexion increases lean tissue of the upper arm (22). Resistance training of the upper arm in prepubescent populations has been evaluated in the literature. Ninety-nine elementary school children were assigned to a training or nontraining group. The training group participated in a resistance training program for 12 weeks consisting of a maximal sustained isometric action of elbow flexion for 10 seconds. Cross-sectional area of the tissue of the upper arm was measured using ultrasound. Maximum isometric and isokinetic strength in elbow flexion/extension was measured. After training, cross-sectional area increased in both the trained and the control group, however the changes were due to increased muscle and bone in the trained group and increased fat in the control group.

## Elderly

Lexell and coworkers (41) reported on the short- and long-term effects of heavy resistance training in older men and women (ages 70–77 years). Elbow flexion increased after 11 weeks of training in both men and women. Strength increased further following an additional 11 weeks of training. Isokinetic testing revealed similar but smaller gains in strength, likely due at least partially to the fact that training was not isokinetic. Older men and women have a high capacity to increase dynamic muscle strength of the elbow flexors. Isokinetic tests are more sensitive to changes due to isokinetic training and not as sensitive to changes that may occur with isoinertial training.

Brown, McCartney, and Sale (8) used isokinetic testing to evaluate dynamic weight training in an elderly population. Dynamic elbow flexion training of one arm resulted in a significant (48%) increase in the maximal 1 RM load, a small (8.8%) improvement in isokinetic torque, and no change in isometric strength. Again this points out that dynamic resistance training causes adaptations that are specific to the type of training. When testing with a different modality than the one used for training, benefits will be less or may not occur at all. Ramsay reported similar results in prepubescent boys, where a dynamic training program produced a 26% increase in isokinetic elbow flexion (67). In the elderly population the primary mechanism of strength gain is increases in cross-sectional area of the muscle, while in the adolescent population the primary mechanism of strength gain is related to neurological adaptations.

## Prepubertal

Hydraulic resistance creates a muscle action of a constant speed of shortening and can be considered isokinetic in nature. Weltman and coworkers (59) examined the effectiveness of hydraulic resistance in improving strength in prepubertal males. Researchers determined the effectiveness of the program by isokinetic testing of elbow flexion/extension at 30 and 90°/s. Eccentric work was not performed. Subjects increased concentric isokinetic strength as a result of the training program. No evidence of epiphyseal damage was seen through evaluation by muscle scintigraphy. The short-term (14-week) program was determined to be safe and effective in adolescent boys.

Abernethy and Jurimae (1) evaluated cross-sectional and longitudinal uses of isoinertial, isometric, and isokinetic dynamometry. All strength-testing methods were sensitive to changes with training, but the adaptations varied greatly within the subjects. These differential effects were thought to be due to differences in muscle structure, neurological function (including learning), and mechanical mechanisms of strength production.

# Isokinetic Wrist Training

As mentioned previously, to draw conclusions on isokinetics and performance based on the current literature, we must consider studies from the rehabilitation field. In one study of women with pain at the lateral epicondyle of the forearm diagnosed as a cumulative trauma disorder, researchers examined isokinetic testing in flexion/extension and pronation/supination (20). A control sample had significantly higher peak torque at 180°/s in wrist extension, flexion, supination, and pronation than the experimental subjects on the injured side. Control subjects also demonstrated higher peak torques than the experimental subjects on the noninjured side in flexion, pronation, and supination. That is, women with cumulative trauma disorder, pain at the lateral epicondyle, demonstrated decreased peak torque in both the symptomatic and asymptomatic wrists. Due to the fact that decreases in peak torque were detected on both sides, the researcher postulated a central nervous system deficiency.

## Summary

The reliability of isokinetic testing, as well as its availability in the clinical sports medicine setting, continues to make it an often-used research tool to document muscle weakness and muscle strength imbalances in specific sports and to measure the effectiveness of specific training programs. Research on isokinetic testing and training is currently focused on either profiling or on rehabilitation, but there is a need for isokinetic research in training athletes to improve performance in upper body sports.

Isokinetic training does not cause muscle action patterns specific to most sporting activities that use the upper body, the exceptions being perhaps swimming and other water sports. The high speeds seen in sports such as tennis and baseball are not reached using typical isokinetic devices. Due to a lack of specificity, isokinetic training should be performed in a preparatory phase of training for these athletes.

Eccentric isokinetic training may be helpful in training the muscles to decelerate the loads experienced in high speed upper body movements, but more research needs to be done in this area. The link between eccentric training and performance should be fully investigated.

Future research should study the effects of concentric and eccentric isokinetic training at a variety of speeds on performance in a variety of sports. The effect of isokinetic training on performance in swimming and related activities should be further evaluated, since the muscle actions in those sports are more similar to isokinetic training than most activities. The effect of eccentric isokinetic and isoinertial training and its relationship to joint range of motion should be evaluated. It is possible that specific eccentric training exercises would modify the loss in range of motion in the upper extremity. It is also possible that specific eccentric training exercises could decrease the amount of flexibility that is lost in high-intensity upper body activities. Differences between isokinetic and isoinertial exercises should be evaluated in this respect.

Studies should be controlled, and should evaluate the difference between eccentric isokinetic training, concentric isokinetic training, and concentric and eccentric dynamic training. Since maximal effort through a full range of motion is theoretically important in isokinetic strength development, methods to insure maximal activation of muscle, such as the amplitude of EMG, should be evaluated in the upper extremity.

# References

1. Abernethy, PJ, and Jurimae, J. 1996. Cross-sectional and longitudinal uses of isoinertial, isometric, and isokinetic dynamometry. *Med Sci Sports Exerc* 28(9): 1180–87.

2. Alway, SE, Stray-Gundersen, J, Grumbt, WH, and Gonyea, WJ. 1990. Muscle cross-sectional area and torque in resistance-trained subjects. *Eur J Appl Physiol* 60(2): 86–90.

3. Amiridis, IG, Cometti, G, Morlon, B, and Van Hoecke, J. 1997. Concentric and eccentric training-induced alterations in shoulder flexor and extensor strength. *J Orthop Sports Phys Ther* 25(1): 26–33.

4. Bartlett, LR, Storey, MD, and Simons, BD. 1989. Measurement of upper extremity torque production and its relationship to throwing speed in the competitive athlete. *Am J Sports Med* 17(1): 89–91.

5. Backman, E. 1988. Methods for measurement of muscle function: Methodological aspects, reference values for children, and clinical applications. *Scand J Rehabil Med Suppl* 20: 9–95.

6. Bronstrom, LA, Kronberg, M, Nemeth, G, and Oxelback, U. 1922. *Scand J Rehabil Med* 24(1): 11–15.

7. Brown, LP, Niehues, SL, Harrah, A, Yavorsky, P, and Hirshman, HP. 1988. Upper extremity range of motion and isokinetic strength of the internal and external shoulder rotators in major league baseball players. *Am J Sports Med* 16(6): 577–85.

8. Brown, AB, McCartney, N, and Sale, DG. 1990. Positive adaptations to weightlifting training in the elderly. *J Appl Physiol* 69(5): 1725–33.

9. Chandler, TJ, Kibler, WB, Uhl, TL, Wooten, B, Kiser, A, and Stone, E. 1990. Flexibility comparisons of junior elite tennis players to other athletes. *Am J Sports Med* 18(2): 134–36.

10. Chandler, TJ, Kibler, WB, Stracener, EC, Ziegler, AK, and Pace, B. 1992. Shoulder strength, power, and endurance in college tennis players. *Am J Sports Med* 20(4): 455–58.

11. Clarkson, PM, Kroll, W, and Melchionda, AM. 1982. Isokinetic strength, endurance, and fiber type composition in elite American paddlers. *Eur J Appl Physiol* 48: 67–76.

12. Codine, P, Pernard, PL, Pocholle, M, Benaim, C, and Brun, V. 1998. Influence of sports discipline on shoulder rotator cuff balance. *Med Sci Sports Exerc* 29(11): 1400–5.

13. Cohen, DB, Mont, MA, Cambell, KR, Vogelstein, BN, and Loewy, JW. 1994. Upper extremity physical factors affecting tennis serve velocity. *Am J Sports Med* 22(6): 746–50.

14. Davison, BL, Engber, WD, and Tigert, LJ. 1996. Long-term evaluation of repaired distal biceps brachii tendon ruptures. *Clin Orthop* 333: 186–91.

15. Davies, GJ. 1995. The need for critical thinking in rehabilitation. *J Sport Rehabil* 4(1): 1–22.

16. Derosiers, J, Rochette, A, Payette, H, Gregoire, L, Boutier, V, and Lazowski, D. 1998. *Can J Rehabil* 11(3): 149–55.

17. Ellenbecker, TS, Davies, GJ, and Rowinski, MJ. 1988. Concentric versus eccentric isokinetic strengthening of the rotator cuff: Objective data versus functional test. *Am J Sports Med* 16(1): 64–69.

18. Ellenbecker, TS. 1991. A total arm strength isokinetic profile of highly skilled tennis players. *Isokinetics Exerc Sci* 1(1): 9–21.

19. Ellenbecker, TS, and Mattalino, AJ. 1997. Concentric isokinetic shoulder internal and external rotation strength in professional baseball pitchers. *J Orthop Sports Phys Ther* 25(5): 323–38.

20. Friedman, PJ. 1998. Isokinetic peak torque in women with unilateral cumulative trauma disorders and healthy control subjects. *Arch Phys Med Rehabil* 79(7): 816–19.

21. Frontera, WR, Hughes, VA, Lutz, KJ, and Evans, WJ. 1991. A cross-sectional study of muscle strength and mass in 45- to 78-year-old men and women. *J Appl Physiol* 71(2): 644–50.

22. Fukunaga, T, Funato, K, and Ikegawa, S. 1992. The effects of resistance training on muscle area and strength in prepubescent age. *Ann Physiol Anthropol* 11(3): 357–64.

23. Gallagher, MA, Cuomo, F, Polonsky, L, Berliner, K, and Zuckerman, JD. 1997. The effects of age, testing speed, and arm dominance on isokinetic strength of the elbow. *Shoulder Elbow Surg* 6(4): 340–46.

24. Greenfield, BH, Donatelli, R, Wooden, MJ, and Wilkes, J. 1990. Isokinetic evaluation of shoulder rotational strength between the plane of the scapula and the frontal plane. *Am J Sports Med* 18(2): 124–28.

25. Griffin, JW. 1988. Differences in elbow flexion torque measured concentrically, eccentrically, and isometrically. *Phys Ther* 67: 1205–8.

26. Hartsell, HD, Hubbard, M, and Van Os, P. 1995. Isokinetic strength evaluation of wrist pronators and supinators: Implications for clinicians. *Physiother Can* 47(4): 252–57.

27. Hartsell, HD, and Forwell, L. 1997. Postoperative eccentric and concentric isokinetic strength for the shoulder rotators in the scapular and neutral planes. *J Orthop Sports Phys Ther* 25(1): 19–25.

28. Heiderscheit, BC, McLean, KP, and Davies, GJ. 1996. The effects of isokinetic vs. plyometric training on the shoulder internal rotators. *J Orthop Sports Phys Ther* 23(2): 125–33.

29. Hislop, HJ, and Perrine, JJ. 1967. The isokinetic concept of exercise. *Phys Ther* 47(2): 114–17.

30. Housh, DJ, and Housh, TJ. 1993. The effects of unilateral velocity-specific concentric strength training. *J Orthop Sports Phys Ther* 17(5): 252–56.

31. Hudak, P, Hannah, S, Knapp, M, and Shields, S. 1997. Reliability of isometric wrist extension torque using the Lido WorkSET for late follow-up of postoperative wrist patients. *J Hand Ther* 10(4): 290–96.

32. Ivey, FM, Calhoun, JH, Rusche, K, and Bierschenk, J. 1985. Isokinetic testing of shoulder strength: Normal values. *Arch Phys Med Rehabil* 66(6): 384–86.

33. Kanehisa, H, and Miyashiti, M. 1983. Effect of isometric and isokinetic muscle training on static strength and dynamic power. *Eur J Appl Physiol* 50(3): 365–71.

34. Keating, JL, and Matyas, TA. 1996. Clinical perspective: The influence of subject and test design on dynamometric measurements of extremity muscles. *Phys Ther* 76(8): 866–89.

35. Kibler, WB, and Chandler, TJ. 1994. Racquet sports. In *Sports injuries, mechanisms, prevention, and treatment*, ed. FH Fu and DA Stone, 531–50. Baltimore: Williams & Wilkins.

36. Kibler, WB, Chandler, TJ, Livingston, BP, and Roetert, EP. 1996. Shoulder range of motion in elite tennis players: Effect of age and years of tournament play. *Am J Sports Med* 24(3): 279–85.

37. Kibler, WB. 1998. Role of the scapula in athletic shoulder function. *Am J Sports Med* 26(2): 325–37.

38. Kibler, WB, and Chandler, TJ. 1998. Changes in range of motion in junior tennis players participating in an injury risk modification conditioning program. Manuscript submitted for publication.

39. Knapik, JJ, and Ramos, MU. 1980. Isokinetic and isometric torque relationships in the human body. *Arch Phys Med Rehabil* 61: 64–67.

40. Leggin, BG, Neuman, RM, Iannotti, JP, Williams, GR, and Thompson, EC. 1996. *J Shoulder Elbow Surg* 5(1): 18–24.

41. Lexell, J, Downham, DY, Larsson, Y, Bruhn, E, and Morsing, B. 1995. Heavy resistance training in older Scandinavian men and women: Short- and long-term effects on arm and leg muscles. *Scand J Med Sci Sports* 5(6): 329–41.

42. Magnusson, SP, Constantini, NW, McHugh, MP, and Gleim, GW. 1995. Strength profiles and performance in master's level swimmers. *Am J Sports Med* 23(5): 626–31.

43. Martin, A, Martin, L, and Morlon, B. 1995. Changes induced by eccentric training on force-velocity relationships of the elbow flexor muscles. *Eur J Appl Physiol* 72(1–2): 183–85.

44. Mikesky, AE, Edwards, JE, Wigglesworth, JK, and Kunkel, S. 1995. Eccentric and concentric strength of the shoulder and arm musculature in college-age baseball pitchers. *Am J Sports Med* 23(5): 638–42.

45. Mont, MA, Cohen, DB, Cambell, KR, Gravare, K, and Mathur, SK. 1994. Isokinetic concentric versus eccentric training of shoulder rotators with functional evaluation of performance enhancement in elite tennis players. *Am J Sports Med* 22(4): 513–17.

46. Motzkin, NE, Cahalan, TD, Morrey, BF, An, KN, and Chao, EYS. 1991. Isometric and isokinetic endurance testing of the forearm complex. *Am J Sports Med* 19: 107–11.

47. O'Hagen, FT, Sale, DG, MacDougall, JD, and Garner, SH. 1995. Response to resistance training in young women and men. *Int J Sports Med* 16(5): 314–21.

48. Otis, JC, and Godbold, JH. 1983. Relationship of isokinetic torque to isometric torque. *J Orthop Res* 1(2): 165–71.

49. Osternig, LR. 1988. Isokinetic dynamometry: Implications for muscle testing and rehabilitation. *Exerc Sport Sci Rev* 14: 45–80.

50. Ozmun, JC, Mikesky, AE, and Surburg, PR. 1994. Neuromuscular adaptations following prepubescent strength training. *Med Sci Sports Exerc* 26(4): 510–14.

51. Page, PA, Lamberth, J, Abadie, B, Boling, R, Collins, R, and Linton, R. 1993. Posterior rotator cuff strengthening using theraband in a functional diagonal pattern in collegiate baseball pitchers. *J Athletic Training* 28(4): 346, 348–50, 352–54.

52. Pappas, AM, Zawacki, RM, Sullivan, TJ. 1985. Biomechanics of baseball pitching: A preliminary report. *Am J Sports Med* 13(4): 216–22.

53. Rokito, AS, Zuckerman, JD, Gallagher, MA, and Cuomo, F. 1996. Strength after surgical repair of the rotator cuff. *J Shoulder Elbow Surg* 5(1): 12–17.

54. Sale, DG, and MacDougall, JD. 1984. Isokinetic strength in weight trainers. *Eur J Appl Physiol* 53(2): 128–32.

55. Sale, DG, MacDougall, JD, and Alway, SE. 1987. Voluntary strength and muscle characteristics in untrained men and women and male bodybuilders. *J Appl Physiol* 62(5): 1767–93.

56. Scoville, CR, Arciero, RA, Taylor, DC, and Stoneman, PD. 1997. End range eccentric antagonist/concentric agonist strength ratios: A new perspective in shoulder strength assessment. *J Orthop Sports Phys Ther* 25(3), 203–7.

57. Timm, KE. 1997. The isokinetic torque curve of shoulder instability in high school baseball pitchers. *J Orthop Sports Phys Ther* 26(3): 150–54.

58. Walmsley, RP. 1993. Movement of the axis of rotation of the glenohumeral joint while working on a Cybex II dynamometer. Part 1: Flexion/extension. *Isokinetics Exerc Sci* 3(1): 16–20.

59. Weltman, A, Janney, C, Rians, CB, Strand, K, Berg, B, Tippitt, S, Wise, J, Cahill, BR, and Katch, FI. 1986. The effects of hydraulic resistance strength training in prepubertal males. *Med Sci Sports Exerc* 18(6): 629–38.

60. Whitcomb, LJ, Kelley, MJ, and Leiper, CI. 1995. A comparison of torque production during dynamic strength testing of the shoulder abduction in the coronal plane and the plane of the scapula. *J Orthop Sports Phys Ther* 21(4): 227–32.

61. Williamson, SC, Hartigan, C, Morgan, RF, Stamp, WG, Chung, JK, and Edlich, RF. 1989. Computerized analysis of isokinetic torque curves for muscle strengthening. *J Burn Care Rehabil* 10(2): 160–66.

62. Wilk, KE, Arrigo, CA, and Andrews, JR. 1992. Isokinetic testing of the shoulder abductors and adductors: Windowed vs. nonwindowed data collection. *J Orthop Sports Phys Ther* 15(2): 107–12.

63. Wilk, KE, Andrews, JR, Arrigo, CA, Keirns, MA, and Erger, DJ. 1993. The strength characteristics of internal and external rotator muscles in professional baseball pitchers. *Am J Sports Med* 21(1): 61–66.

64. Wilk, KE, and Arrigo, C. 1993. Current concepts in the rehabilitation of the athletic shoulder. *J Orthop Sports Phys Ther* 18(1): 365–78.

65. Wilk, KE, Andrews, JR, and Arrigo, CA. 1995. The abductor and adductor strength characteristics of professional baseball pitchers. *Am J Sports Med* 23(3): 307–11.

66. Wilson, GJ, and Murphy, AJ. 1996. The use of isometric tests of muscular function in athletic assessment. *Sports Med* 22(1): 19–37.

67. Ramsay, JA, Blimkie, CJ, Smith, K, Garner, S, MacDougall, JD, Sale, DG. 1990. Strength training effects in prepubescent boys. *Med Sci Sports Exerc* 22(5): 605–14.

# Chapter 8

# Testing and Training the Lower Extremity

John E. Kovaleski and Robert J. Heitman

**L**ess commonly used in the athletic population than variable resistance and other forms of free weight exercise, lower body isokinetic resistance exercise and testing has received considerable attention in the applied research setting. Academic interest has led to research that provides support for the use of open and closed kinetic chain isokinetic resistance exercise for sport performance. Isokinetic resistance exercise in the lower extremity may be used for

- concentric and eccentric muscle loading,
- improving muscular strength and power,
- functional evaluation and profiling of athletes,
- maximal dynamic muscle loading,
- neural activation and muscle fiber adaptations,
- specificity of joint angle effects,
- velocity spectrum training, and
- reproducibility of muscle function testing.

The purpose of this discussion is to provide the strength and conditioning specialist with an understanding of the principles that govern isokinetic resistance training for the lower body. If the specialist is knowledgeable of the physiological responses and applications of isokinetic resistance training, then he or she can develop safe and effective exercise programs that will meet an individual's physiological needs and improve athletic performance.

## The Resistance Training Program

The first step when accurately prescribing resistance exercise is to understand the components of the resistance exercise prescription. Table 8.1 outlines the component requirements of the resistance exercise program (22, 43, 44).

## Table 8.1  Components of the Resistance Exercise Program

| Component | Description |
| --- | --- |
| Acute program variables | Choice of exercise; the order of exercise; the resistance or load used during the exercise; the number of sets performed for each exercise; the number of repetitions performed during each set; and the length of the rest period between each set. |
| Chronic program variables | Changing acute program variables at regular intervals to stimulate physiological changes within the muscle "periodization". |
| Administrative variables | Involves the available equipment and exercise time the individual has for performing the resistance training. |
| Choice of exercise | Applies the "principle of specificity" when determining the appropriate resistance exercise. The movement patterns and energy systems of the exercise should resemble the movement patterns and energy systems of the activity. |
| Determining exercise order | Involves ways to arrange the order in which the exercise routine is performed to maximize strength, power, size. |
| Length of the rest period | Can significantly influence the degree to which the metabolic systems contribute to the energy needs of the working muscle. |

The specialist should complete a needs analysis prior to the start of the exercise program to ensure maximal safety of the exerciser and effectiveness of the resistance training program. The needs analysis provides information concerning the individual's physical strengths and weaknesses, basic energy system requirements for athletic events, movement patterns that are employed during athletic events, and the common injuries that result from those activities or events (22, 74). Muscular strength, power, and endurance and flexibility of the lower extremities are some of the qualities that should be tested, along with body composition and oxygen consumption, prior to beginning the training program. It is beyond the purpose of this discussion to elucidate further on the specifics of the fitness assessment. However, if additional information is needed the reader is referred to the American College of Sports Medicine's *Guidelines for exercise testing and prescription* (2).

As a part of the needs analysis, the exercise specialist must factor in the load, intensity, and duration of the training when considering the muscular responses to resistance training. The specialist can develop a resistance training program for an individual, which, as a result of specificity of training and the need for maintaining muscular strength and power, will meet his or her physiological needs and improve fitness and athletic performance.

# Lower Body Isokinetic Training

Improving lower body muscular strength and power improves athletic performance; this has been documented in the literature. Isokinetic resistance exercise, a popular training method, improves the strength, power, and endurance characteristics of skeletal muscle (27, 37, 71). Investigators have examined isokinetic training protocols and shown variations in intensity, frequency, duration, and type of muscle action and the effects of each on muscle strength, power, and endurance (23, 29, 58, 59). Investigators also have compared various strength-training methods including concentric and eccentric torque comparisons, concentric and eccentric versus isometric actions, as well as training at slow and fast isokinetic velocities, while others have studied torque-velocity and power-velocity relationships, muscle fiber composition and cross-sectional areas of muscle in elite athletes, and strength-training motor neuron excitability in human leg musculature.

## Effects of Velocity on Isokinetic Strength and Power

There are various reasons for training at varying velocities during isokinetic resistance loading for lower body testing and training. Isokinetic resistance exercise provides

- maximal loading throughout the ROM,
- velocity spectrum exercise,
- concentric/eccentric muscle action, and
- open and closed kinetic chain movements.

Slow velocity training of the knee extensors has been reported to result in greater strength gains over a wide range of angular velocities than fast velocity training (19, 65). Faster velocities create training demands on the muscle that promote maximal force and power development at high velocities of movement, improved motor-learning responses, and decreased joint compressive forces. By utilizing isokinetic exercise, the exercise specialist is able to vary velocities to more closely model activities performed at various velocities (see figure 8.1). This theory is supported by the principle of specificity of exercise, which states that one should create training demands that develop those particular aspects of neuromuscular function necessary to perform a motor task.

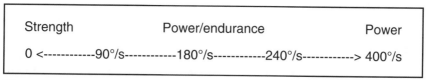

| Strength | Power/endurance | Power |
|---|---|---|
| 0 <------------90°/s------------180°/s------------240°/s------------> 400°/s | | |

**Figure 8.1**  The isokinetic resistance-velocity continuum. Shown is a continuum that depicts velocity ranges for the development of muscle strength, power, and endurance using isokinetic loading.

Studies that examined knee extensor strength, power, and endurance changes after training at different isokinetic velocities have produced conflicting results. In an early study, Moffroid and Whipple (53) reported that the strength and endurance effects of training at a specific isokinetic velocity are limited to that velocity or to lower velocities. Other studies (13, 49) using high velocity isokinetic training have reported that the strength "overflow" training effects reach higher velocities. Caiozzo, Perrine, and Edgerton (8) reported that torque increased throughout all velocities tested when subjects trained at a slower velocity and torque increased only at faster velocities for subjects who trained at a faster velocity. Vitti (77) concluded that increases in average leg power resulting from variable training velocities were not great enough to differentiate in favor of low, high, or low/high speed isokinetic training. Clearly, velocity-specific adaptations to resistance training are complex and are very likely mediated by morphological, biochemical, and neural factors that may or may not follow similar time courses over short-term training programs. Since changes in the adaptive mechanisms responsible for changes in strength performance may be different and velocity dependent, use of high and low velocity training for athletes who perform at a variety of angular velocities appears appropriate. In addition, use of velocity-specific training to maximize strength and power gains at a specific velocity of movement is probably appropriate for the athlete at some point in his or her training as well.

## Physiological Mechanisms

Controversy exists concerning the physiological mechanisms responsible for increasing muscular strength and power during lower body isokinetic exercise. Many studies have examined the effects of training velocity for torque-velocity performance, muscle enzyme activity and fiber areas, and neurological adaptations. Increased strength, as the result of concentric isokinetic knee extension and flexion training, has been reported (11, 13, 49, 56, 60). Some authors have reported an increased muscle cross-sectional area (CSA) (13, 20, 26, 56), others have found no increases in muscle CSA (11, 19, 49, 60). The difference in results among these studies may be due to factors such as genetics, training status of the subjects, differences in training protocols, or differences in the techniques used to determine muscle CSA.

## Muscle Adaptations

Weight training results in an increase in type IIa muscle fibers with transitions moving from type IIb to type IIa with resistance exercise training (47, 75). It appears that as soon as a type IIb muscle fiber is stimulated it starts a process of transformation toward the type IIa profile by changing the quality of proteins and expressing different types and amounts of mATPase (44). Interestingly, this shift from type IIb to type IIa has been observed following concentric isokinetic training in the leg. Ewing and coworkers (20) studied two groups that trained at different velocities. A slow speed group trained at 60°/s with

3 sets of 8 maximal repetitions. A fast speed group trained at 240°/s with 3 sets of 20 repetitions. Both groups were tested before and after the training at 60°/s, 180°/s, and 240°/s. Peak torque and power test results are presented in table 8.2, which shows that only the group that trained at the 60°/s speed increased ($p < .05$) peak torque and power at that speed. At the 180°/s speed, both groups increased peak torque and power with no differences between groups. The group that trained at the 240°/s speed was the only group to show a significantly increased peak torque after training, with no change in power for either group.

This study and others (13, 31) show that concentric isokinetic training is effective in enhancing peak torque and power, but the velocity of training and testing affects the gains that can be expected. This is important to understand in light of the changes in muscle fiber areas. Both the slow and fast speed training groups showed significant increases in type I and type IIa fiber areas but no change in the type IIb fiber area. Even though the fast speed training was four times that of the slow, the former was still only about 35% of the maximal velocity of unresisted muscle (17). These results imply that gains are dependent upon the velocity at which one trains and the speed at which testing is conducted, and the total work performed during training may not be as important as the type of repetition performed (i.e., fast versus slow velocity) (20).

Costill and coworkers (11) and Lesmes and associates (49) reported that performing 6 s or 30 s bouts of maximal isokinetic exercise resulted in similar gains in peak torque, power, and changes in muscle fiber area ratios after 7 weeks of isokinetic training. They found an increase in the type IIa-to-I and type IIa-to-IIb fiber area ratios of both the 6 s and 30 s trained muscles. However, only

### Table 8.2   Pre-Post Percentage Increases in Peak Torque and Power for Isokinetic Knee Extension Following 10 Weeks of Isokinetic Training

| Test velocities | % Peak torque increases | | % Power increases | |
|---|---|---|---|---|
| 60°/s | [Slow | Fast] | [Slow | Fast] |
|  | 8.5* | −2.7 | 12.0* | 2.4* |
| 180°/s | [Slow | Fast] | [Slow | Fast] |
|  | 10.9* | 17.5* | 19.2* | 24.9* |
| 240°/s | [Slow | Fast] | [Slow | Fast] |
|  | 3.2 | 19.7* | 5.1 | 6.9 |

Slow speed training group = 60°/s; fast speed training group = 240°/s. (*$p < .05$). These results indicate that muscular strength and power can be increased through isokinetic training, but the gains accrued are dependent upon the training velocity and the speed at which testing is conducted (20).

the 30 s exercise program resulted in elevated glycolytic, ATP-CP, and mito-chondrial enzyme activities. Thorstensson (76) also observed a selective hyper-trophy of the fast twitch (type II) fibers after 8 weeks of maximal isokinetic training. These studies of strength training demonstrate significant enzymatic changes and modifications in the composition of skeletal muscle after isokinetic resistance training. These data suggest that regardless of the angular velocity used, the stimulus responsible for increasing muscle enzyme activities appears related to the duration of each isokinetic exercise bout and not the quantity of work performed by the muscle. Therefore, exercise sets of at least 30 s are recommended to produce muscle enzymatic adaptations that enhance perfor-mance.

Esselman and coworkers (19) also examined torque gains and muscle fiber and enzyme changes after 12 weeks of isokinetic concentric knee extensions and reported different results. Subjects were placed into training groups that exercised both legs at either 36°/s with 20 or 60 repetitions (group 1), 20 repe-titions at 36°/s with one limb and 60 repetitions at 108°/s contralaterally (group 2), and 108°/s with 20 or 60 repetitions (group 3). Subjects were tested for peak torque production before, after, and every 2 weeks during training at velocities between 0°/s to 234°/s. Subjects who trained at 36°/s made signifi-cant overall gains in torque and showed significantly greater torque gains than those training at 108°/s. No significant increases in muscle fiber areas in re-sponse to training were observed, but there were significant increases in gly-colytic and mitochondrial enzyme activities. However, torque gains were not uniformly made during the 12 weeks of training. They occurred primarily during the initial 4 to 8 weeks with the greatest torque gains observed at the slower testing velocity. These findings suggest that the critical variable for developing strength (maximal torque) during isokinetic training is exercising at a slow velocity where greater torque can be developed. In addition, the absence of changes in muscle fiber size illustrates the dominant role of in-creased neural activation in the early phase of training. The neurological vari-ables consistent with the pattern of torque gains early in the training program probably involved increased levels of motor neuron recruitment, increased synchronization of motor units, and improved coordination and learning (36, 46, 55).

Only recently has the relationship between training and strength perfor-mance with respect to the eccentric component of the traditionally used isokinetic concentric resistance exercise been studied for its effects on strength and muscle fiber area. Petersen and coworkers (66) investigated the effects of isokinetic concentric training on isokinetic concentric and eccentric torque outputs using the knee extensors. Subjects trained 3 days weekly for 6 weeks, completing 5 sets of 10 maximal effort knee extensions at 60°/s. Significant ($p < .01$) increases in peak and average concentric torque (11% and 12%, respec-tively), peak and average eccentric torque (18% and 21%, respectively), and muscle cross-sectional area (3.2%) were observed for training group subjects. These data suggest that isokinetic concentric training results in significant improvements in both concentric and eccentric torque outputs and that resistance training effects may not be as specific to the training mode as has been thought. These findings support the long-time use of isokinetic concentric resistance exercise training.

Other studies have investigated increased peak torque and strength-related performance using protocols consisting of combined concentric and eccentric muscle actions versus using concentric muscle actions only (9, 48). Colliander and Tesch (9) reported significant increases in peak torque, vertical jump height, and 3 repetition maximum half-squats for both groups. However, peak torque gains (17% to 45%) were significantly greater only in the groups that trained using a combination of eccentric and concentric actions compared to the concentric-only groups. Nonsignificant increases in muscle fiber areas between groups were also observed in these studies, suggesting that short-term increases in muscle strength are mainly due to neural adaptations within the neuromuscular system as well as in motor unit activation.

It is possible that isokinetic velocity spectrum training protocols cited in the literature do not provide sufficient duration of exercise to promote muscle size adaptations (12). This may partially explain the differences in the magnitude of strength and power gains sometimes observed between isokinetic and isotonic constant load training (42). In addition, individuals who exercise isokinetically to improve muscular strength and power may need to use larger volumes of training as compared to those who train with constant loads. Pearson and Costill (60) compared the training-induced hypertrophy of the quadriceps before and after 8 weeks of constant load and isokinetic resistance exercise. Constant load training produced hypertrophy of the thigh, whereas the leg trained isokinetically showed no change in muscle size. The number of constant load (36 reps) and isokinetic (65 reps) repetitions necessary to produce equal work bouts (based on total torque produced) was also significantly different. In comparison to concentric isokinetic resistance training, the two phases of dynamic action for constant load training (concentric and eccentric) resulted in a greater amount of torque and a greater intensity of training when performed on a set and repetition basis. This study illustrates the importance of incorporating eccentric actions into the standard concentric isokinetic training program if both size and strength increases are desired.

## Neural Adaptations

Neurological adaptations are important to strength gains and have been shown to contribute to the time course of torque gains during training. Isokinetic velocity spectrum training advocates claim that recruitment of both type I (slow twitch) and type II (fast twitch) muscle fibers occurs by varying the velocity of the movement over the course of the exercise session (11, 13, 34, 37). This method of training is practiced to promote an optimal neuromuscular response. It does not mean that slow velocity exercise recruits primarily type I fibers and high velocity exercise recruits primarily type II fibers (34, 54, 65).

Muscle fiber recruitment depends on the tension requirements of a given muscular action and not the velocity. The literature seems to support the idea of recruitment of both fibers rather than selective recruitment of type I and type II muscle fibers based on exercise velocity. Training adaptations caused by varying the velocity during isokinetic exercise are more likely related to variations in the order of motor unit recruitment than to the recruitment of one fiber type in the absence of activation of another type (61).

# Functional Performance

In response to resistance training, changes within skeletal muscle are an important and perhaps the major adaptation. However, voluntary strength performance is determined not only by the quantity of the involved muscle mass but also by the extent to which the muscle mass has been activated. Further, the expression of voluntary strength often is expressed through the performance of a motor act. Thus, the method of resistance training may play a role in the expression of strength as observed through the learning, acquisition, and performance of a motor skill. Because training improvements in neuromuscular power may be related to enhanced recruitment of motor units as well as hypertrophy of individual muscle fibers, it is important to understand how isokinetic strength training contributes to improvements in neuromuscular power and the learning and performance of a motor task.

The contributions of the ankle, knee, and hip musculature to successful athletic performance are essential considerations when designing a lower body training program. To produce the most efficient movement, maximal muscular actions must occur at each joint to allow the individual to perform the functional task. Thus, the method of strength training is obviously important to developing strength. Resistance training often involves both free weight and resistance machine training to increase muscle strength and power. Both constant load and isokinetic machines serve to enhance performance, especially as an adjunct to an already existing training program. Functional strength and functional performance are ways to discuss the amount of force produced by the extremity in a movement specific to a sport or a weight-bearing movement. Functionality and direct application to sport activities are most important for optimal performance gains.

Most strengthening programs for the lower extremity involve resistance training in the form of a squat or leg press exercise (both closed chain movements involving multiple joints) or knee flexion/extension exercises (open chain movements involving a single joint). Increases in training loads are often observed regardless of the mode of resistance training, with improvements explained by neural, biochemical, and morphological adaptations. Making comparisons between specific training studies is difficult due to differences in training conditions, trying to equate total volume of training, total work, and total training time. In addition, there is debate as to whether isokinetic or isotonic resistance training results in greater increases in muscle strength and power. Following six weeks of knee extension training, isotonic resistance training was found to be superior to isokinetic resistance training in terms of increasing muscle strength (+52% versus +11%) and power (+44% versus +10%) and eliciting full range of motion strength development (42). Based on these findings, the strength and conditioning professional should consider an integrated approach that uses different modes of training to ensure optimal results.

Specificity of training suggests that the different modes of resistance training will influence the motor performance tests (i.e., vertical jump). Colliander and Tesch (9) observed an 8% increase in vertical jump height after a 12-week isokinetic resistance training period, which is comparable to the 13% improvement reported for a group of subjects who performed barbell squat resistance training (3). Knapik and coworkers (33) compared the relationships among isometric, isotonic, and isokinetic strength measurements in knee flexion and extension and found a generally high correlation among torque measurements. They concluded that one mode of strength testing may be an adequate predictor of maximal voluntary strength of the other testing modes.

Muscular strength and power are two parameters that are recognized as influencing sport performance. Study of both of these muscular characteristics has acquired even more importance in the functional evaluation and profiling of athletes, in training control, and in the prevention of sport injury (69). Two methods of dynamic muscle force determination that are used frequently in the lower body are isokinetic dynamometry, which gives information about the strength of specific muscles or muscle groups at a specific velocity (62), and a vertical jump test from a contact or force plate platform (5), which provides information about the mechanical work accomplished by the whole kinetic extensor chain (68).

Both methods have been utilized and validated in the sporting field (69). However, they have been used by preference in different situations. The vertical jump test has been shown to be useful for measurement of directly applied inferior limb force in athletic movement, whereas isokinetic dynamometry has been used for quantitative measurement, strength and power training, and for profiling specific strength characteristics of different sports (68). Wiklander and Lysholm (78) studied elite runners for isokinetic thigh muscle strength and in the vertical jump, standing 5-step jump, and long jump. Good correlation for the quadriceps ($r$ = .83–.84) and fair correlation for the hamstrings ($r$ = .61–.77) were found between the three jump tests and the strength measurements. Knowing there exist different muscle tests for strength, which have good reproducibility, may be important if the exercise specialist wants to accurately measure an individual's abilities and conditioning progress.

Smith and Melton (73) compared the effects of constant load variable resistance training with low and high speed isokinetic knee extension and flexion resistance training on isokinetic and isotonic constant load strength and functional tests that included the standing broad jump, vertical jump, and the 40-yard dash. The exercised groups showed good gains in strength when tested isometrically, with constant load, and isokinetically. However, when tested for motor performance, the high speed isokinetic group dominated. The high speed isokinetic group showed a 5.38% gain in the vertical jump versus 3.87% for the slow isokinetic group and 1.57% for the constant load variable resistance group; they showed a 9.14% gain in the standing broad jump versus 0.42% and 0.28%, respectively, for the slow speed isokinetic and constant load trained groups; and they showed a 10.11% gain in the 40-yard dash versus 1.12% and 1.35%, respectively, for the slow speed isokinetic and constant load trained groups. The authors suggested that strength increases after isokinetic training are attributed to the nature of the accommodating resistance and to greater work performed in the same time as compared to the work done during the constant resistance exercise.

Other studies, both observational and training, have compared both methods of force analysis to establish a correlation to performance. Cordova and associates (10) conducted a functional training study that compared isokinetic and constant load strength to one-legged jump reaction force. Two groups trained using a leg press exercise 3 days a week for 5 weeks, while the control group did not train. The isokinetic extremity was trained using a velocity spectrum (2 sets of 10 repetitions at speeds of 60°/s, 180°/s, and 240°/s). The constant load extremity was trained using the 4-set daily adjustable progressive resistive exercise (DAPRE) technique. Data analysis revealed no difference between the three groups for change in one-legged jump force (see table 8.3). Strength increased in both the isokinetic and constant load groups after training, but these changes did not correlate with changes in one-legged jump reaction force. These results suggest that changes in neither isokinetic force nor constant load weight lifted in a nonweight-bearing closed kinetic chain directly translate into increased force production during a functional activity.

In contrast, two groups of athletes (junior and senior Spanish alpine skiers and high jumpers) were studied to compare isokinetic peak torque at speeds between 60°/s and 300°/s with vertical jump force using squat jumps, countermovement jumps, and squat jumps with additional weights of 20 and 40 kg (68). The correlation between isokinetic peak torque and the vertical jump tests was significant, with the strongest relationships observed at 120°/s and

### Table 8.3    Isokinetic Versus Constant Load CKC Training Effects on Vertical Jump (VJ) Performance

| Variable | # Weeks training | Pre-post % strength | Task | Pre-post % change | r value | p value |
|---|---|---|---|---|---|---|
| Isok CKC | 5 | +50.0 | VJ | 3.8 ± 5.5 | .134 | .66 |
| Isot CKC | 5 | +64.0 | VJ | 2.4 ± 4.3 | −.470 | .09 |

Study suggests that changes in neither isokinetic force nor constant load weight lifted directly translate into increased force production during a functional activity (10).

240°/s with the squat jump that included the 20 kg weight ($r > .80, p \leq .001$). Both methods satisfactorily measured the dynamic force of the knee extensor muscles, but in different ways. The differences observed between the methods may be discussed in terms of the relative utilization of the elastic and reactive components of dynamic force and the participation of other muscle groups in the movement. A potentiation of the stretch-shortening cycle takes place in the jump with a load, and there is evidence of some muscle stretching due to elastic and reactive components of the muscle during activation in this type of muscular action. It may be speculated that the motor unit recruitment process is not velocity dependent but acceleration independent. This phenomenon does not occur in isokinetic movements (4, 35). In the isokinetic movement no acceleration exists as it does in a ballistic movement like jumping. Since the torque value decreases with increases in isokinetic speed, it may be obtained from a force-velocity curve of an isokinetic evaluation. The latter could be a useful tool to control force during each training cycle, if the characteristics of this type of action are taken into account (5, 57, 63, 68).

Both isokinetic dynamometry and functional tasks such as the vertical jump may be used satisfactorily to measure the dynamic force of the extensor and flexor muscle groups of the knee. However, the differences between the methods should be appreciated. Isokinetic dynamometry allows a better standardization of the test protocol. The method also gives information about the characteristics of the force-velocity curve, the strength generated at every angle of movement, the power and the work accomplished, and the relationship between agonist and antagonist muscle groups. It also provides comparison between the contralateral limbs and may be used to assess isolated muscular movements. Vertical jump tests represent a functional method of evaluation of the dynamic force of the whole kinetic chain through the inferior limb. This test permits evaluation of the intervention of muscle elastic and reactive components, whereas isokinetic dynamometry measures muscle contractile and recruitment capacity (68).

Single-test observational studies show low to good correlation between isokinetic strength and performing motor performance tasks. Table 8.4 presents a summary of observational studies that examine the correlation between isokinetic strength and motor performance. Several training studies have also evaluated the extent and transferability of improvements in strength elicited by constant load and isokinetic exercise (3, 10, 51). Augustsson and coworkers (3) compared closed versus open chain weight training of the thigh muscles to determine which mode resulted in the greatest performance changes measured using the squat, isokinetic knee extension, and vertical jump tests. Improvements in constant load strength as the result of the 6-week training, but no transfer to the isokinetic test, were reported (see table 8.5). In contrast, Mannion, Jakeman, and Willan (51) reported that, after 16 weeks of either slow (60°/s) or fast (240°/s) isokinetic strength training of the knee extensors, neither group differed significantly from the other in the training response to maximal voluntary action, peak pedal velocity, and peak power output during all-out cycling. The posttraining increases in average peak power output (7%)

## Table 8.4    Single Open Kinetic Chain (OKC) Test Correlation Studies

| Author | Peak force | Muscle | Testing subjects | Task | r value |
|---|---|---|---|---|---|
| Jameson et al. (28) | Isok OKC 180°/s | Knee ext. | All (n = 51) | VJ | .57 |
| | | | Sedentary (n = 11) | VJ | .79 |
| | | | Active (n = 24) | VJ | .26 |
| | | | Trained (n = 16) | VJ | .85 |
| | Isot OKC | Knee ext. | All (n = 51) | VJ | .68 |
| | | | Sedentary (n = 11) | VJ | .82 |
| | | | Active (n = 24) | VJ | .56 |
| | | | Trained (n = 16) | VJ | .82 |
| Greenberger & Paterno (25) | Isok OKC 240°/s | Knee ext. Knee ext. | Dominant (n = 20) Nondom. (n = 20) | HT HT | .78 .65 |
| Wiklander & Lysholm (78) | Isok OKC 180°/s | Knee ext. | Elite runners (n = 39) | VJ SLJ 5-step jump | .84 .84 .83 |
| Pincivero et al. (67) | Isok OKC 60°/s 180°/s 60°/s 180°/s | Dom. quads Dom. hams | College (n = 37) | SLH SLH SLH SLH | .39 .42 .55 .55 |

In the Jameson group's study isokinetic, constant load, and isometric knee extension strength measurements only moderately correlated to one-legged vertical jump (VJ) and cannot be used independently to predict vertical jump ability.

In Greenberger and Paterno's study the relationship between knee extensor strength and the one-legged hop performance test (HT) did not correlate strongly, which supports the belief that isokinetic strength does not correlate strongly with functional tasks.

In Wiklander and Lysholm's study there was good correlation between the results in 3 jump tests (vertical jump [VJ], standing long jump [SLJ], and 5-step jump) and isokinetic strength measurement at 180°/s.

In the Pincivero group's study low to moderate significant relationships were found to exist between the single leg hop (SLH) for distance test and isokinetic variables for the quadriceps and hamstring muscle groups at each test velocity.

and peak pedal velocity (6%) during the cycle tests were each significantly different from the control group response. The authors concluded that 16 weeks of isokinetic strength training of the knee extensors significantly improves peak power output and pedal velocity during sprint cycling, an activity that demands considerable involvement of the trained muscle group but with a different pattern of coordination. This type of training may be able to induce changes within the muscle that are beneficial to the performance of other tasks that employ the trained muscle group at a similar work intensity but in a different pattern of coordination from the training movement.

**Table 8.5    Constant Load Training Effects on Squat, Isokinetic Knee Extension Strength, and Vertical Jump (VJ) Performance**

| Variable | # Weeks training | Pre-post % strength | Task | Pre-post % change | p value |
|---|---|---|---|---|---|
| Isot CKC | 6 | +50 | Squat | 31[a] | .0001 |
| | | | Isokinetic | 5[b] | n.s. |
| | | | VJ | 10[c] | .005 |
| Isot OKC | 6 | +100 | Squat | 13 | .0001 |
| | | | Isokinetic | 2[b] | n.s. |
| | | | VJ | 7[c] | n.s. |

[a]Both groups increased significantly in barbell squat test, but constant load closed kinetic chain (CKC) increased significantly greater than constant load open kinetic chain (OKC).
[b]Constant load weight training did not transfer ($p > .05$) to isokinetic movements.
[c]In the vertical jump test, the CKC group improved significantly; no significant changes were observed for the OKC group.
Data from Augustsson et al. (3).

It is apparent that training-induced improvements are frequently confined to the performance of tasks that closely simulate the training task in their mode of action and velocity. This specificity of training is particularly noticeable when training is conducted for a relatively short period of time. In view of the known neural adaptations to training, which account for the gains in strength and power during the early weeks of training, it is not surprising that the improvements displayed during performance of the training task are not always transferable to other activities. Few training studies are conducted beyond the initial weeks or "learning phase" and those that are seldom have examined the transferability to other tasks of the newly acquired strength and power. This is somewhat surprising, since the majority of individuals who undertake strength-training programs do so in the belief that their improved strength will enhance performance in their own particular sporting activity (51).

## Specificity of Isokinetic Exercise

The issues related to specificity of training and testing of the lower extremity are important when assessing sport- or performance-related activities. For example, when examining a squat or a vertical jump, the activation of the stretch-shortening cycle is inherent to the performance of the movement. During single-joint testing and training such as isokinetic knee extensions, even though the stretch-shortening cycle may not be activated, advantages such as greater control over velocity of motion, technique, and extraneous movements that contribute to measurement reliability and objectivity are found with isokinetic testing (1, 3).

Identifying the specificity of each resistance training task is essential to ensure that any improvement in size, strength, or power can be translated to an improvement in athletic performance (44). Various studies have reported that weight-training strength improvements do not transfer to isokinetic movements (72, 79). This specificity of the response to resistance training is understandable because strength improvement is related to the adaptations that occur both in the muscle fiber itself and in the neural organization and excitability for a particular pattern of voluntary movement (70, 75). However, even though the results of most training studies support the concept of specificity, the exceptions are often overlooked (52). In one study, two groups of subjects trained by performing upright squats for 12 weeks using either free weight eccentric and concentric muscle actions or concentric-only hydraulic (isokinetic) resistance. Testing before and after training showed that the free weight trained group made large increases in concentric squat strength (+35%), but these increases were not significantly different from those of the group that trained using only concentric muscle actions (+39%). When squat strength was assessed with eccentric and concentric actions, both groups improved about 30%. Although the specificity principle in resistance training may encompass joint angle or muscle length specificity, velocity specificity, and task or movement pattern specificity, the principle may not be totally applicable to the type of muscle action or test mode (30, 52, 64). It is possible that the resistance training with free weights or isokinetic devices was not distinct enough in terms of muscle action to elicit highly specific training adaptations. Unlike isokinetic training, free weight exercise includes both eccentric and concentric muscle actions. During an exercise that incorporates both eccentric and concentric muscle actions, the limiting factor in overcoming resistance is the concentric and not the eccentric muscle force. Despite differences between the muscle actions used for free weight and most isokinetic exercise, both subject groups may still have used the same training stimulus via the concentric load. There exists a distinct possibility that any form of concentric or combined concentric plus eccentric resistance training should result in comparable gains in muscle strength as long as similar movement patterns and velocities are employed for training and testing (50, 52). More importantly, the design of resistance training programs, where possible, should employ the types and velocities of muscular actions encountered in the sport.

Since dynamic strength-training methods produce significant strength increases, the crucial consideration is the intended purpose of the newly acquired strength. To increase physical performance through resistance training, muscles must be trained in movements as close as possible to the movement or actual skill that is to be improved. This coordination could be accomplished with supplemental training that uses isokinetic resistance without disrupting the mechanics of the particular performance.

# Isokinetic Assessment and Training: Applications to Performance

Isokinetic resistance testing and training programs can play a significant role in the preparation of the athlete before, during, and after a training period and may serve as a basis for identifying specific muscle weaknesses that predispose the athlete to injury. Isokinetic exercise concepts are applied to resistance training methods and technology in an attempt to improve muscular strength, power, and functional performance. We discuss several of these applications in the following section.

## Principles of Isokinetic Assessment

Isokinetic assessment provides reliable measures of lower extremity muscle function using both open and closed kinetic chain dynamometry (6, 7, 16, 21, 40). Assessment of the components of lower body muscle performance is made by assessing muscle action (concentric/eccentric) and muscle function parameters such as peak torque (strength), power, work and endurance, force-velocity relationships, and peak torque relative to body weight and by comparing bilateral muscle groups and reciprocal muscle groups (14, 61).

Standard open (OKC) and closed kinetic chain (CKC) isokinetic evaluation protocols for the lower extremity are presented in table 8.6. Selection of the assessment protocol is based on the muscle group to be tested, the stage of progression through the training program, and the overall physical status of the athlete. CKC isokinetic testing permits assessment of the entire lower limb in either the weight-bearing (squat) or nonweight-bearing (leg press) position. CKC positioning allows coactivation of muscles around the joint and axial loading in the joint, and it provides controlled ROM and testing speeds (see figure 8.2). OKC isokinetic testing is performed because the tester can isolate individual muscles in the selected portion of the kinetic chain (i.e., ankle, knee, or hip). Since most functional activities involve positioning the lower extremity in the closed kinetic chain, measurement of an individual's strength in both the OKC and CKC positions appears to be appropriate when determining functional strength.

The standard OKC isokinetic test protocol for concentric knee extension/ flexion focuses on muscle force (torque), power, and work (fatigability). Standard procedure is 6 repetitions for slow velocity strength analysis and 6 repetitions for higher velocity strength and power analysis. The use of 20 to 40 repetitions is the standard protocol when fatigue analysis is performed, using testing velocities between 180°/s and 240°/s with athletes. Normal peak torque should be observed at approximately 72° to 55° toward normal knee extension and at 20° to 45° of flexion for the hamstring muscles. Unilateral comparisons should reveal quadriceps-to-hamstring torque ratios of 60 to 65% at the 90°/s speed and an 80 to 90% ratio at 300°/s. The male athlete quadriceps peak torque development should be approximately 90 to 100% of body weight at slow

## Table 8.6    Isokinetic Evaluation Protocols

**Open (OKC) testing (two or four speeds)**

|  | Speeds | Parameter | Reps |
|---|---|---|---|
| Ankle plantarflexion/ dorsiflexion | 30 to 240°/s | Strength | 3–6 |
| Ankle inversion/eversion | 30 to 120°/s | Strength | 3–6 |
| Knee flexion/extension | 60 to 400°/s<br>180 to 300°/s | Strength/power<br>Work/endurance | 3–6<br>20–40 |
| Hip flexion/extension | 30 to 240°/s | Strength | 3–6 |
| Hip abduction/adduction | 30 to 180°/s | Strength | 3–6 |

**Closed (CKC) testing (two speeds)**

|  | Speeds | Parameter | Reps |
|---|---|---|---|
| Bilateral extremity leg press (linear ROM) | 10 to 30"/s<br>20 to 30"/s | Strength/power<br>Work/endurance | 3–6<br>20–30 |
| Single extremity leg press (linear ROM) | 10 to 15"/s | Strength/power | 3–6 |

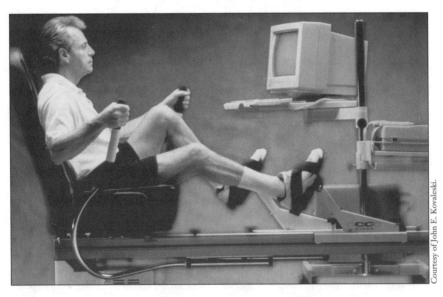

**Figure 8.2**   Lower leg-press exercise using the Closed Chain Rider System (Mettler Electronics, Anaheim, CA).

contractile velocities of 60°/s to 90°/s. Females have been observed to produce an average quadriceps peak torque about 75 to 80% of body weight. Obviously, individual activity level and sport participation may vary these percentages. When measuring muscle endurance at least 20 repetitions must be performed for total work output to be a valid parameter of muscle function. The overall drop in the percentage of work output is called the fatigue index. The higher the percentage the better the performance (61).

Standard CKC isokinetic testing is relatively new and very little is known about muscle function comparisons using this type of testing. The few studies published on this topic show that the standard muscle function parameters of force, power, and work commonly used in OKC isokinetic testing are also used in both squat and leg press CKC isokinetic testing (15, 16, 40). Descriptive data for CKC computerized isokinetic test data for female and male athletes' lower extremities are described in table 8.7. Closed kinetic chain isokinetic test data provide the clinician with information relative to the full weight-bearing position, which allows for controlled functional assessment.

**Table 8.7    Descriptive Closed Kinetic Chain Computerized Isokinetic Data for Athletes' Lower Extremity (Linear Pattern)**

Force/Body Weight

| Speed | Males | Females |
|---|---|---|
| Slow (10"/s) | ~3.0 × BW | ~2.5 × BW |
| Medium (20"/s) | ~2.5 × BW | ~2.0 × BW |
| Fast (30"/s) | ~2.0 × BW | ~1.5 × BW |

BW = body weight. Reprinted from Andrews, Harrelson, and Wilk 1998.

## Principles of Isokinetic Training

Isokinetic training studies have examined and shown variations in velocity, frequency, and duration and effects on muscle strength, endurance, and power. Frequently used protocols cover a range of angular velocities, which has been termed velocity spectrum exercise (table 8.8). This method of training is practiced to promote an optimal neuromuscular response and is supported by current theory with regard to velocity-specific resistance training. Velocity spectrum exercise in which the velocity of movement is varied during the course of a series of repetitions has been reported (14, 61). One variation of velocity spectrum exercise is in the logical order of velocity progression from slow to fast speeds in given increments.

Power is the product of force and velocity, and the speed of exercise appears to be an important consideration when determining an exercise protocol. Traditional heavy resistance weight training and slow velocity isokinetic training

### Table 8.8  Velocity Spectrum Exercise Protocols

**Slow velocity training protocol**

| Set #:    | 1   | 2   | 3   | 4   | 5   | 6   | 7   | 8   | 9   | 10  |
|-----------|-----|-----|-----|-----|-----|-----|-----|-----|-----|-----|
| Velocity: | 60  | 90  | 120 | 150 | 180 | 180 | 150 | 120 | 90  | 60  |
| Reps:     | 10  | 10  | 10  | 10  | 10  | 10  | 10  | 10  | 10  | 10  |

**Fast velocity training protocol**

| Set #:    | 1   | 2   | 3   | 4   | 5   | 6   | 7   | 8   | 9   | 10  |
|-----------|-----|-----|-----|-----|-----|-----|-----|-----|-----|-----|
| Velocity: | 180 | 210 | 240 | 270 | 300 | 300 | 270 | 240 | 210 | 180 |
| Reps:     | 10  | 10  | 10  | 10  | 10  | 10  | 10  | 10  | 10  | 10  |

lead primarily to improvements in maximum strength. Plyometric training and other forms of dynamic weight training such as loaded jump squats maximize explosive power. Since the isokinetic dynamometer controls acceleration and deceleration of the limb, fast speed isokinetic resistance exercise should also be considered in muscle power development because momentum changes will be controlled.

Muscle power production has not often been the focus of attention in the determination of specific velocities and progressions for isokinetic velocity spectrum exercise. Kovaleski and coworkers (38, 39, 41) compared changing the progression order of velocities during velocity spectrum exercise using the knee extensor muscles. Significantly greater power was produced when the faster velocities were performed before progressing to the slower velocities. This observation was explained by the force-velocity and power-velocity curvilinear relationships reported in the physiological literature. That is, when exercising at faster velocities the potential for producing power is greatest, and when exercising at slower velocities force production is greatest. Since slower velocities are performed under greater resistance than the faster velocities the muscle may fatigue more quickly. This may partially explain why slow velocity training performed before progressing to the fast velocity training generally produced less power production. The faster velocity sets, which are associated with greater power production, should be performed early in the exercise session before fatigue becomes a factor. Thus, if an individual exercises isokinetically to increase power, performance of fast speed training prior to progressing to slow speed training is recommended. Other studies support this finding of enhancement of muscle power output by high velocity training (13, 58, 59).

# Metabolic Specificity of Isokinetic Training

Strength-power type activities that receive energy primarily from ATP hydrolysis include performing a power lift, high jump, and long jump. Examples of sustained activities in which the predominance of energy is supplied by the ATP-CP system include power lifting, sprints, fast breaks, and football line play. Examples of anaerobic power-endurance activities in which anaerobic glycolysis is the primary supplier of energy include wrestling, 100-meter swimming, and 200- and 400-meter runs.

By knowing the intensity and duration of a specific event, one should be able to understand which system contributes to energy production. The energy system(s) can then be enhanced through the resistance training program, which provides an overload to that system. For example, the specialist may determine that the athletic event consists of short (30–60 s), high-intensity work bouts followed by 60 to 90 s of rest (e.g., 200–400 m sprints). By knowing the work and rest intervals, the specialist will better understand how energy is supplied to the working muscle. Thus, in order to maximize improvements in performance using isokinetic resistance training, the appropriate energy system must be overloaded during the resistance training program. For the above example, this would be best accomplished through the use of high velocity maximal exercise with work bouts lasting 30 to 40 s (11, 49).

While the duration and intensity of the work bout will determine energy utilization during the initial sets, a proper rest period length ensures maximal overload during subsequent sets in the resistance training session. For instance, if a rest period is too short it will not allow for maximal ATP-CP repletion, which would decrease the contribution of anaerobic glycolysis in meeting the energy demands in the later workouts (sets). Instead, anaerobic glycolysis would be required to supply a larger percentage of the needed energy to the working muscles. Thus, if the rest period length is inappropriate to provide overload to the specific energy system used during competition, then maximal performance enhancement will not occur. Likewise, if too much time is allowed between work bouts, total ATP-CP repletion will lessen the overload on anaerobic glycolysis. Table 8.9 outlines ATP-CP repletion rates while table 8.10 highlights the relationship between work bout and rest period length. If the individual is resistance training for reasons other than the improvement of athletic performance, then the length of the rest period becomes a less important issue. In

### Table 8.9   Muscle ATP-CP Repletion Rates During Passive Rest

| Time, s | % ATP-CP repletion |
| --- | --- |
| 20 s | 50% |
| 40 s | 75% |
| 60 s | 88% |
| 180 s* | 100% |

*To maximize the ATP-CP system involvement during high-intensity activity, rest periods should be at least 3 minutes. Adapted from *National Strength and Conditioning Journal* 1982.

**Table 8.10    Relationship Between Work Bout and Rest Period Length With Anaerobic Metabolic System Enhancement**

| Metabolic system | Work bout length | Rest period length |
|---|---|---|
| ATP-PC | 0–45 s | 3 min |
| Glycolysis | 45–180 s | 1 min |

Adapted from *National Strength and Conditioning Journal* 1982.

this case, the specialist should determine the length of the rest period based on the administrative constraints of time and equipment availability.

# Summary

The strength and conditioning specialist involved with a resistance training program should be knowledgeable of the physiology and principles of isokinetic resistance training for those in need of improving muscular strength or endurance. The specialist performs a needs analysis before an individual begins training, to ensure the prescription of a safe and effective exercise program. Muscle action, exercise velocity, and volume of the training performed are essential factors when considering the muscular responses to isokinetic resistance training. As a result of specificity of training and the need for improving muscular strength, power, and endurance, isokinetic resistance training can be developed and used for individuals that will meet their physiological needs and improve their athletic performance.

# References

1. Abernethy, P., G. Wilson, and P. Logan. 1995. Strength and power assessment. *Sports Medicine* 19: 401–17.

2. American College of Sports Medicine. 1995. *Guidelines for exercise testing and prescription.* 5th ed. Baltimore: Williams & Wilkins.

3. Augustsson, J., A. Esko, R. Thomee, and U. Svantesson. 1998. Weight training of the thigh muscles using closed versus open kinetic chain exercises: A comparison of performance enhancement. *Journal of Orthopaedic and Sports Physical Therapy* 27: 3–8.

4. Bosco, C., and P.V. Komi. 1979. Potentiation of the mechanical behavior of the human skeletal muscle through prestretching. *Acta Physiologica Scandinavica* 106: 467–72.

5. Bosco, C., P. Luhtanen, and P.V. Komi. 1983. A simple method for measurement of mechanical power in jumping. *European Journal of Applied Physiology* 50: 273–82.

6. Brown, L.E., M. Whitehurst, and J.R. Bryant. 1992. Reliability of the Lido active isokinetic dynamometer concentric mode. *Isokinetic Exercise Science* 2: 191–94.

7. Burdett, R.G., and J. Van Swearingen. 1987. Reliability of isokinetic muscle endurance tests. *Journal of Orthopaedic and Sports Physical Therapy* 8: 484–88.

8. Caiozzo, V.J., J.J. Perrine, and V.R. Edgerton. 1981. Training-induced alterations of in vivo force-velocity relationship of human muscle. *Journal of Applied Physiology* 51: 750–54.

9. Colliander, E.B., and P.A. Tesch. 1990. Effects of eccentric and concentric muscle actions in resistance training. *Acta Physiologica Scandinavica* 140: 31–39.

10. Cordova, M.L., C.D. Ingersoll, J.E. Kovaleski, and K.L. Knight. 1995. A comparison of isokinetic and isotonic predictions of a functional task. *Journal of Athletic Training* 30: 319–22.

11. Costill, D.L., E.F. Coyle, W.F. Fink, G.R. Lesmes, and F.A. Witzmann. 1979. Adaptations in skeletal muscle following strength training. *Journal of Applied Physiology: Respiratory and Environmental Exercise Physiology* 46: 96–99.

12. Cote, C., J.A. Simoneau, P. Lagasse, and M. Boulay. 1988. Isokinetic strength training protocols: Do they induce skeletal muscle fiber hypertrophy? *Archives of Physical Medicine and Rehabilitation* 69: 281–85.

13. Coyle, E.F., D.C. Feiring, T.C. Rotkis, F.B. Roby, W. Lee, and J.H. Wilmore. 1981. Specificity of power improvements through slow and fast isokinetic training. *Journal of Physiology and Respiratory and Environmental Exercise Physiology* 51: 1437–42.

14. Davies, G.J. 1992. *A compendium of isokinetics in clinical usage and rehabilitation techniques.* 4th ed. Onalaska, WI: S & S.

15. Davies, G.J., and T.S. Ellenbecker. 1998. Application of isokinetics in testing and rehabilitation. In *Physical rehabilitation of the injured athlete,* ed. J.R. Andrews, G.L. Harrelson, and K.E. Wilk, 219–59. Philadelphia: Saunders.

16. Davies, G.J., and B.C. Heiderscheit. 1997. Reliability of the Lido Linea closed kinetic chain isokinetic dynamometer. *Journal of Orthopaedic and Sports Physical Therapy* 25: 133–36.

17. deKoning, F.L., R.A. Binkhorst, J.A. Vos, and M.A. van't Hoff. 1985. The force-velocity relationship of arm flexion in untrained males and females and arm-trained athletes. *European Journal of Applied Physiology* 54: 89–94.

18. Dudley, G.A., R.T. Harris, M.R. Duvoisin, B.M. Hather, and P. Buchanan. 1990. Effect of voluntary vs. artificial activation on the relationship of muscle torque to speed. *Journal of Applied Physiology* 69: 2215–21.

19. Esselman, P.C., B.J. de Lateur, A.D. Alquist, K.A. Questad, R.M. Giaconi, and J.F. Lehmann. 1991. Torque development in isokinetic training. *Archives of Physical Medicine and Rehabilitation* 72: 723–28.

20. Ewing, J.L., D.R. Wolfe, M.A. Rogers, M.L. Amundson, and G.A. Stull. 1990. Effects of velocity of isokinetic training on strength, power, and quadriceps muscle fiber characteristics. *European Journal of Applied Physiology* 61: 159–62.

21. Farrell, M., and J.G. Richards. 1986. Analysis of the reliability and validity of the kinetic communicator exercise device. *Medicine and Science in Sports and Exercise* 18: 44–49.

22. Fleck, S.J., and W.J. Kraemer. 1997. *Designing resistance training programs.* 2d ed. Champaign, IL: Human Kinetics.

23. Gettman, L.R., L.A. Culter, and T.A. Strathman. 1980. Physiological changes after 20 weeks of isotonic vs. isokinetic circuit training. *Journal of Sports Medicine and Physical Fitness* 20: 265–73.

24. Golnick, P.D., J. Karlsson, K. Piehl, and B. Saltin. 1974. Selective glycogen depletion in skeletal muscle fibers of man following sustained contraction. *Journal of Physiology* 241: 59–67.

25. Greenberger, H.B., and M.V. Paterno. 1995. Relationship of knee extensor strength and hopping test performance in the assessment of lower extremity function. *Journal of Orthopaedic and Sports Physical Therapy* 22: 202–6.

26. Housh, D.J., T.J. Housh, G.O. Johnson, and W.K. Chu. 1992. Hypertrophic response to unilateral concentric isokinetic resistance training. *Journal of Applied Physiology* 73: 65–70.

27. Ivy, J.L., W.M. Sherman, J.M. Miller, B.D. Maxwell, and D.L. Costill. 1982. Relationship between muscle $QO_2$ and fatigue during repeated isokinetic contractions. *Journal of Applied Physiology* 53: 470–74.

28. Jameson, T.D., K.L. Knight, C.D. Ingersoll, and J.E. Edwards. 1997. Correlation of isokinetic, isometric, isotonic strength measurements with a one-leg vertical jump. *Isokinetics and Exercise Science* 6: 203–8.

29. Jenkins, W.L., M. Thackaberry, and C. Killian. 1984. Speed-specific isokinetic training. *Journal of Orthopaedic and Sports Physical Therapy* 6: 181–83.

30. Johnson, B.L. 1976. A comparison of concentric and eccentric muscle training. *Medicine and Science in Sports and Exercise* 8: 35–39.

31. Kanehisa, H., and M. Miyashita. 1983. Specificity of velocity in strength training. *European Journal of Applied Physiology* 52: 104–6.

32. Kawakami, M. Training effect and electromyogram. I. Spatial distribution of spike potentials. *Japanese Journal of Physiology* 51: 1–8.

33. Knapik, J.J., J.E. Wright, R.H. Mawdsley, and J.M. Braun. 1983. Isokinetic, isometric, and isotonic strength relationships. *Archives of Physical Medicine and Rehabilitation* 64: 77–80.

34. Komi, P.V. 1979. Neuromuscular performance: Factors influencing force and speed production. *Scandinavia Journal of Sports Science* 1: 2–15.

35. Komi, P.V., and C. Bosco. 1978. Utilization of stored elastic energy in leg extensor muscles by men and women. *Medicine and Science in Sports and Exercise* 10: 261–65.

36. Komi, P.V., and E.R. Buskirk. 1972. Effect of eccentric and concentric muscle conditioning on tension and electrical activity of human muscle. *Ergonomics* 15: 417–34.

37. Kovaleski, J.E., B.W. Craig, D.L. Costill, A.J. Habansky, and L.J. Matchett. 1988. Influence of age on muscle strength and knee function following arthroscopic meniscectomy. *Journal of Orthopaedic and Sports Physical Therapy* 10: 87–92.

38. Kovaleski, J.E., and R.J. Heitman. 1993. Interaction of velocity and progression order during isokinetic velocity spectrum exercise. *Isokinetics and Exercise Science* 3: 118–22.

39. Kovaleski, J.E., and R.J. Heitman. 1993. Effects of isokinetic velocity spectrum exercise on torque production. *Sports Medicine, Training, and Rehabilitation* 4: 67–71.

40. Kovaleski, J.E., R.J. Heitman, L.R. Gurchiek, J.W. Erdmann, and T.L. Trundle. 1997. Reliability and effects of leg dominance on lower extremity isokinetic force and work using the Closed Chain Rider System. *Journal of Sports Rehabilitation* 6: 319–26.

41. Kovaleski, J.E., R.J. Heitman, F.M. Scaffidi, and F.B. Fondren. 1992. Effects of isokinetic velocity spectrum exercise on average power and total work. *Journal of Athletic Training* 27: 54–56.

42. Kovaleski, J.E., R.J. Heitman, T.L. Trundle, and W.F. Gilley. 1995. Isotonic preload versus isokinetic knee extension resistance training. *Medicine and Science in Sports and Exercise* 27: 895–99.

43. Kraemer, W.J. 1985. Exercise prescription: Chronic program variables (periodization of training). *National Strength and Conditioning Journal* 7: 45–47.

44. Kraemer, W.J., N.D. Duncan, and J.S. Volek. 1998. Resistance training and elite athletes: Adaptations and program considerations. *Journal of Orthopaedic and Sports Physical Therapy* 28: 110–19.

45. Kraemer, W.J., and S.J. Fleck. 1982. Anaerobic metabolism and its evaluation. *National Strength and Conditioning Journal* 4: 20–21.

46. Kraemer, W.J., S.J. Fleck, and W.J. Evans. 1996. Strength and power training: Physiological mechanisms of adaptation. *Exercise and sports sciences review*. Vol. 23. Baltimore: Williams & Wilkins.

47. Kraemer, W.J., J. Patton, S.E. Gordon, E.A. Harman, M.R. Deschenes, K. Reynolds, R.U. Newton, N.T. Triplett, and J.E. Dziados. 1995. Compatibility of high intensity strength and endurance training on hormonal and skeletal muscle adaptations. *Journal of Applied Physiology* 78: 976–89.

48. Lacerte, M., B.J. deLateur, A.D. Alquist, and K.A. Questad. 1992. Concentric versus combined concentric-eccentric isokinetic training programs: Effect on peak torque of human quadriceps femoris muscle. *Archives of Physical Medicine and Rehabilitation* 73: 1059–62.

49. Lesmes, G.R., D.L. Costill, E.F. Coyle, and W.J. Fink. 1978. Muscle strength and power changes during maximal isokinetic training. *Medicine and Science in Sports and Exercise* 10: 266–69.

50. Manning, R.J., J.E. Graves, D.M. Carpenter, S.H. Leggett, and M.L. Pollock. 1990. Constant vs. variable resistance knee extension training. *Medicine and Science in Sports and Exercise* 22: 397–401.

51. Mannion, A.F., P.M. Jakeman, and P.L.T. Willan. 1992. Effects of isokinetic training of the knee extensors on isometric strength and peak power output during cycling. *European Journal of Applied Physiology* 65: 370–75.

52. McArdle, W., F. Katch, and V. Katch. 1996. *Exercise physiology: Energy, nutrition, and human performance*. 4th ed. Philadelphia: Lea & Febiger.

53. Moffroid, M.T., and R.H. Whipple. 1970. Specificity of speed of exercise. *Physical Therapy* 50: 1692–99.

54. Moffroid, M., R. Whipple, J. Hofkosh, E. Lowman, and H. Thistle. 1969. A study of isokinetic exercise. *Physical Therapy* 49: 735–46.

55. Moritani, T., and H.A. deVries. 1979. Neural factors versus hypertrophy in the time course of muscle strength gain. *American Journal of Physical Medicine* 58: 115–30.

56. Narici, M.V., G.S. Roi, L. Landoni, A.E. Minetti, and P. Cerretelli. 1989. Changes in force, cross-sectional area, and neural activation during strength training and detraining of the human quadriceps. *European Journal of Applied Physiology* 59: 310–19.

57. Osternig, L.R. 1986. Isokinetic dynamometry: Implications for muscle testing and rehabilitation. *Exercise and Sports Science Reviews* 14: 45–80.

58. Osternig, L.R. 1975. Optimal isokinetic loads and velocities producing muscular power in human subjects. *Archives of Physical Medicine and Rehabilitation* 56: 152–55.

59. Osternig, L.R., J. Hamill, J.A. Sawhill, and B.T. Bates. 1983. Influence of torque and limb speed on power production in isokinetic exercise. *American Journal of Sports Medicine* 62: 163–71.

60. Pearson, D.R., and D.L. Costill. 1988. The effects of constant external resistance exercise and isokinetic exercise training on work-induced hypertrophy. *Journal of Applied Sport Science and Research* 2: 39–41.

61. Perrin, D.H. 1993. *Isokinetic exercise and assessment.* Champaign, IL: Human Kinetics.

62. Perrine, J.J. 1968. Isokinetic exercise and the mechanical energy potential of muscle. *Journal of Health, Physical Education, and Recreation* 39: 40–48.

63. Perrine, J.J., and Edgerton, V.R. 1978. Muscle force-velocity relationships under isokinetic loading. *Medicine and Science in Sports and Exercise* 10: 159–66.

64. Petersen, S.R. 1988. The influence of isokinetic concentric resistance training on concentric and eccentric torque outputs and cross-sectional area of the quadriceps femoris. *Canadian Journal of Sport Science* 13: 76–80.

65. Petersen, S.R., K.M. Bagnall, H.A. Wenger, D.C. Reid, W.R. Castor, and H.A. Quinney. 1989. The influence of velocity-specific resistance training on the in vivo torque-velocity relationship and the cross-sectional area of quadriceps femoris. *Journal of Orthopaedic and Sports Physical Therapy* 10: 456–62.

66. Petersen, S.R., J. Wessel, K. Bagnall, H. Wilkins, A. Quinney, and H. Wenger. 1990. Influence of concentric resistance training on concentric and eccentric strength. *Archives of Physical Medicine and Rehabilitation* 71: 101–5.

67. Pincivero, D.M., S.M. Lephart, and R.G. Karunakara. 1997. Relation between open and closed kinematic chain assessment of knee strength and functional performance. *Clinical Journal of Sports Medicine* 7: 11–16.

68. Riera, J., F. Drobnic, and P.A. Galilea. 1994. Comparison of two methods for the measurement of the extensor muscle dynamic force of the inferior limb: Isokinetic dynamometry and vertical jump tests. *Sports Medicine, Training, and Rehabilitation* 5: 137–43.

69. Sale, D.G. 1990. Testing strength and power. In *Physiological testing of the high-performance athlete*, ed. J.D. MacDougall, H.H. Wenger, and H.S. Green, 21–106. Champaign, IL: Human Kinetics.

70. Sale, D.G., J.D. MacDougall, A.R.M. Upton, and A.J. McComas. 1983. Effect of strength training upon motoneuron excitability in man. *Medicine and Science in Sports and Exercise* 15: 57–62.

71. Sherman, W.M., M.J. Plyley, D.A. Vogelgesang, D.L. Costill, and A.J. Habansky. 1981. Isokinetic strength during rehabilitation following arthrotomy: Specificity of speed. *Athletic Training* 16: 138–41.

72. Sleivert, G.G., R.D. Backus, and H.A. Wenger. 1995. The influence of a strength-sprint training sequence on multijoint power output. *Medicine and Science in Sports and Exercise* 27: 1655–65.

73. Smith, M.J., and P. Melton. 1981. Isokinetic versus isotonic variable-resistance training. *The American Journal of Sports Medicine* 9: 275–79.

74. Soukup, J.T., T.S. Maynard, and J.E. Kovaleski. 1994. Resistance training guidelines for individuals with diabetes mellitus. *The Diabetes Educator* 20: 129–37.

75. Staron, R.S., D.L. Karapondo, J. Kraemer, A.C. Fry, S.E. Gordon, J.E. Falkel, F.C. Hagerman, and R.S. Hikida. 1994. Skeletal muscle adaptations during the early phase of heavy resistance training in men and women. *Journal of Applied Physiology* 76: 1247–55.

76. Thorstensson, A. 1977. Observations on strength training and detraining. *Acta Physiologica Scandinavica* 100: 491–93.

77. Vitti, G.J. 1984. The effects of variable training speeds on leg strength and power. *Athletic Training* 19: 26–29.

78. Wiklander, J., and J. Lysholm. 1987. Simple tests for surveying muscle strength and muscle stiffness in sportsmen. *International Journal of Sports Medicine* 8: 50–54.

79. Wilson, G.J., R.U. Newton, A.J. Murphy, and B.J. Humphries. 1993. The optimal training load for the development of dynamic athletic performance. *Medicine and Science in Sports and Exercise* 25: 1279–86.

# Chapter 9

# Multiple-Joint Performance Over a Velocity Spectrum

Lawrence W. Weiss

Physical activities ranging from everyday tasks to elite athletic performances involve a myriad of movements, from simple to complex. For activities in which strength deficits hinder performance, specific strength and power tests may provide useful information to assist in selecting members of teams or other organizations, to identify performance deficits needing remediation, or to serve as a guide in evaluating the effectiveness of a particular intervention strategy.

Often, strength and power tests consist of single components of more complex endeavors (e.g., isolated joint actions). This approach to testing permits us to limit the number of factors influencing performance at a given time. Thus, testing portions of a larger, more complex activity enables us to isolate factors thought to contribute to overall variability in performance. This type of information is particularly helpful in allowing us to identify specific weaknesses and strengths. Unfortunately, strength performance on selected aspects of a given activity will likely not provide us with information on the "whole" action, especially when the action involves a multiple-link kinetic chain. Multiple-joint strength and power tests may be more beneficial in this regard.

## What Strength and Power Testing Reveals

The primary goal of strength and power testing is to provide the most meaningful and objective information concerning how well a person is likely to perform on related tasks in which the level of strength and power is critical to success. Unfortunately, strength and power are frequently oversimplified on a conceptual level. Although not easily answered, the following questions exemplify germane considerations often overlooked in the process of test selection and interpretation when a simplistic view of strength is embraced:

- How related are single-joint tests to multiple-joint activities?
- How related are open kinetic chain tests to closed kinetic chain performances and vice versa?
- How related are isokinetic tests to performances involving constant or variable external loads?
- How related are slow velocity strength tests to fast velocity and "explosive" activities?
- How related are peak, average, and angle-specific torque, force, and power to various types of activities?
- How related are timing variables such as peak time, peak hold time, and pulse duration to various types of activities?
- How trustworthy are the numbers emanating from computerized "black boxes"?

# Single-Joint Tests and Multiple-Joint Activities

Isolated single-joint tests are often used to evaluate the current status of individuals for whom the level of strength and power has been deemed to be important. Evidence suggests that singling out an isolated joint action from sequential joint activities will not always produce performance that is highly related to the combined effects of multiple-joint actions. For example, knee extension strength does not highly relate to vertical jumping performance (1, 11). Although single-joint tests of strength and power provide information concerning an individual's capabilities for performing apparently related multiple-joint tasks, the addition of an appropriate multiple-joint test would provide a more complete profile. The information provided by single- and multiple-joint tests is complimentary with neither test being fully capable of replacing the other.

# Open Kinetic Chain Tests
# and Closed Kinetic Chain Performance

In 1955, Steindler described diarthrodial (freely movable) joint actions as falling into one of two categories, "open" and "closed kinetic chains" (22). These categories were useful in differentiating joint actions when strength was considered as a simple construct. In recent years, however, conflicting interpretations and applications of these particular terms have resulted in confusion. In his original recitation, Steindler wrote the following:

*A kinetic chain is a combination of several successively arranged joints constituting a complex motor unit. We designate as open kinetic chain a combination in which the terminal joint is free. The waving of the hand is an open kinetic chain in which the action of the shoulder joint, the elbow joint, and the wrist joint are successively involved. A closed kinetic chain, on the other hand, is one in which the terminal joint meets with some considerable external resistance which prohibits or restrains its free motion. Eventually, the external resistance may be overcome and the peripheral portion of the joint may move against this resistance, for instance, in pushing a cart or lifting a load; or the external resistance is absolute, in which case the proximal part moves against the peripheral, as for instance, in chinning oneself on a horizontal bar; or the limitations of the muscular effort may assert itself both peripherally and proximally and may be unsurmountable, in which case no visible motion is produced. Only in the latter instance is the kinetic chain strictly and absolutely closed. However in common use we apply the term to all situations in which the peripheral joint of the chain meets with overwhelming external resistance. (p. 63)*

Later on in the same text he wrote the following:

*In the standing body the lower extremity is a closed kinetic chain, i.e., a system of articulations joined to an external resistance. This resistance is the superincumbent weight or, rather, the gravitational reaction of the floor which it produces. These reactions are transmitted from below to the subastragalar, the ankle, the knee, and the hip joints. In such a closed kinetic chain, where the limb is not moving freely because of the external resistance, the action of the muscles is quite different from what it is when the muscle operates on a free lever arm which is unencumbered except by its own weight. In a closed kinetic chain the muscle often develops a rotatory effect upon a remote joint which lies outside of the muscle. (p. 436)*

And further on, he said the following:

*There are situations in which the upper extremity moves against an external resistance large enough to interfere with the free peripheral motion of the extremity or even to arrest visible motion altogether. This resistance forms then with the extremity a closed kinetic chain. When one lifts a heavy weight or moves a very heavy object, it furnishes the external resistance, which closes the kinetic chain. . . . On the whole, the characteristic feature of the closed kinetic chain is the display of force, whereas the creation of speed or acceleration is the central effort of the open kinetic chain. (pp. 563–64)*

The recent confusion with Steindler's original concepts of open and closed kinetic chains appears to be due to multiple interpretations of the original features of each term together with expanded characterizations of each based upon new insights. As noted above, the open kinetic chain was originally characterized as a series of joints in which

- the terminal joint is free,
- the muscle operating on a free lever arm is unencumbered except by its own weight, and
- speed or acceleration is a predominant characteristic.

On the other hand, the closed kinetic chain was originally characterized as a system in which

- the terminal joint meets with considerable resistance that prohibits or restrains free motion,
- articulations are joined to an external resistance,
- the muscle often develops a rotatory effect upon a remote joint that lies outside the muscle,
- the resistance is large enough to interfere with the free peripheral motion of the extremity, and
- force is a predominant characteristic.

More recently, open kinetic chain systems have been characterized as normally producing substantial shear forces at involved joints while closed kinetic chains are thought normally to produce substantial compressive forces (3, 14), even though a substantial amount of shear force may exist during activities normally considered closed (9, 23).

Exercises often referred to as being "open," according to contemporary convention, may in some instances be considered "closed" by following Steindler's original descriptions of the two kinetic chain categories (see table 9.1).

The examples found in table 9.1 illustrate why Steindler's kinetic chain model no longer appears to be tenable. In all cases, the display of force against a

### Table 9.1    Classification of Various Exercises Using Contemporary* and Original Interpretations of Steindler

| Exercise | Contemporary approach | | Original approach | |
|---|---|---|---|---|
| | Open KC | Closed KC | Open KC | Closed KC |
| Leg press w/fixed feet & movable torso | | X | | X |
| Leg press w/movable feet & fixed torso | X | | | X |
| Push-up | | X | | X |
| Bench press | X | | | X |
| Chin-up | | X | | X |
| Lat pull-down | X | | | X |
| Squat | | X | | X |
| Knee extension against resistance | X | | | X |

*Universal agreement nonexistent.

considerable external resistance is evident; therefore, *all* of the exercises could be considered examples of closed kinetic chains. Furthermore, with the advent of isokinetic devices, it is unclear at what point in a velocity spectrum that the exercises noted above would be performed sufficiently slow to "interfere with the free peripheral motion of the extremity." Dillman, Murray, and Hintermeister (6) thoroughly addressed the confusion associated with the multiple interpretations of open and closed chain exercises with particular reference to the shoulder, while Smidt (21) addressed it more generally in an editorial. Both of these reports eloquently point out a number of impediments to continued use of Steindler's classifications. In short, although Steindler's efforts in this regard were laudable for 1955, his simplified model no longer serves us well regardless of whether the movement involves a constant external resistance or a constant velocity. At this time, it appears the original multifaceted and somewhat vague definitions (by today's standards) confuse rather than clarify how investigators and clients interpret them. In that light, I recommend that it is time to abandon his two-component classification scheme in favor of defining both the joint actions and the concurrent types of muscular actions involved in particular movements. If sufficient information is available, joint actions from past and future investigations may be described without using the currently ambiguous open and closed kinetic chain designations. Much remains to be determined concerning the relationship between specific movements performed during both testing and real-life situations, and it would be unfortunate for semantic differences to hamper progress in this area.

# Isokinetic Tests Versus Variable Velocity Performances

Isokinetic exercise involves performing a specified movement at a constant velocity using a specialized dynamometer. Within the limits of a particular device, this may provide the capability of assessing muscular output at a velocity that mimics that which occurs during a designated performance, a concept referred to as velocity specificity (16).

Various modality studies suggest that a change in performance in one strength-developing device will often not be reflected in concomitant changes in another, especially as it pertains to strength measures such as torque, force, or the load lifted (2, 10, 30). If the movement pattern for a particular strength or power test corresponds to that of another strength-related activity, and changes in one are not reflected in concomitant changes in the other, then the test may be inappropriate for that situation.

The exclusive use of single-joint tests of strength or power to represent capabilities for multiple-joint activities would seem to compound this apparent problem regardless of the testing modality. If a person's ability to perform a multiple-joint activity is dependent on the ability to summate internal forces generated in the various links of a particular kinetic chain, it stands to reason that a similar multiple-joint strength test might be able to provide us with a more comprehensive assessment of a person's capabilities than if only single-joint tests are performed.

Furthermore, if the velocity of the strength test corresponds to that of a particular type of related activity, then it also stands to reason that the strength and power information may be more meaningful than that of a test performed at substantially faster or slower velocities. And finally, if the load or resistance for a particular activity is reasonably constant (e.g., putting a shot), then for a corresponding single- or multiple-joint strength test the most meaningful variables might be things such as the velocity at which the load can be moved, the elapsed time to peak velocity, and the power generated while moving a specified load in a particular manner.

The fact that isokinetic tests frequently do not reflect training responses similar to those found via dynamic constant external resistance testing suggests that they measure unique performance characteristics. The crucial consideration, then, is to determine which tests are most indicative of performance for a designated situation.

A general drawback to isokinetic testing is the fact that it is rare to find strength and power activities performed at a constant velocity. It is much more common to find velocity varying either against a constant external load or against a variable one. Furthermore, it is unclear if velocity-matched isokinetic tests will reflect concomitant performance changes in other activities. It may be more meaningful in some circumstances to use a device that enables us to specify constant external loads while we measure velocity. Obviously, comparative studies are needed to sort out the association between these phenomena.

It may very well be that we are focusing in some activities on strength variables that are not as important as we think. Instead of focusing on only peak force or torque, average force or torque, or angle-specific force or torque, expressions of power or timing variables may be of greater importance. For example, we have determined the relationship between vertical jumping performance and isokinetic squatting performance and found that peak power generated at a moderately fast velocity and expressed relative to body weight is the best predictor of vertical jumping capability (24, 27). It follows that training interventions designed to enhance relative power output at moderately fast squatting velocities will also enhance vertical jumping ability. We are currently assessing this via a series of investigations in our lab. The first study is designed to compare the effects of deep versus shallow squats, while the second will compare the effects of power lifts such as hang cleans and high pulls versus strength lifts such as squats on jumping performance and related factors. If changes in our predictors do not correspond to those in jumping performance, then they would be useless in evaluating the effectiveness of our training interventions, and we will need to reevaluate our predictors.

In our zeal to conceptually simplify and standardize testing, we seem to be overlooking that our tests of strength and power do not universally apply to all situations. It is analogous to the television commercial in which a banker recommends his institution's Super CD (certificate of deposit) for all clients, regardless of their individual financial circumstances. We need to be much more objective and flexible in approaching strength testing. We need to take advantage of the fact that many tools are now available that provide us with unique insights into a person's ability to perform. Our mistake appears to be that we are not doing our utmost to match the tool or tools to the situation. Much more research in this area is needed, however, in order for this to be possible.

# Slow Velocity Strength Tests and Fast Velocity Activities

It has been well documented that maximal force output decreases with increasing velocities (4, 12, 25, 26, 29). Power, on the other hand, is low at slow velocities, increases to a maximum at intermediate velocities, and then decreases progressively as velocity continues to increase (19, 20, 26). However, the relative change in strength and power with increasing velocity varies from one person to the next (18). Consequently, maximal strength and power performance at one velocity are not necessarily related to strength and power at substantially faster or slower velocities. Therefore, only two logical approaches appear to exist to comprehensively represent strength and power for a given movement pattern: (1) assess maximal strength and power over a velocity spectrum (isokinetics) or (2) assess maximal velocity over a load spectrum. Similar curves should emerge regardless of the variable manipulated as long as the lifts are similar.

# Peak, Average, and Angle-Specific Measurements

Cases have been advanced for the efficacy of peak, average, and angle-specific measurements of force or torque and power in association with isokinetic testing and for determining the weakest point in the range of motion as is characteristic of strength assessments using dynamic constant external resistance (DCER). Thus, in all four of the preceding measurements, a different aspect of strength performance is measured. At the present time, I generally dismiss arguments about the relative merit of one approach versus another unless it has been demonstrated for a specific scenario that one is more highly related to a particular type of performance. Generally speaking, each of the expressions represents a unique variable. As long as the measurements are valid and clearly defined, and we restrain ourselves from overgeneralizing the nature of the variables (i.e., strength), then we stand a far better chance of eventually gaining an understanding of force and power development and performance.

# Peak Time, Rise Time, Peak Hold Time, and Pulse Duration

Peak time is the elapsed interval between the initiation of the motion and the point at which peak force or torque occurs. Rise time is the elapsed interval at which force or torque increases from 10% to 90% of the peak value. Peak hold time is the elapsed interval at which force or torque is maintained at or above 90% of the peak value. Pulse duration is the elapsed interval at which force or torque is maintained at or above 50% of the peak value. All four of these variables provide unique information that may be used to characterize and distinguish performances, although there is probably nothing magical about the percentages used for the latter two. It remains to be seen how related any of these timing variables are to various types of performances.

Unfortunately, at this time, we have been unable to establish sufficient reliability to have confidence in the timing variables during multiple-joint isokinetic testing over a velocity spectrum (28). For squat exercises performed over a velocity spectrum and repeated in the identical test sequence subsequent to 48 h of inactivity, our reliability coefficients ranged from .59 to .88. Especially if change in performance is to be evaluated, higher reliability coefficients would be desirable. If a high level of reliability is eventually attained, however, we suspect these or similar measurements will be very useful in specific circumstances.

# Infallable Measurements and Meaningful Calibration Checks

Technological developments in the strength-testing arena have been taking place at an ever increasing pace. All too often, experimental subjects and even researchers are enamored with flashy devices having a great capacity to produce data and video graphics. This is a wonderful phenomenon as long as researchers take the time to thoroughly evaluate and then monitor the quality of the information gathered. To assume all is well may be a dreadful mistake.

## Equipment and Data Evaluation

It is imperative to initially evaluate the validity of new strength assessment devices as well as new or unique protocols. The data emanating from the devices should be comparable to some type of standard. Subsequently, anyone using a testing device should assess the reliability of the data collected for each protocol used. The device itself or the manner in which it is used may adversely affect reliability. The device should be calibrated, or at the very least tested for calibration, so that the tester will know if a problem exists that requires correction prior to attempting to collect data.

Data establishing the level of validity are often either meager or assumed to exist for many strength-testing devices. A healthy level of skepticism appears to be absent in the professional community as we have not demanded accountability on this issue. The level of validity may be established over time and should emanate from multiple independent laboratories. Ignoring this issue may lead to serious problems and confusion due to inaccurate or misleading data generated in experimental studies.

A high level of reliability is required of valid tests although it does not guarantee validity. Strength data should be consistent when nothing intervenes to alter performance; otherwise, change will be difficult to detect. Testing protocols or devices may yield erratic output that would adversely affect reliability. However, unless this is assessed, machine malfunctions and performance irregularities may go undetected. The reliability levels for single-joint isokinetic assessments have been firmly established for many years (17). Although validity has not been firmly established, a number of investigators have reported reasonable reliability values for specific multiple-joint strength tests using equipment that can function in an isokinetic mode (5, 7, 8, 13, 15, 25, 28).

In our lab, for example, we have established that the Ariel Multifunction dynamometer may be used over a substantial velocity spectrum to produce reliable force and power data for concentric-only squats and bench presses (25, 28). Squatting performances by young men and women at 0.51, 0.82, 1.12, 1.43, 1.73, and 2.04 m/s were found to have reliability coefficients ranging from .94 to .99 (28). Although force and power data were highly reliable, it is likely that few of our subjects attained a load range at either 1.73 or 2.04 m/s; therefore, it would be difficult to attribute any particular velocity to the actual performances at the two fastest squatting tests. For that reason, we are using the squats up to a velocity of only 1.43 m/s at this time.

Bench press force and power outputs by young men at 0.0, 0.124, 0.496, and 0.868 m/s were found to have reliability coefficients ranging from .95 to .99 (25). Although load ranges were obtained at all velocities for all subjects, the absence of a reduction in power output at the fastest velocity, as would be expected based upon typical power-velocity curves, suggests that one or more faster velocities should have been attempted. Although highly reliable, the zero velocity bench press was performed at a less than optimal bar angle, which resulted in relatively low force output (power is 0.0 watts at 0.0 m/s). In subsequent studies, we will perform isometric tests at bar angles that come closer to optimizing performance.

## Calibration Evaluation

Calibration checks are often convenient ways to determine if the testing device is producing consistent data that concurrently fall within an acceptable range of values. This information should be obtained on a frequent and regular basis and reported in research reports. Unfortunately, calibration checks are not routinely performed in all laboratories and are not required for research published in many journals. The effect of this omission can be critical. For example, if a device loses its calibration for a posttest subsequent to some type of intervention, the tester may mistakenly report that a person has gained, lost, or not changed in strength when, in fact, the contrary has occurred.

Technological developments in recent years have resulted in much progress in our understanding of skeletal muscle performance. However, as professionals, we need to guard against the complacent assumption that we will never see bad data. To aid in combating this problem, calibration checks should be performed routinely, as well as at times when values for variables of interest fall outside what you as an experienced tester sense is actually occurring. As long as you are thoroughly familiar with your strength-testing device, you will likely be able to detect aberrations from the norm that should prompt you to check the calibration of the equipment. All isokinetic strength-testing equipment will have specified acceptable ranges of values, and a calibration check should yield values within the respective ranges. A scientific approach to data collection will go a long way in instilling confidence in anyone "consuming" the information we report.

In our lab, we check dynamic force calibration for our dynamometer in the desired direction as part of our routine start-up procedures (25, 28). At the present time, our multiple-joint exercises consist of concentric-only squats and bench presses, so we test calibration only in the upward direction. This is accomplished using a special calibration bar that functions as a continuation of the exercise bar but is on the opposite side of the axis of rotation. Therefore, when we hang weights from it, the exercise bar moves in an upward direction similar to what occurs during the squat and bench press. Since most of our exercises are dynamic in nature, a dynamic calibration check seems to be appropriate, although I would not be averse to complimenting that with the more conventional static measurements. Failure of either approach to yield data within the respective unit's acceptable accuracy range would signal the existence of a calibration problem. Since errant readings from a pressure transducer may occur at times, the fact that values were or were not corrected should be reported.

We use one low and one high standardized load for the Ariel Multifunction dynamometer and perform calibration checks in duplicate. Subsequent to each investigation we also use the results from the force calibration checks to calculate intra- and intertest coefficients of variation to assess the consistency of our device to recognize standardized loads. Our values have routinely been less than 2%, and we would not accept anything beyond 5%, as these procedures assess only the machine's ability to recognize a load (25, 28). Once a human performs a particular exercise on the testing device, additional variability is introduced, which would make change in performance more difficult to detect. I have observed at least one other investigation reporting force calibration results for a testing apparatus used for multiple-joint exercise (5). However, a bar angle as well as a velocity check should also be a routine procedure in calibration verification. Velocity, bar angle, and force output are certainly critical outputs of these isokinetic devices, and we must insure that the values are correct. As I noted previously, we jeopardize real progress in our discipline when we do not require these simple preliminary assessments prior to data collection.

## Multiple-Joint Isokinetic Testing

Unfortunately, the vast majority of isokinetic tests have involved isolated joint actions. As pointed out previously, although this approach is relevant in identifying some of the component strengths and weaknesses a person may have in performing a particular task, it appears to be much less useful in reflecting performance capabilities on multiple-joint activities. Our focus has been on determining predictors of two different styles of vertical jumping performance. In both cases, the variable most highly related to jumping performance was squatting peak power expressed relative to body weight when performed at 1.43 m/s during the ascension phase, which started at 90° of knee flexion (24, 27). We have thus far been able to account for between 68% and 80% of the variability in jumping performance and are working toward identifying other independent factors that will enable us to account for most of the remainder. When multiple independent factors are responsible for performance, it may be possible to tailor training to meet the specific needs of an individual, but this can only be done if the variables have been objectively identified.

## Summary

A combination of testing approaches using single- and multiple-joint protocols over a spectrum of standardized velocities and loads is likely to produce the most meaningful and comprehensive strength and power profiles of individuals so that performance capabilities may be projected for a variety of activities. Although single-joint isokinetic testing devices and protocols have been standardized and evaluated for the major diarthrodial joints in the body, the same cannot be said for multiple-joint approaches. This omission is minimizing the utility of many of our research studies and needs to be vigorously addressed by the myriad of professionals evaluating functional musculoskeletal capabilities.

## References

1. Anderson M, J Gieck, D Perrin, A Weltman, A Rutt, and C Denegar. 1991. The relationship among isometric, isotonic, and isokinetic concentric and eccentric quadriceps and hamstring force and three components of athletic performance. *J Ortho Sports Phys Ther* 14: 114–20.
2. Augustsson J, A Esko, R Thomee, and U Svantesson. 1998. Weight training of the thigh muscles using closed vs. open kinetic chain exercises: A comparison of performance enhancement. *J Ortho Sports Phys Ther* 27: 3–8.
3. Bynum B, R Barrack, and A Alexander. 1995. Open versus closed chain kinetic exercises after anterior cruciate ligament reconstruction. *Am J Sports Med* 23: 401–6.
4. Caiozzo V, J Perrine, and V Edgerton. 1981. Training-induced alterations of the in vivo force-velocity relationship of human muscle. *J Appl Physiol: Respirat Environ Exer Physiol* 51: 750–54.
5. Davies G and B Heiderscheit. 1997. Reliability of the Lido Linea closed kinetic chain isokinetic dynamometer. *J Ortho Sports Phys Ther* 25: 133–36.

6. Dillman C, T Murray, and R Hintermeister. 1994. Biomechanical differences of open and closed chain exercises with respect to the shoulder. *J Sport Rehab* 3: 228–38.

7. Dvir Z. 1996. An isokinetic study of combined activity of the hip and knee extensors. *Clin Biomech* 11: 135–38.

8. Engle B. 1983. Clinical use of an isokinetic leg press. *J Ortho Sports Phys Ther* 5: 148–49.

9. Escamilla R, G Fleisig, N Zheng, S Barrentine, K Wilk, and J Andrews. 1998. Biomechanics of the knee during closed kinetic chain and open kinetic chain exercises. *Med Sci Sports Exer* 30: 556–69.

10. Fry A, W Kraemer, and C Weseman. 1991. The effect of an off-season strength and conditioning program on starters and nonstarters in women's intercollegiate volleyball. *J Appl Sport Sci Res* 5: 174–81.

11. Genuario S and F Dolgener. 1980. The relationship of isokinetic torque at two speeds to the vertical jump. *Res Q Exer Sport* 51: 593–98.

12. Gregor R, V Edgerton, J Perrine, D Campion, and C deBus. 1979. Torque-velocity relationships and muscle fiber composition in elite female athletes. *J Appl Physiol: Respirat Environ Exer Physiol* 47: 388–92.

13. Hortobagyi T and F Katch. 1990. Reliability of muscle mechanical characteristics for isokinetic and isotonic squat and bench press exercise using a multifunction computerized dynamometer. *Res Q Exer Sport* 61: 191–95.

14. Jenkins W, S Munns, G Jayaraman, K Wertzberger, and K Neely. 1997. A measurement of anterior tibial displacement in the closed and open kinetic chain. *J Ortho Sports Phys Ther* 25: 49–56.

15. Levine D, A Klein, and M Morrissey. Reliability of isokinetic concentric closed kinematic chain testing of the hip and knee extensors. 1991. *Isokinetic Exer Sci* 1: 146–52.

16. Morrissey M, E Harman, and M Johnson. 1995. Resistance training modes: Specificity and effectiveness. *Med Sci Sports Exer* 27: 648–60.

17. Perrin D. 1993. *Isokinetic assessment and exercise*, 112–14, 168–73. Champaign, IL: Human Kinetics.

18. Perrine J. 1986. The biophysics of maximal muscle power outputs: Methods and problems of measurement. In *Human muscle power*, ed. N Jones, N McCartney, and A McComas, 16. Champaign, IL: Human Kinetics.

19. Perrine J and V Edgerton. 1978. Muscle force-velocity and power-velocity relationships under isokinetic loading. *Med Sci Sports* 10: 159–66.

20. Rizzardo M, G Bay, and J Wessel. 1988. Eccentric and concentric torque and power of the knee extensors of females. *Can J Sport Sci* 66: 707–13.

21. Smidt G. 1994. Current open and closed kinetic chain concepts—clarifying or confusing? *Ortho Sports Phys Ther* 20: 235.

22. Steindler A. 1955. *Kinesiology of the human body under normal and pathological conditions*. Springfield, IL: Charles C Thomas.

23. Stuart M, D Meglan, G Lutz, E Growney, and K An. 1996. Comparison of intersegmental tibiofemoral joint forces and muscle activity during various closed kinetic chain exercises. *Am J Sports Med* 24: 792–99.

24. Weiss L, G Relyea, C Ashley, and R Propst. In press. Predicting depth vertical jumping distance. *Isokinetics Exer Sci.*

25. Weiss L, A Fry, E Gossick, J Webber, and E Barrow. 1998. Reliability of bench press velocity-spectrum testing. *Meas Phys Educ Exer Sci* 2: 243–52.

26. Weiss L and G Relyea. 1997. Velocity-spectrum testing using a closed kinetic chain. *Isokinetics Exer Sci* 6: 197–202.

27. Weiss L, G Relyea, C Ashley, and R Propst. 1997. The use of velocity-spectrum squats and body composition to predict standing vertical jump ability. *J Strength Cond Res* 11: 14–20.

28. Weiss L, G Relyea, C Ashley, and R Propst. 1996. Reliability of selected measures of musculoskeletal function obtained during closed kinetic chain exercises at multiple velocities. *J Strength Cond Res* 10: 45–50.

29. Wickiewicz T, R Roy, P Powell, J Perrine, and V Edgerton. 1984. Muscle architecture and force-velocity relationships in humans. *J Appl Physiol: Respirat Environ Exer Physiol* 57: 435–43.

30. Wilson G, R Newton, A Murphy, and B Humphries. 1993. The optimal training load for the development of dynamic athletic performance. *Med Sci Sports Exer* 25: 1279–86.

# Chapter 10

# Control of Voluntary Contraction Force

Tammy M. Owings and Mark D. Grabiner

Isokinetic dynamometry, which has entered its third decade, has become widely used in the research arena. By design, isokinetic instrumentation provides a safe exercise environment; the devices offer a desirable level of control over variables such as the range of joint motion, the minimum and maximum speeds that can be obtained during joint motion, the minimum and maximum forces that are allowed during joint motion, and the type of muscle contraction that can be performed. The instruments have the capacity to store digital signals representing angular displacement, angular speed, and force or moment. These clinically attractive qualities are no less attractive in a research environment.

The most popular application of isokinetic instrumentation in the research environment has been to acquire quantitative information about the strength and power capabilities of a particular skeletal muscle group under the specific conditions of the test. Underlying the expression of muscle strength and power are the anatomical, physiological, and contractile properties of the involved skeletal muscle. Anatomical properties include the cross-sectional area of the muscle, the orientation of muscle fibers within the muscle, and the relationship between the length of the muscle and the muscle tendons. Physiological factors include the fiber composition of the muscle. Contractile properties of muscle derive from force-velocity and length-tension relationships. Further, neural factors (9), which include the ability to deliver appropriately coordinated activation signals to the agonist, synergistic, and antagonistic elements of a muscle group, make a large contribution to strength. Ultimately the control of motor units via recruitment and rate coding is reliant upon these neural factors.

The purpose of this chapter is to provide an introduction to the anatomy and physiology that underlie the control of submaximum voluntary force, to present the results of a recent research undertaking related to the control of submaximum voluntary force that has used isokinetic dynamometry and that has immediate functional application, and lastly, to serve as a catalyst for those who implement isokinetic dynamometry to undertake further systematic study of the ability to control submaximum voluntary force.

# Overview of Motor Units

A motor unit is the functional component of skeletal muscle. The structural elements of a motor unit are an alpha ($\alpha$) motoneuron, the cell body of which resides in the ventral horn of the spinal cord, a single motor axon, and all of the muscle fibers activated by the motor axon. The number of muscle fibers innervated by a motor axon, the innervation ratio, varies widely among muscles by over two orders of magnitude, from 15 to 1900, and dictates the level of fine control muscle force that may be exerted. The innervation ratio is thus inversely related to fine muscle force control. The number of motor units within muscles also can vary over a range of at least an order of magnitude, from 100 to 1000.

The basic mechanical output of the motor unit is the twitch force. A single impulse that descends the nerve axon causes an activation of the muscle fibers in the motor unit and gives rise to a twitch that may be characterized by three values. These values are the peak twitch force, the elapsed time from the twitch force onset to the peak force, referred to as contraction time, and the elapsed time required for the force level to diminish from its peak value to one-half of the peak value, referred to as the half-relaxation time. These aspects of a motor unit twitch force are illustrated in figure 10.1 with data generated using a mathematical model of a motor unit pool consisting of 100 motor units (14).

A series of impulses descending the nerve axon causes the individual twitch forces to sum temporally. The maximum force so generated, called the peak tetanic force, is generally much larger than the twitch force, depending on the twitch/tetanus ratio of the particular motor unit. Figure 10.2, *a* through *c*, illustrates the influence on the force output of increased neural drive to a motor unit. In figure 10.2*a*, motor unit number 10 of 100, having a peak twitch force of 10 units, is receiving activation associated with 10% of the maximum neural drive available. Because the frequency of motor unit discharge is low, the motor unit twitch forces do not summate to a large extent. In figure 2*b* the neural drive has been increased to 30%. One of the effects of the increased discharge frequency of the motor unit is that the twitch forces sum nearly to the maximum extent, generating a nearly constant force of approximately 100 units. However, there are significant oscillations in the force level that represent the insufficiency of the discharge frequency to fully fuse the twitch forces. The insufficiency in neural drive is practically eliminated in figure 10.2*c* in which the level of neural drive is 50% of maximum. A decrease in the elapsed time to reach the maximum force output is also evident in comparing figure 10.2, *b* and *c*.

The variety of structural and physiological differences among motor units gives rise to an extraordinary number of degrees of freedom over which the

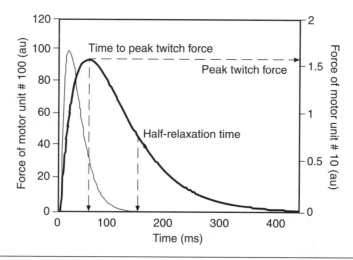

**Figure 10.1**   Two motor units from a simulation of a motor unit pool consisting of 100 motor units. Motor unit twitch forces, in arbitrary units, are modeled as second order critically damped functions. The smaller of the two motor units shown with the thick line is plotted on the right vertical axis and is labeled to include three descriptive variables of motor unit twitch forces.

See Grabiner et al. (14).

central nervous system must exert control to control muscle force. This represents a potentially huge computational problem to be solved by the central nervous system. The problem, simply stated, is Which motor units should be activated given a desired mechanical output? This problem requires the central nervous system to control two processes: recruitment and discharge frequency. Recruitment refers to the number of motor units that are activated. Discharge frequency refers to rate, expressed in Hz, at which a particular motor unit receives neural impulses. To underscore the nature of the problem that must be solved, consider a muscle composed of 100 motor units. Further, for this example, consider that the central nervous system has 100 discrete levels of neural drive with level 100 being that at which all 100 motor units are recruited and are discharging at their maximum discharge frequency. The total number of combinations of active units that are possible under conditions of free and unsequenced selection is

$$N = \sum_{k=1}^{100} (100! \, / \, k!(100-k)!)$$

Thus, unless the central nervous system invokes some type of simplifying rule, it is faced with $10^{30}$ combinations of active motor units for a single, small muscle composed of 100 motor units (17). Imagine the magnitude of the overall control problem when the coordination of numerous agonist, synergist, and antagonist muscles is required to generate even simple functional joint motion. The central nervous system solves the problem essentially by taking advantage of the spectrum of structural and physiological differences between motor units. Denny-Brown and Pennybacker (6) reported that a specific task was always initiated by activation of the same motor unit and that larger force was achieved by activation of inactive motor units in a particular sequence. Further, it was observed that the early recruitment of small motor units was followed by recruitment of larger motor units. Henneman (16) proposed the "size principle" to explain the phenomenon of orderly recruitment. The size principle states that the order in which motor units are recruited is reliant on the size of the motor unit. The size of the motor unit may be represented in a number of ways, including the amount of neural drive required to initiate motor unit discharge, the number muscle fibers innervated by the α-motoneuron, and the histological and contractile properties of the muscle fibers.

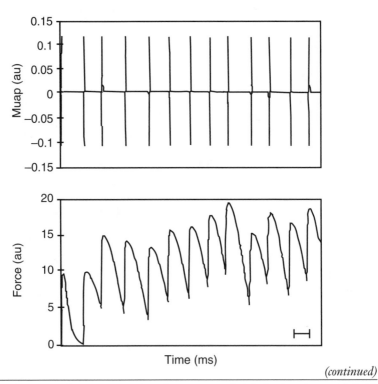

a                                   Time (ms)

(continued)

**Figure 10.2**   A single motor unit (number 10 out of 100) discharging at (*a*) 5, (*b*) 10, and (*c*) 30 Hz. The horizontal bar represents 150 ms. The vertical axes are in arbitrary units. With increased discharge frequency the changes in maximum force, the rate of force generation, and the oscillations in the constant force phase, especially in panels *b* and *c* are notable.

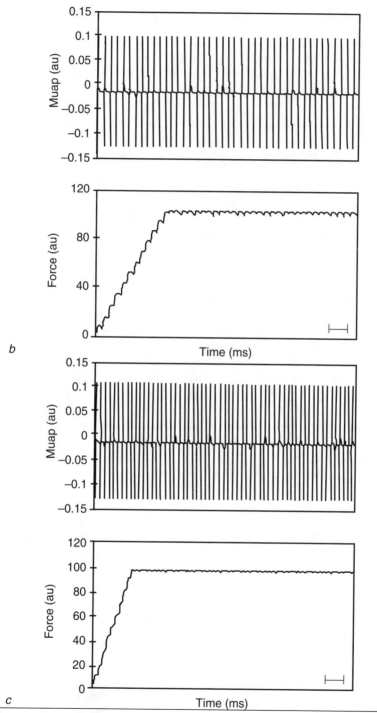

*b*

*c*

**Figure 10.2** *(continued)*

# Changes to Motor Units With Aging

Aging represents a model system for the study of the relationships between changes in motor function and underlying motor unit behavior. The age-related loss of muscle mass and muscle strength has long been recognized, although not entirely understood. For example, the age-related decrease in maximum voluntary strength does not necessarily parallel that predicted by the age-related loss of muscle mass (13, 21). Another set of independent observations have been made in conjunction with space-science in which muscle strength loss generally tends to be larger than that accounted for by muscle atrophy (1, 3, 8, 20). At least part of the age-related loss of muscle mass, referred to as sarcopenia, relates to the atrophy of muscle fibers, which is particularly prevalent in the fibers of large, or type II, motor units. However, aging is also associated with a reduction in the number of muscle fibers, which is likely related to spinal motoneuron apoptosis (10, 12) and also seems prevalent in type II motor units (18). The death of spinal motoneurons, beginning perhaps in the sixth decade and particularly marked by age 70 (7), may not necessarily be associated with the loss of all of the muscle fibers innervated by their axons. Surviving motoneurons may reinnervate the abandoned muscle fibers. At least in animal models, re-innervation of muscle fibers by the motoneurons of small, or type I, motor units appears to be particularly prevalent. This process, called collateral re-innervation, results in an increase in the innervation ratio of the surviving motor units, the result of which is to alter the relationship between the neural drive to the reorganized motor unit and the force output of the motor unit.

There have been a number of investigations related to the effects of age on the mechanical output of human upper and lower extremity motor units. The results seem consistent with expected outcomes of collateral reinnervation of muscle fibers by the motoneurons of small, type I motor units. On average, peak tension time decreases 31% and contraction time (measured as the sum of time to peak tension plus the half-relaxation time) increases 28% (21, see their table 1).

Age-related changes in the innervation ratio of motor units that are associated with these contraction changes led Galganski, Fuglevand, and Enoka (12) to hypothesize that the ability to finely grade, or control, muscle force would be diminished in older adults. Younger and older adults were required to maintain an isometric contraction of the first dorsal interosseous muscle (this muscle abducts the index finger). Four levels of isometric contraction were studied: 5, 20, 35, and 50% of the measured maximum voluntary force. A target force level was displayed on an oscilloscope and the subjects were instructed to develop voluntary force and maintain the level as close as possible to the target level for 20 s. The results of the study revealed that compared to younger adults, older adults demonstrated diminished ability to maintain steady submaximum isometric index finger abduction force. Further, the force output measured for single motor units discharging at low frequencies was larger in the older adults. Thus, this study linked age-related reorganization of motor units to a diminished functional outcome. This finding offered an alternative to that offered by Cole (4), who reported that older subjects exert larger grip forces compared to younger adults during tasks requiring small object manipulation.

Keen, Yue, and Enoka (15) extended the results of Galganski and coworkers (12) by testing the hypothesis that increasing motor unit force would further decrease the ability of older adults to maintain a constant isometric index finger abduction force. In that study, younger and older adults participated in a 12-week program designed to increase the strength and size of the first dorsal interosseous muscle. At the end of the training period, the younger and older adults had increased their isometric index finger abduction maximum voluntary contraction (MVC) by 37% and 41%, respectively. The hypothesis that the increase in MVC would be associated with a diminished ability to maintain constant isometric index finger abduction force was not supported, however. Indeed, the ability to maintain the constant force improved.

# Research Methods

Despite the potential functional implications, the ability to control voluntary force, and the underlying physiological changes that impair control such as aging, disease, and injury, has not been well studied. We have conducted a study using younger and older adults to investigate the utility of a technique to provide answers to questions about motor control that are not provided using other existing isokinetic procedures. Based on the previously described research, in the presently reported study, we expected that compared to younger subjects, older adults would demonstrate diminished ability to accurately and smoothly control submaximum isokinetic knee extension moments.

## Subjects

Ten healthy, community dwelling older men and women, average age 75 yr, were recruited to participate in this study. Ten healthy younger adults, average age 30.3 yr, also participated in the study.

## Pretest-Posttest Protocol

Each subject participated in a pretest and posttest session, separated by a 4-wk training program. The pretest and posttest consisted of measuring maximum voluntary isokinetic contractions (MVC) of the knee joint extensor muscles performed concentrically and eccentrically and measuring the ability to generate a voluntary submaximum knee extension force to a designated, constant target level during concentric and eccentric isokinetic contractions. The pre- and posttests as well as the training sessions were conducted on a Kin-Com isokinetic dynamometer. All tests and training were conducted at an isokinetic velocity of 15°/s through a 50° range of knee joint motion (from approximately 90° of knee flexion to 40° of knee flexion). Based on the absence of reports in the published literature, the task appears to be a novel application of isokinetic dynamometry but one for which the instrumentation is perfectly suited.

The testing protocol consisted of conditions during which knee extension MVCs were performed concentrically and eccentrically followed by conditions during which the ability to control dynamic knee extension moment was measured. The intent of the task in these conditions was to assess the extent to which subjects could develop and maintain a constant level, target knee extension moment through the range of motion. Four target knee extension moments, performed both concentrically and eccentrically, were used. The target knee extension moments were 15%, 30%, 45%, and 60% of the previously established MVC.

To assist the subjects in performing the task, real-time visual feedback of the target knee extension moment and the voluntary knee extension moment was provided during each trial using an oscilloscope placed in front of the subject. On the oscilloscope were displayed two traces. One trace displayed the target knee extension moment, and the second trace displayed the actual knee extension moment generated by the subject. The subjects were instructed to generate a knee extension force that would remain as close as possible to the displayed target throughout the entire range of knee extension motion.

The activation signal from the vastus lateralis was collected using a pair of surface electrodes. The detected signal was digitized at 1 kHz and stored with the digitized force, position, and velocity signals from the dynamometer.

The protocol is quite different from those experiments discussed in a previous section in which subjects maintained a constant level isometric moment. In those experiments the oscillations of the generated moment about the target force were measured and from those measurements an index of steadiness was derived. In those experiments, however, because the contractions were static there were no influences exerted on the muscle moment by the changes in moment arm expected with dynamic contractions. Further, there were no influences exerted on the muscle moment by the force-velocity and length-tension properties of skeletal muscle. For example, during knee flexion, the moment arm of the quadriceps femoris component changes in a nonlinear manner. Figure 10.3 displays the variation in the anatomical moment arms of the knee extensors as a function of the knee flexion angle. These relationships were computed as fifth order polynomials based upon a weighted average of the model data of Delp (5) and the tendon travel data of Fick (11), Spoor and van Leeuwen (22), and Visser and coworkers (23). To maintain a steady knee extension moment through a range of motion requires the ability to change the level of neural drive to the muscle to accommodate the changes in moment arm.

In addition to the influence on knee extension moment by the quadriceps moment arm, the changes in knee joint angle impose subsequent changes in muscle length and, therefore, independently affect the maximum force potential of the quadriceps components. During concentric contractions, the quadriceps muscles decrease in length. Because of the tendency of shortened muscle

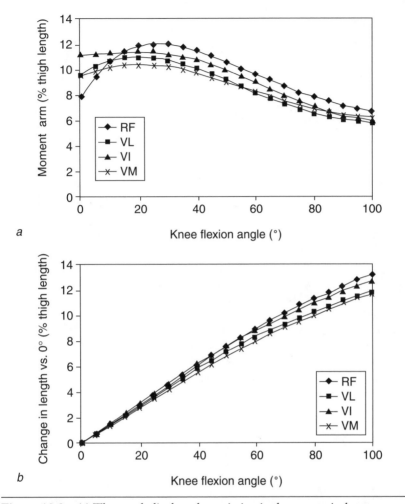

**Figure 10.3** (*a*) The graph displays the variation in the anatomical moment arms of the knee extensors as a function of the knee flexion angle. Data comprised moment arm estimates at each 5° interval, with cubic spline interpolation and linear extrapolation employed for graphical data sources and a hip position of 0° assumed for the model data. Moment arms were normalized to a percentage of thigh length before averaging, with the average of the male and female median thigh lengths from Webb Associates (24) used for the data of Fick (11). In combining the data from different sources, the model and tendon travel data were weighted equally and each source of tendon travel data was weighted equally. As little reliable data existed for the moment arms of the vastii across the full range of knee motion, the rectus femoris data of Fick (11) was included in the vastii moment arm calculations but with a weighting half that of the other tendon travel data. (*b*) The change in muscle length as a function of knee joint flexion angle.

to generate less active force, described by the length-tension relationship, maintaining constant force output would be expected to require an increase in neural drive. The contrary is true during eccentric contractions in which increasing knee flexion angle causes the quadriceps components to increase in length. Thus, to maintain a steady knee extension force, neural drive must be reduced. Because the changes in moment arm and the changes in muscle length are not parallel, the modulation of neural drive to accommodate the mechanical effects and maintain a steady dynamic knee extension moment becomes somewhat of a complex problem to solve.

## Data Analysis

The outcome variables were the accuracy of submaximum contraction control and the maximum moment that could be generated during an MVC. The accuracy of submaximum contraction control was analyzed during the middle one-third of the range of knee extension motion. The middle one-third of the range of motion was identified using a custom algorithm that operated on the digitized data obtained from the position sensor of the Kin-Com. The stored data, digitized at 1000 Hz, was smoothed using a recursive Butterworth filter prior to analysis. Analysis of the smoothed force data was performed point by point in the analysis window, which was the middle one-third of the range of motion. Analysis consisted of comparing the target moment value to the voluntarily generated moment value and computing an RMS error term. The RMS represents the average absolute error between the target and actual moments and is computed in the following manner:

$$RMS_{error} = \sum_{i=1}^{n} \sqrt{\frac{(x_i - t \arg et)^2}{n}}$$

The accuracy with which a knee extension moment can be generated is not necessarily related to the "smoothness" with which the knee extension moment can be generated. This is highlighted in figure 10.4. In the figure, the two curves, $M_1$ and $M_2$, each of which is sampled at the instant of a hash mark on the time line, have the same RMS error with regard to the target value, given as the dashed line at $t_m$. However, the difference in the smoothness of the two curves is obvious, demonstrating that the accuracy and smoothness of the curves need not be related. To compute the smoothness of the isokinetic knee extension moments, the analysis window used for computation of the RMS error was used. The smoothness of the knee extension moment was represented by the square root of the differentiated, squared, summed, and averaged signal in the analysis window. The resulting value was referred to as the smoothness index.

$$Smoothness\ index = \sqrt{\left( \sum_{i=1}^{n} [dM / dt]_i^2 / n \right)}$$

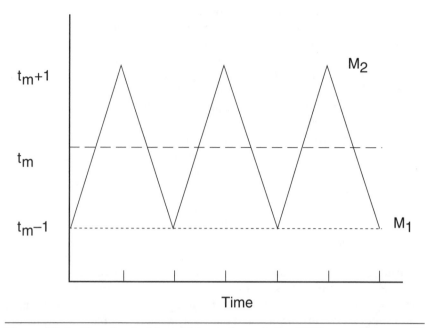

**Figure 10.4**   Two signals, $M_1$ and $M_2$, can have similar RMS errors but very different smoothness indexes thereby suggesting that these two descriptors can provide different information regarding motor control.

## *Training*

The training period was four weeks in length. Each week included two training sessions separated by at least one day. The four-week training period was anticipated to be adequate to induce the neurally mediated changes associated with the motor skill of controlling submaximum knee joint extension moment. However, the short duration of the training period was sufficient to substantially reduce the possibility of there being a trophic effect on the knee joint musculature. Each training session consisted of a series of submaximum concentric and eccentric isokinetic knee extension contractions during which visual feedback was provided. The instructions to the subject were to maintain knee extension force as close as possible to the visually specified target value. The target values were 15, 30, 45, and 60% of the pretest maximum concentric or eccentric knee extension force for weeks one, two, three, and four, respectively. For the 15, 30, 45, and 60% MVC conditions, the subject performed 25, 25, 20, and 15 repetitions, respectively, for both the concentric and eccentric contractions.

Analysis of the digitized EMG signal consisted of full wave rectification followed by integration in the analysis window. The resulting values were expressed as a percentage of the value obtained during the concentric MVC.

Statistically, the design for the RMS error and the smoothness index was treated as a between group (younger adult vs. older adult) 2 by 2 by 4 (pretest/

posttest by concentric/eccentric by submaximum contraction level) repeated measures analysis of variance. The maximum isokinetic knee extension strength was analyzed as a between group 2 by 2 (pretest/posttest by concentric/eccentric) repeated measures analysis of variance. The EMG data were analyzed for the posttest using a between group 2 by 4 (concentric/eccentric by submaximum contraction level) repeated measures analysis of variance. A correlation analysis was conducted to determine the extent to which the RMS error and the smoothness index were codependent. All analyses were conducted using SPSS V7.0. Reporting of the results is presently limited to the between group differences relative to the above mentioned experimental factors without consideration of the higher order interaction effects.

# Test Results

Not unexpectedly, the younger adults were significantly stronger than the older adults for both concentric and eccentric MVC at the time of the pretest and the posttest (see tables 10.1 and 10.2). Following the four-week training program the young adults registered small changes in concentric and eccentric MVC, increases of 3.0% and 8.2%, respectively, but these changes were not significant ($p > .05$). In contrast, and quite surprisingly, the older adults demonstrated significant increases in both concentric and eccentric MVC following the training program of 32% and 11%, respectively.

As indicated by the overall significant main effect of group ($p = .011$), the younger adults tended to have smaller RMS errors than the older adults (see

### Table 10.1    Measures of Knee Extension Strength for Younger Adults (n = 10)

|          | Concentric MVC   | Eccentric MVC    |
|----------|------------------|------------------|
| Pretest  | 219.9 ± 63.0     | 279.6 ± 90.3     |
| Posttest | 226.4 ± 55.1     | 302.7 ± 102.0    |

The values are means ± standard deviations given in pounds.

### Table 10.2    Measures of Knee Extension Strength for Older Adults (n = 10)

|          | Concentric MVC   | Eccentric MVC    |
|----------|------------------|------------------|
| Pretest  | 80.2 ± 45.8      | 136.53 ± 61.3    |
| Posttest | 105.66 ± 50.3    | 150.9 ± 63.4     |

The values are means ± standard deviations given in pounds.

figures 10.5 and 10.6). The interactions between group and submaximum contraction intensity, pretest/posttest, and concentric/eccentric, were significant ($p < .001$, =.004, and <.001, respectively). This was particularly evident for the eccentric contractions.

With regard to the smoothness index, the overall effect of group did not achieve significance ($p = .078$). This result was reflected in the computed power value, 0.423. However, even qualitatively, with possibly one exception, the differences in smoothness of the knee extension moments do not appear to display any systematic age-related differences (see figures 10.7 and 10.8). The interactions between group and submaximum contraction intensity, pretest/posttest, and concentric/eccentric, were significant ($p = .001$, .004, and .001, respectively). The one exception may be reflected in the relationship between smoothness and contraction intensity. For the younger subjects, figure 10.7 illustrates that for both concentric and eccentric contractions, and for the data collected during the pretest and the posttest, the mean values of the smoothness index increase as a function of contraction intensity. This relationship is noticeably different for the older adults.

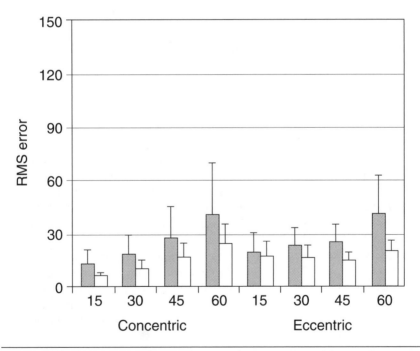

**Figure 10.5**   The RMS error of the younger adults collected during the pretest (shaded bars) and posttest (clear bars) for concentric and eccentric contractions performed at four levels of normalized contraction intensity. For comparison to the data of the older adults (see figure 10.6) the vertical scales are similar. The data represent the mean ± standard deviation (n = 10).

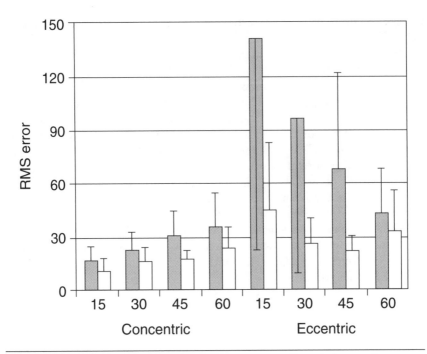

**Figure 10.6**   The RMS error of the older adults collected during the pretest (shaded bars) and posttest (clear bars) for concentric and eccentric contractions performed at four levels of normalized contraction intensity. The data represent the mean ± standard deviation (n = 10). To maintain similar vertical scales for figures 10.5 and 10.6, some standard deviations have been placed in downward direction.

Correlation analysis revealed that the relationships between RMS error and the smoothness indexes were mostly weak to moderate (.05 < $r$ < .50, see tables 10.3 and 10.4) although some relationships were strong ($r$ > .75). Only 7 of the 32 correlations computed achieved statistical significance and there was no distinct pattern that emerged and to which a functional relevance might be attributed.

A striking difference in the pattern of vastus lateralis activation was found (see figure 10.9). For the younger subjects, the activation levels during eccentric contractions were lower than the activation levels during the concentric contractions. This is generally an expected observation. In contrast, for the older adults, the activation levels during the eccentric contractions were larger than those of the concentric contractions. This pattern was the source of the significant group by concentric/eccentric interaction term ($p$ = .004). For the younger subjects, the concentric activation levels were significantly larger than the eccentric activation levels for the 45% and 60% MVCs ($p$ = .028 and .032, respectively). For the older adults, the eccentric activation levels were significantly larger than the concentric activation levels for the 45% and 60% MVCs ($p$ = .031 and .037, respectively).

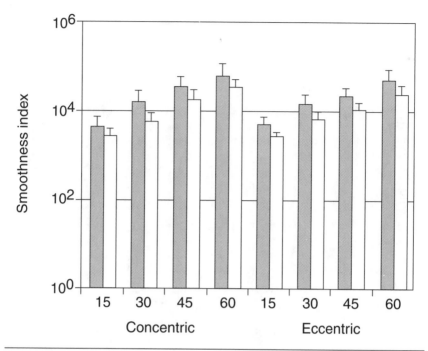

**Figure 10.7** The smoothness index of the data for younger adults collected during the pretest (shaded bars) and posttest (clear bars) for concentric and eccentric contractions performed at four levels of normalized contraction intensity. Note that the vertical scale is logarithmic. The data represent the mean ± standard deviation (n = 10).

In summary, the results generally suggest the following:

- Accurately generating submaximum isokinetic knee extension moments appears to be a more difficult task for older adults compared to younger adults, particularly during eccentric contractions.

- During eccentric contractions older adults demonstrate larger vastus lateralis activation than is observed during concentric contractions of similar magnitude.

- Smoothly generating submaximum isokinetic knee extension moments appears to be an easier task for older adults than for younger adults.

- The described methods of quantifying accuracy and smoothness represent different aspects of isokinetic knee extension motor control.

# Test Conclusions

Using a small muscle of the hand, Galgansky and coworkers (12) and Keen and coworkers (15) demonstrated that expected age-related changes in the organization

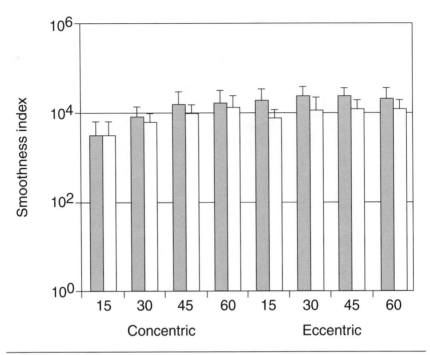

**Figure 10.8** The smoothness index of the data for the older adults collected during the pretest (shaded bars) and posttest (clear bars) for concentric and eccentric contractions performed at four levels of normalized contraction intensity. Note that the vertical scale is logarithmic. The data represent the mean ± standard deviation (n = 10).

and control of motor units is associated with a potentially important functional outcome—diminished ability to accurately control isometric contraction force. Using an isokinetic dynamometer, we extended the experimental paradigm of those authors to study a locomotor muscle group, the knee extensor muscles, and to include concentric and eccentric contractions. Based on the prior work, we expected that compared to younger subjects, older adults would demonstrate diminished ability to accurately and smoothly control submaximum isokinetic knee extension moments. The results were mixed relative to our expectations but nevertheless have increased our enthusiasm for further developing this application of isokinetic dynamometry. Our expectations with regard to the accuracy of control were supported in that the older adults were generally less accurate in their control than younger adults, a finding that was amplified during eccentric contractions. Our expectations were not supported relative to the smoothness of control. However, this may reflect to a greater extent the fact that the study was underpowered to detect differences of this size, rather than indicating the absence of between group differences. The correlation analysis between RMS error and smoothness index, which suggested that these variables represent different aspects of isokinetic knee extension motor control, provides a motivation to further

## Table 10.3 Correlation Matrix Between the Pretest and Posttest RMS Error and Smoothness Indices (SI) for the Concentric Contractions

| | SIpre C15 | SIpre C30 | SIpre C45 | SIpre C60 | SIpost C15 | SIpost C30 | SIpost C45 | SIpost C60 |
|---|---|---|---|---|---|---|---|---|
| **RMSpre C15** | .13(.07) | | | | | | | |
| **RMSpre C30** | | −.06(.41) | | | | | | |
| **RMSpre C45** | | | −.16(.54) | | | | | |
| **RMSpre C60** | | | | .08(.75*) | | | | |
| **RMSpost C15** | | | | | .48(.70*) | | | |
| **RMSpost C30** | | | | | | .58(.04) | | |
| **RMSpost C45** | | | | | | | .47(.70*) | |
| **RMSpost C60** | | | | | | | | .58(.61) |

Correlations were computed using the data from the older adults (younger adults). $p < 0.05$.

## Table 10.4 Correlation Matrix Between the Pretest and Posttest RMS Error and Smoothness Indices (SI) for the Eccentric Contractions

| | SIpre E15 | SIpre E30 | SIpre E45 | SIpre E60 | SIpost E15 | SIpost E30 | SIpost E45 | SIpost E60 |
|---|---|---|---|---|---|---|---|---|
| **RMSpre E15** | .75*(.96)* | | | | | | | |
| **RMSpre E30** | | .51(.73*) | | | | | | |
| **RMSpre E45** | | | .07(.32) | | | | | |
| **RMSpre E60** | | | | .26(.48) | | | | |
| **RMSpost E15** | | | | | .68*(.06) | | | |
| **RMSpost E30** | | | | | | .80(.55) | | |
| **RMSpost E45** | | | | | | | −.07(.26) | |
| **RMSpost E60** | | | | | | | | .07(.69) |

Correlations were computed using the data from the older adults (younger adults). $p < 0.05$.

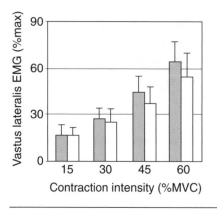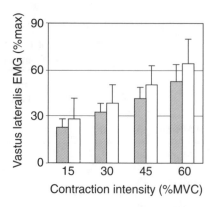

**Figure 10.9**    The normalized EMG acquired during the posttest from the vastus lateralis during concentric (shaded bars) and eccentric (clear bars) isokinetic knee extension at four levels of normalized contraction intensity. The left panel is the data of the younger adults and the right panel is the data from the older adults. The data represent the mean ± standard deviation (n = 10).

explore this variable and methods by which it may be better quantified. The solutions to these technical questions, hardware and software, may enhance data collection and analysis methods. Improved methods will allow more accurate quantification of the underlying physiological mechanisms that give rise to the observed age-related differences and the functional outcome of these changes.

There were two interesting outcomes of the present study, one of which had not been previously reported in the literature. The first was that older adults demonstrated improved concentric and eccentric knee extension strength as a result of a short-term training protocol emphasizing accurate control of knee extension moment (19). During the training protocol the contraction intensities did not exceed 60% of the MVC measured at the time of the pretest. Thus, a training protocol consisting of entirely submaximum contractions was effective in increasing knee extension strength. This observation seems to merit further systematic study.

Secondly, the older adults demonstrated a different pattern of activation during eccentric contraction than would normally be expected. Specifically, for an eccentric contraction that creates a similar knee extension moment magnitude as a concentric contraction, the level of activation was larger than for the concentric contraction. Two questions are thus raised. First, is this activation pattern related to the differences observed between the younger and older adults relative to the ability to accurately and smoothly generate knee extension moment? Second, what are the underlying changes to the morphology and control of motor units that result in the activation pattern?

## Summary

An isokinetic dynamometer was used to test the ability of younger and older adults to accurately control the magnitude of a voluntary knee extension moment performed concentrically and eccentrically. This application of the dynamometer was an outcome of a number of published studies demonstrating that, compared to younger adults, older adults have a diminished capability to maintain a steady isometric contraction of a hand muscle. An underlying contention of these studies is that the ability to finely control contraction force is an important aspect of motor function. The results of the present study suggest that the smoothness index may represent a different aspect of motor control than the accuracy of control. This possibility merits further systematic investigation. The results of the present study confirmed that older adults demonstrate reduced control of isokinetic knee extension contraction, especially eccentric contraction. This was accompanied by an unexpected and novel finding of larger levels of muscle activation during eccentric contraction than concentric contraction at the same contraction level. Although the study was not designed to investigate the underlying age-related mechanisms that result in these observations, the consistency of the findings with those of previous investigators using a different model system and the novel characteristics of some of the findings provide a level of enthusiasm for the further development and utilization of isokinetic dynamometry for the explicit purpose of studying motor control.

# References

1. Adams GR, Hather BM, and Dudley GA. 1994. Effect of short-term unweighting on human skeletal muscle strength and size. *Aviation, Space, and Environmental Medicine* 65: 1116–21.

2. Bennett JG and Stauber WT. 1986. Evaluation and treatment of anterior knee pain using eccentric exercise. *Medicine and Science in Sports and Exercise* 18: 526–30.

3. Berg HE, Larsson L, and Tesch PA. 1997. Lower limb skeletal muscle function after six weeks of bed rest. *Journal of Applied Physiology* 82: 182–88.

4. Cole KJ. 1991. Grip force control in old age. *Journal of Motor Behavior* 23: 251–58.

5. Delp SL. 1990. Surgery simulation: A computer graphics system to analyze and design musculoskeletal reconstruction of the lower limb. PhD dissertation, Stanford University.

6. Denny-Brown D and Pennybacker JB. 1938. Fibrillation and fasciculation in voluntary muscle. *Brain* 61: 311–33.

7. Doherty TJ, Vandervoort AA, and Brown WF. 1993. Effects of aging on the motor unit: A brief review. *Canadian Journal of Applied Physiology* 18: 331–58.

8. Dudley GA, Duvoisin MR, Covertino VA, and Buchanan P. 1989. Alterations in the in vivo torque-velocity relationship of human skeletal muscle following 30 days exposure to simulated microgravity. *Aviation, Space, and Environmental Medicine* 60: 659–63.

9. Enoka RM and Fuglevand AJ. 1993. Neuromuscular basis of the maximum voluntary force capacity of muscle. In *Current issues in biomechanics*, ed. M.D. Grabiner, 215–35. Champaign, IL: Human Kinetics.

10. Enoka RM. 1997. Neural strategies in the control of muscle force. *Muscle and Nerve* 5(Suppl.): S66–69.

11. Fick AE. 1879. Uber zweigelenkige muskeln. *Arch Anat Physiol (Anat Abt)* 201–39.

12. Galganski M, Fuglevand AJ, and Enoka RM. 1993. Reduced control of motor output in a human hand muscle of elderly subjects during submaximal contractions. *Journal of Neurophysiology* 69: 2108–15.

13. Grabiner MD and Enoka RM. 1995. Changes in movement capabilities with aging. In *Exercise and sport science reviews*, ed. JO Holloszy, 65–104. Baltimore: Williams & Wilkins.

14. Grabiner MD, Owings TM, George M, and Enoka RM. July 1995. Eccentric contractions are specified a priori by the CNS. Proceedings of the 15th Congress of the International Society of Biomechanics at Jyvaskyla, Finland.

15. Keen DA, Yue GH, and Enoka RM. 1994. Training-related enhancement in the control of motor output in elderly humans. *Journal of Applied Physiology* 77: 2648–58.

16. Henneman E. 1957. Relation between the size of neurons and their susceptibility to discharge. *Science* 126: 1345–46.

17. Henneman E. 1990. Comments on the logical basis of muscle control. In *The segmental motor system*, ed. MD Binder and LM Mendell, vii–x. New York: Oxford University Press.

18. Larsson L, Sjödin B, and Karlsson J. 1978. Histochemical and biochemical changes in human skeletal muscle with age in sedentary males age 22 to 65 years. *Acta Physiologica Scandinavica* 103: 31–39.

19. Owings TM and Grabiner MD. August 1995. Submaximum stimulus intensity increases maximum strength in the elderly. Paper presented at the American Society of Biomechanics in Palo Alto, California.

20. Ploutz-Snyder LL, Tesch PA, Crittenden DJ, and Dudley GA. 1995. Effect of unweighting on skeletal muscle use during exercise. *Journal of Applied Physiology* 79: 168–75.

21. Roos MR, Rice CL, and Vandervoort AA. 1997. Age-related changes in motor unit function. *Muscle and Nerve* 20: 679–90.

22. Spoor CW and van Leeuwen JL. 1992. Knee muscle moment arms from MRI and from tendon travel. *Journal of Biomechanics* 25: 201–6.

23. Visser JJ, Hoogkamer JE, Bobbert MF, and Huijing PA. 1990. Length and moment arm of human leg muscles as a function of knee and hip joint angles. *European Journal Applied Physiology* 61: 453–60.

24. Webb Associates. 1978. *Anthropometry for designers*, Volume I. NASA Reference Publication No. 1024. Washington, DC: National Aeronautics and Space Administration.

# Acknowledgments

The authors wish to express gratitude to Michael J. Pavol for supplying the data on quadriceps components moment arms and muscle excursion found in figure 10.3. The authors also gratefully acknowledge funding provided for this work by Bauerfiend, USA and The Chattanooga Group.

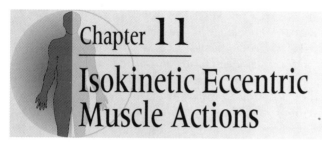

# Chapter 11
## Isokinetic Eccentric Muscle Actions

William R. Holcomb

Originally, isokinetic dynamometers provided resistance for only concentric muscle actions. However, the Kinetic Communicator (Kin-Com) was modified to provide the necessary movement that is resisted during eccentric muscle actions as well. Today, a number of isokinetic dynamometers are available that provide for eccentric muscle actions (e.g., Kin-Com, Cybex, Biodex). This chapter is devoted to a discussion of the characteristics of isokinetic eccentric muscle actions and the specific implications of strength training with this unique type of resistance. It defines eccentric muscle actions, describes the plyometric effect, addresses the concepts of mode, speed, and joint angle specificity, and discusses implications for effective resistance training. This should provide the reader with information required for using isokinetic eccentric muscle actions for strength training.

## Characteristics of Eccentric Muscle Actions

An eccentric muscle action occurs when a muscle is required to lower a load with a controlled movement in the direction of the force of gravity. Practical examples of eccentric muscle actions include descending stairs or lowering a child into a crib. Eccentric muscle actions also occur in free weight training when the weight is lowered prior to lifting. In this case the muscle is lengthened while actively producing tension. Conversely, lifting a load against the force of gravity requires a concentric muscle action. Here, the muscle shortens while producing sufficient tension to overcome the resistance provided by the weight being lifted. It is important to compare and contrast eccentric and concentric muscle actions in order to understand the unique benefits of eccentric training.

### Physiology

In order to understand the physiology of eccentric and concentric muscle actions, an understanding of muscle anatomy is required. The muscle is composed of two mechanical components: a contractile component (CC) and a noncontractile component. The noncontractile component is composed of two elastic components that are named based on their relationship to the CC. These are the series elastic component (SEC), which consists primarily of the tendon, and the parallel elastic component (PEC), which consists of the connective tissue sheath and sarcolemma. During an isolated concentric muscle action, the force required to raise the load is provided entirely by the myofibrils that constitute the CC. However, when a load is lowered with an eccentric muscle action, the force is provided by the sum of the active contraction of the CC and by the passive resistance to stretch provided by the SEC and PEC (2).

# Efficiency of the Elastic Component

Because of the passive contribution of the noncontractile elastic component, the tension required by the CC to lower a given load is less than required by the CC to raise the same load. Due to the need for less tension, fewer motor units are activated during the eccentric muscle action. Thus for a given force output, the energy required for an eccentric muscle action is less than that required for a concentric muscle action. Consequently, eccentric muscle actions are considered more efficient. This has been observed by using electromyography (EMG), which measures electrical activity that is indicative of the relative number of muscle fibers being recruited (11, 22).

# Force Production

In addition to improved efficiency, the contribution of the elastic component enables a greater maximum force output during eccentric muscle actions when compared to concentric muscle actions or isometric muscle actions (production of tension within a muscle without a change in muscle length). This has been observed in a number of studies with several muscle groups. Two early studies demonstrated this using the elbow flexors. Doss and Karpovich (3) developed a dynamometer that continuously measured isotonic force throughout the range of motion (ROM) during both concentric and eccentric muscle actions. They then measured force production during isometric muscle actions at various increments in the ROM. The average force productions were then compared and Doss and Karpovich reported the eccentric force output to be 13.5% greater and concentric force output to be 23% less than the isometric force output of the elbow flexors. These results were supported by the results of Singh and Karpovich (16) using a similar dynamometer that measured force throughout the ROM. They found the eccentric force output of the elbow flexors to be 32.7% greater than the concentric force output. In more recent studies, the isokinetic dynamometer was used to compare force production during different muscle actions at various speeds. Walmsley, Pearson, and Stymiest (20) showed greater force output during eccentric muscle actions of the wrist extensors at all test velocities when compared to force output during an isometric muscle action. The mean isometric peak torque was 0.89 kg as compared to mean eccentric peak torques ranging from .99 kg to 1.12 kg across three test velocities. Westing and Seger (23) further investigated force production with different muscle actions and velocities using the knee joint in both male and female subjects. Westing and Seger measured force produced during concentric and eccentric knee flexion and extension at velocities ranging from 60°/s to 360°/s using female subjects. Mean concentric torques were significantly lower than the corresponding eccentric torques at each test velocity. In a similar study, Westing, Cresswell, and Thorstensson (22) supported these findings using only knee extension in male subjects. For each test velocity, eccentric torque was greater than concentric torque. This difference in force production ranged from 20% to 146%.

# The Force-Velocity Relationship

A relationship exists between force output and the rate by which muscles change length. This has been called the force-velocity relationship and is best described graphically (see figures 11.1 and 11.2). Two important points are illustrated with these figures. First, the forces produced during eccentric muscle actions are greater than the forces produced during isometric muscle actions, and the forces produced during concentric muscle actions are the smallest. Secondly, there is a direct relationship between increasing velocity of lengthening (eccentric muscle action) and maximum force output, while there is an inverse relationship between increasing velocity of shortening (concentric muscle action) and maximum force output. The classic force-velocity curve (see figure 11.1) was produced from in vitro isolated animal muscle. This relationship between force and velocity of eccentric muscle actions was reproduced using the human wrist extensors. Walmsley, Pearson, and Stymiest (20)

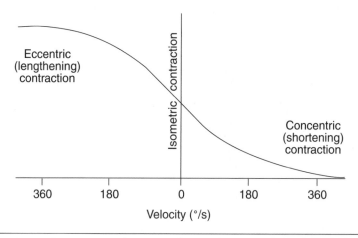

**Figure 11.1**   Concentric and eccentric force-velocity curve resulting from in vitro isolated animal muscle.

From Perrin 1993.

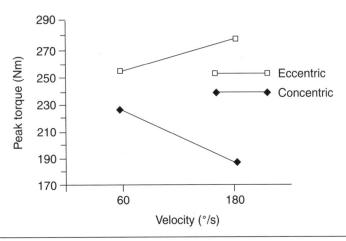

**Figure 11.2**   Concentric and eccentric peak torque of the hamstring muscle group at two test velocities.

From Perrin 1993. Data from *Journal of Orthopaedic and Sports Physical Therapy* 1991.

reported units of measure that are not those typically used to describe the velocity of joint movement or torque output. However, the change in force with increasing velocity is apparent by the reported torque values. The test velocities used were 0.36 cm/s, 0.93 cm/s, and 1.12 cm/s. The corresponding torque values produced during eccentric muscle actions increased with increasing velocity and were reported as 0.99 kg, 1.06 kg, and 1.12 kg, respectively. The force-velocity curve was produced using the human hamstrings and is shown in figure 11.2 (26). The relationship is similar in each figure except the intact hamstring shows less eccentric force increase with increasing velocity. This leveling off of eccentric force is likely due to neural inhibition that serves to prevent muscular injury.

Several studies by Westing and coworkers (22–25) have demonstrated a more pronounced deviation from the classic force-velocity relationship. The first of those studies measured force production with increased velocity using the knee extensors in male subjects. No significant increase in torque was reported as velocity increased. The peak torques at 30°/s, 120°/s, and 270°/s were 287 (± 52.7) Nm, 288 (± 59.0) Nm, and 299 (± 52.7) Nm, respectively (24). It was suspected that a restricting neural mechanism was present that prevented maximum torque output even though a maximum voluntary eccentric action was performed. To test this idea a similar study was conducted with the addition of EMG analysis. In this case neither an increase in torque production nor an increase in EMG activity resulted from an increase in movement velocity (22). The Westing group's conclusions from the first study were further supported by an experiment utilizing maximum voluntary muscle actions superimposed with electrical stimulation. The superimposed muscle actions were compared to isolated maximum voluntary muscle actions to identify any neurological recruitment reserve. An increased torque output was seen with superimposed eccentric muscle actions, but no increased torque output was seen with superimposed isometric or concentric muscle actions (25). Therefore, this restricting neural mechanism appears to affect only eccentric muscle actions of high tension, particularly those that occur at rapid movement velocities.

You can test this force-velocity relationship in a laboratory setting using the isokinetic dynamometer:

1. After a thorough warm-up, have a subject complete three repetitions of concentric knee extension and concentric knee flexion at 60°/s, 120°/s, and 180°/s.

2. Record peak torque for extension and flexion at each speed.

3. Repeat the procedure using eccentric knee extension and eccentric knee flexion.

4. Once again, record peak torque for extension and flexion at each speed.

5. Plot the values for extension and flexion on two separate graphs. It is important to allow sufficient time between sets to insure full recovery. Compare your figure to figure 11.1. The expected result is that your figure will closely match figure 11.1 with the exception of a leveling of eccentric torque with increasing velocity.

6. Repeat the procedures with a different subject, and compare results.

## The Plyometric Effect

During a rapid eccentric muscle action, potential energy is stored in the SEC of the lengthening muscle. If a concentric muscle action immediately follows the eccentric muscle action, the potential energy developed during lengthening can be used by the CC to provide a more forceful muscle contraction. In addition, the muscle spindle will be stretched and stimulated during the rapid eccentric muscle action, which will trigger a reflex contraction of the muscle being stretched. This reflex contraction is called the myotatic or stretch reflex. The more forceful contraction characterized as the plyometric effect is the summation of the voluntary concentric muscle action energized with stored elastic energy and the involuntary contraction provided by the stretch reflex (7).

Early isokinetic dynamometers allowed only concentric muscle actions, where concentric extension was followed by concentric flexion. These protocols could not take advantage of storage and utilization of elastic energy. The isokinetic dynamometer of today will allow manipulation of the type of muscle action used in an exercise bout. If a subject follows a protocol that allows an eccentric muscle action to be followed immediately by a concentric muscle action, elastic energy will be stored during the eccentric muscle action and used during the concentric muscle action for a more forceful contraction. The storage and utilization of elastic energy will increase as the speed of movement increases.

The plyometric effect can be observed in a laboratory setting using the isokinetic dynamometer:

1. After a thorough warm-up, have a subject complete three repetitions of concentric knee extension preceded by concentric knee flexion at 30°/s and 180°/s, and three repetitions of concentric knee extension preceded by eccentric knee flexion at 30°/s and 180°/s.

2. Record peak torque for each of the four conditions and compare torque output. The expected findings will be greater torque output when concentric muscle actions are preceded by eccentric muscle actions. The difference in torque should be greater between conditions at the faster speed of 180°/s than at the slower speed of 30°/s.

# Effectiveness of Eccentric Training

Isokinetic training with only eccentric muscle actions has been shown effective in significantly increasing eccentric strength in as little as six weeks of training. Ryan, Magidow, and Duncan (15) trained the hamstrings with eccentric muscle actions and showed a significant increase in eccentric strength when compared to a control group that did not train. The training group increased peak torque by 52.7 Nm while the control group increased by only 13.5 Nm. Tomberlin and coworkers (19) had similar findings using the hamstrings in female subjects. Subjects trained with eccentric muscle actions at 120°/s and then were tested at 60°/s, 120°/s, and 180°/s. Significantly greater increases were seen in the group that trained versus the control group at each test velocity. The mean percentage of torque increase at each test velocity for the eccentric training group was 18.5%, 22.8%, and 23.0%, respectively. A more recent study examined both the effect of eccentric training and detraining on eccentric strength. It was shown that eight weeks of eccentric-only training resulted in significant eccentric strength gains. The mean strength increase was reported as 29%. Follow-up strength testing indicated that strength gains were retained during eight weeks of detraining (8). The benefit of incorporating eccentric muscle actions in training has been further supported using constant load exercise. Kaminski, Wabbersen, and Murphy (10) found that eccentric-only constant load training improved the one repetition maximum (1 RM) during a constant load knee curl exercise by 28.8%, whereas concentric-only constant load training improved the 1 RM under identical testing procedures by only 19.0%. Eccentric-only training had a significantly greater effect on concentric strength than did concentric-only training.

Closer examination of the results of studies using isokinetic training with eccentric muscle actions has revealed that benefits are not limited to specific eccentric strength gains. This has led researchers to a complex investigation of specificity of training.

# Specificity of Training

The evolution of resistance training equipment has created a variety of exercise parameters that can be manipulated for optimal training. Therefore, the concept of specificity of training has become increasingly important. Specificity of training refers to the degree to which strength gains under certain testing parameters are specific to the parameters used during training. To illustrate, consider an athlete who trains under condition A and then is tested for strength under conditions A and B. Significant strength gains only under test condition A would be indicative of specificity of training. Ideally a training protocol would not show specificity but would produce strength gains that overflow to other strength performance conditions. Three types of training specificity should be considered when training with isokinetics: mode, speed, and joint angle specificity.

## Mode Specificity

The mode of exercise refers to the exercise type. The mode of interest with isokinetic training is the type of muscle action being performed. Concentric, eccentric, and isometric muscle actions will be considered here. Several studies have examined mode specificity with isokinetic training in healthy subjects. Pavone and Moffat (13) studied the effect of training with each of the three muscle actions on isometric strength of the quadriceps. The results showed a significant increase in isometric strength with each training mode, but no significant difference in strength gains was found between the individual training modes. The mean percentage increases for the training groups were 18.7%, 22.8%, and 20.7% for the eccentric, concentric, and isometric training groups, respectively. Ellenbecker, Davies, and Rowinski (5) examined the effect of concentric and eccentric training of the muscles of the rotator cuff on concentric and eccentric strength gains. Subjects trained with concentric or eccentric muscle actions at 60°/s, 180°/s, and 210°/s for six weeks. Subjects were then tested both concentrically and eccentrically at all three training velocities. The results showed a significant increase in both concentric and eccentric strength regardless of the muscle action used during training. Petersen and coworkers (14) conducted a similar study but used the quadriceps and only trained with concentric muscle actions at 120°/s. The results again showed a significant increase in both concentric and eccentric strength. Concentric peak torque increased 11% while eccentric peak torque increased by 18%. These studies support the concept that there is an overflow from the mode of training to strength gains experienced under other testing modes. However, a more recent study that used concentric and eccentric training of the quadriceps reported conflicting results. In this study, Tomberlin and coworkers (19) assigned subjects to one of three groups: concentric training, eccentric training, or no training. After six weeks of training, concentric and eccentric strength gains were assessed at the training speed of 100°/s. Concentric torque gains were twofold in the concentric training group when compared to the eccentric training group. Likewise, eccentric torque gains were twofold in the eccentric training group when compared to the concentric training group. Significantly greater strength gains were seen when strength testing utilized the same mode as that used during training, thus supporting the concept of mode specificity.

To further complicate matters there has been some evidence to suggest that the degree of mode specificity is dependent upon the mode of training. Eccentric training has been shown to be more highly mode specific than concentric training (4). Further research is needed to provide evidence that will answer this important question regarding mode specificity.

## Speed Specificity

The isokinetic dynamometer allows the strength and conditioning professionals to control the speed of exercise used during training. The angular velocity used during training typically ranges from 30°/s to 300°/s. A number of studies have investigated the effect of training at various speeds on strength and power. Significant improvement has been shown with isokinetic training at both high and low speeds (1, 9, 18). With regard to velocity specificity of these improvements, there appears to be a difference when training with concentric versus training with eccentric muscle actions. Concentric training at fast speeds tends to increase strength at both fast and slow speeds, whereas training at slow speeds only increases strength at and slightly above the training speed (1). Eccentric training appears to show even less speed specificity than concentric training does. Eccentric training at one speed has been shown to increase strength at both slower and faster speeds. Duncan and coworkers (4) trained the quadriceps of subjects with either concentric or eccentric muscle actions at 120°/s for six weeks. Subjects were then tested for strength gains concentrically and eccentrically at 60°/s, 120°/s, and 180°/s. Results showed that the eccentric training group had significant gains in eccentric force at all three testing speeds. Conversely, the concentric training group only had significant gains at the highest testing speed of 180°/s. Ryan, Magidow, and Duncan (15) conducted a similar study using only eccentric training of the hamstrings at 120°/s. After six weeks of training, strength testing was conducted at 60°/s, 120°/s, and 180°/s. The results showed that eccentric training at 120°/s significantly increased eccentric force at all three testing speeds. As with mode specificity, the ideal training tool would not demonstrate speed specificity. This would allow training at a single speed with strength improvements that overflow to a variety of testing speeds. A lack of speed specificity would be beneficial in a rehabilitation setting where athletes could train only at the less tension producing higher speeds (concentric) or less tension producing lower speeds (eccentric). This would also be beneficial in a situation where time permitted training at only one speed.

## Joint Angle Specificity

Joint angle specificity has long been a concern when training with isometric muscle actions. Significant strength gains will be seen only within 10° of the angle used during training. A recent study suggests a response to eccentric training that is also specific to joint angle. In this study, subjects trained for eight weeks with eccentric muscle actions through a full ROM. Subjects were tested for maximum isometric strength at three joint angles (15°, 45°, and 75°). Significant strength gains were found at 45° and 75° but not at 15°, which indicated that the effects of eccentric weight training were joint angle specific (21). Further research is needed to answer the question of joint angle specificity.

# Delayed Onset Muscle Soreness (DOMS)

The only down side to eccentric training would appear to be exercise-induced muscle injury, which leads to delayed onset muscle soreness (DOMS). The injury occurs to the myofibril and is therefore considered a microinjury (6, 11). The underlying mechanism is unknown but is thought to be related to a loss of intracellular calcium homeostasis (11). When compared to concentric and isometric training, eccentric training was shown to cause significantly greater DOMS. In addition, a significant decrease in strength has been observed after eccentric training that persists as long as does the soreness (17). The soreness is transient, however, and the athlete will become accustomed to the muscular breakdown associated with subsequent eccentric training bouts. Therefore, muscular soreness is not a tremendous concern for the strength and conditioning professional unless the pain or decreased strength impairs performance.

# Summary

Eccentric isokinetic training is a unique form of resistance training that differs significantly from concentric training in a number of ways. The contribution from the elastic component during eccentric muscle actions allows for more forceful maximum contractions than with concentric muscle actions. In addition, less energy is consumed by the CC to move the same load, which makes eccentric muscle actions more efficient than concentric muscle actions. The elastic component is capable of storing energy during the eccentric muscle action that can be used by the CC in a subsequent action. The force-velocity relationship is reversed with eccentric muscle actions so that the force output increases with increasing velocity of lengthening.

These physiological differences have implications in strength training. The strength and conditioning professional has the ability to use isolated concentric and eccentric muscle actions with isokinetics or in combination. Because almost all sports and activities involve both concentric and eccentric muscle actions, it is recommended that athletes train with both types of muscle action. However, the preponderance of evidence suggests that isokinetic training is not very specific to mode or speed. Therefore, if an athlete has limitations that prevent the performance of all types of resistance, an overflow of strength gains from a specific exercise parameter to other strength performance parameters is likely.

# References

1. Coyle, E.F., D.C. Feiring, T.C. Rotkis, R.W. Cote, F.B. Roby, W. Lee, and J.H. Wilmore. 1981. Specificity of power improvements through slow and fast isokinetic training. *Journal of Applied Psychology* 51: 1437–42.

2. Dean, E. 1988. Physiology and therapeutic implications of negative work: A review. *Physical Therapy* 68: 233–37.

3. Doss, W.S., and P.V. Karpovich. 1965. A comparison of concentric, eccentric, and isometric strength of elbow flexors. *Journal of Applied Physiology* 20: 351–53.

4. Duncan, P.W., J.W. Chandler, D.K. Cavanaugh, K.R. Johnson, and A.G. Buehler. 1989. Mode and speed specificity of eccentric and concentric exercise training. *Journal of Orthopedic and Sports Physical Therapy* 11: 70–75.

5. Ellenbecker, T.S., G.J. Davies, and M.J. Rowinski. 1988. Concentric versus eccentric isokinetic strengthening of the rotator cuff. *American Journal of Sports Medicine* 16: 64–69.

6. Friden, J., M. Sjostrom, and B. Ekblom. 1983. Myofibrillar damage following intense eccentric exercise in man. *International Journal of Sports Medicine* 4: 170–76.

7. Holcomb, W.R., J. Lander, R. Rutland, and G. Wilson. 1996. Biomechanical analysis of the vertical jump and three modified plyometric depth jumps. *Journal of Strength and Conditioning Research* 10: 83–88.

8. Housh, T.J., D.J. Housh, J.P. Weir, and L.L. Weir. 1996. Effects of eccentric-only resistance training and detraining. *International Journal of Sports Medicine* 17: 145–48.

9. Jenkins, W.L., M. Thackaberry, and C. Killian. 1984. Speed-specific isokinetic training. *Journal of Orthopedic and Sports Physical Therapy* 6: 181–83.

10. Kaminski, T.W., C.V. Wabbersen, and R.M. Murphy. 1998. Concentric versus enhanced eccentric hamstrings strength training: Clinical implications. *Journal of Athletic Training* 33: 216–21.

11. Kibler, W.B. 1990. Initial events in exercise-induced muscular injury. *Medicine and Science in Sports and Exercise* 22: 429–35.

12. Knuttgen, H.G. 1986. Human performance in high-intensity exercise with concentric and eccentric muscle contractions. *International Journal of Sports Medicine* 7(Suppl.): 6–9.

13. Pavone, E., and M. Moffat. 1985. Isometric torque of the quadriceps femoris after concentric, eccentric, and isometric training. *Archives of Physical Medicine and Rehabilitation* 66: 168–70.

14. Petersen, S., J. Wessel, K. Bagnall, H. Wilkins, A. Quinnei, and H. Wenger. 1990. Influence of concentric resistance training on concentric and eccentric strength. *Archives of Physical Medicine and Rehabilitation* 71: 101–5.

15. Ryan, L.M., P.S. Magidow, and P.W. Duncan. 1991. Velocity-specific and mode-specific effects of eccentric isokinetic training of the hamstrings. *Journal of Orthopedic and Sports Physical Therapy* 13: 33–39.

16. Singh, M., and P.V. Karpovich. 1966. Isotonic and isometric forces of forearm flexors and extensors. *Journal of Applied Physiology* 21: 1435–37.

17. Talag, T.S. 1973. Residual muscular soreness as influenced by concentric, eccentric, and static contractions. *Research Quarterly* 44: 458–69.

18. Thomee, R., P. Renstrom, G. Grimby, and L. Peterson. 1987. Slow or fast isokinetic training after knee ligament surgery. *Journal of Orthopedic and Sports Physical Therapy* 8: 475–79.

19. Tomberlin, J.P., J.R. Basford, E.E. Schwen, P.A. Orte, S.G. Scott, R.K. Laughman, and D.M. Listrup. 1991. Comparative study of isokinetic eccentric and concentric quadriceps training. *Journal of Orthopedic and Sports Physical Therapy* 14: 31–36.

20. Walmsley, R.P., N. Pearson, and P. Stymiest. 1986. Eccentric wrist extensor contractions and the force-velocity relationship in muscle. *Journal of Orthopedic and Sports Physical Therapy* 8: 288–93.

21. Weir, J.P., D.J. Housh, T.J. Housh, and L.L. Weir. 1995. The effect of unilateral eccentric weight training and detraining on joint angle specificity, cross training, and the bilateral deficit. *Journal of Orthopedic and Sports Physical Therapy* 22: 207–15.

22. Westing, S.H., A.G. Cresswell, and A. Thorstensson. 1991. Muscle activation during maximal voluntary eccentric and concentric knee extension. *European Journal of Applied Physiology* 62: 104–8.

23. Westing, S.H., and J.Y. Seger. 1989. Eccentric and concentric torque-velocity characteristics, torque output comparisons, and gravity effect torque corrections for the quadriceps and hamstring muscles in females. *International Journal of Sports Medicine* 10: 175–80.

24. Westing, S.H., J.Y. Seger, E. Karlson, and B. Ekblom. 1988. Eccentric and concentric torque-velocity characteristics of the quadriceps femoris in man. *European Journal of Applied Physiology* 58: 100–104.

25. Westing, S.H., J.Y. Seger, and A. Thorstensson. 1990. Effects of electrical stimulation on eccentric and concentric torque-velocity relationships during knee extension in man. *Acta Physiologica Scandinavica* 140: 17–22.

26. Worrell, T.W., D.H. Perrin, B.M. Gansneder, and J.H. Gieck. 1991. Comparison of isokinetic strength and flexibility measures between hamstring-injured and noninjured athletes. *Journal of Orthopedic and Sports Physical Therapy* 13: 118–25.

# Chapter 12
# Functional Lift Capacity

John C. Bruno and Scott D. Minor

Aggressive conditioning of athletes and treatment of athletic injuries has been a philosophy of athletic training for more than 30 years. By the 1980s, industry began treating occupational musculoskeletal injuries with the same aggressive approach used in treating athletic injuries. Subsequently, testing and conditioning of workers was implemented to prevent occupational injuries. The philosophy of aggressive conditioning and treatment is based on the premise that well-conditioned people are less prone to injury and more likely to recover from injury. Isokinetic dynamometers provide a method of quantifying results for both testing and conditioning.

This chapter focuses on using isokinetic dynamometry to determine functional capacity of musculature in a systematic manner. Measuring functional capacity of musculature in an occupational environment determines a job candidate's ability to perform specified job tasks safely. Such tests quantify muscle performance and may be performed prior to offering a job candidate employment, after offering employment to a candidate before job placement is determined, and during or following recovery from an injury. Each situation has certain legal constraints under different laws and regulations.

## Definitions

The following terms are used in our discussion of applying isokinetic testing to the evaluation of occupational activities.

**Disability:** The inability to engage in age-specific, gender-related, and sex-specific roles in a particular social context and physical environment (1).

**Evaluation:** A dynamic process in which clinical judgments are based on data gathered during an examination (3).

**Examination:** The process of obtaining a history, performing relevant systems reviews, and selecting and administering specific tests and measures (1).

**Function:** Relates to those activities identified by an individual as essential to support physical, social, and psychological well-being and to create a personal sense of meaningful environment (1).

**Functional capacity evaluation (FCE):** A detailed examination that objectively measures a client's current level of function, primarily within the context of the demands of competitive employment. Measurements of function from an FCE are compared to the physical demands of a job or other functional activities. An FCE measures the ability of an individual to perform functional or work-related tasks and predicts the potential to sustain these tasks over a defined time frame (2).

**Functional limitation:** The restriction of the ability to perform a physical action, activity, or task in an efficient, typically expected, or competent manner (1).

**Impairment:** A loss or abnormality of physiological, psychological, or anatomical structure or function (1).

**Injury or illness:** Refers to the occurrence of work-related pathology, pain, impairment, or loss of function. The categorization of an incident to injury or illness may be different depending upon the regulations or regulatory agency involved (1).

**Medical examination:** A procedure or test that seeks information about an individual's physical or mental impairments or health. At the pre-offer stage, an employer cannot require examinations that seek information about physical or mental impairments or health. It is not always easy to determine whether something is a medical examination (23).

**Pre-offer testing:** Entails an examination in which a series of criteria are applied by employers to determine a job candidate's qualifications to perform a specific job function before a bona fide offer of employment is made. Disability-related questions (questions likely to elicit information about a disability) are not permitted at the pre-offer stage. Physical fitness tests, in which an applicant's performance of physical tasks is measured, are not considered a medical examination and are therefore permitted at the pre-offer stage. Measurement of a job candidate's physiological or biological responses (heart rate, blood pressure, respiration, etc.) to activity are considered medical measurements and thus are not permitted (23).

**Post-offer testing:** Entails an examination in which a series of criteria are applied by employers to determine a job candidate's qualifications to perform a specific job function after a bona fide offer of employment is made. Following a bona fide offer of employment, an employer may ask disability-related questions and perform medical examinations. A job offer may be conditional on the results of post-offer disability-related questions or medical examinations and their impact on whether a new employee can perform the essential physical demands of a job. All similarly situated employees within the same job category must be subjected to the same testing or inquiry process. Medical information must be kept confidential (23).

# Quantifying Torque-Generating Capability

Static, or isometric, tests have been used to measure back strength (4, 5). Isometric testing occurs in one position without movement. This type of testing does not measure changes that occur during joint loading or through the spectrum of muscle length/tension ratios that accompany functional activity (6). Isokinetic testing examines "other physiological factors . . . by optimizing neuromuscular responses to exercise, the promotion of motor unit synchrony, the facilitation of maximal muscular activity at each point in the range of motion, and the stimulation of both slow and fast twitch muscle fiber types as related to the principles of accommodating resistance across a variable spectrum of fixed exercise velocities" (21). As a result, isokinetic testing promotes objectivity when measuring muscle performance, the ability to quantify functional components of joint motion, and the parameters of joint motion during dynamic movement.

There is extensive literature concerning the reliability, validity, accuracy, and precision of isokinetic testing. While many of the original investigations were performed on athletes, evaluation of isokinetic testing has also been done in the realm of occupational health applications. Hazard and coworkers (9) present the benefits of isokinetic testing for quantifying the legitimacy of work-related injury. Mayer and colleagues (13, 14, 19) present data that validate isokinetic dynamometer systems for measuring trunk extension and flexion and torso rotation in the presence of occupational injury. Timm (20) and Porterfield and colleagues (17) present data that demonstrate the validity and reliability of an isokinetic lifting platform. In sum, the technology itself has been demonstrated to be reliable, valid, precise, and accurate. The same is true for the application of the technology to the area of occupational health.

# Isokinetic Test Safety

Isokinetic testing is recognized as an extremely safe method of loading the musculoskeletal system, provided testing is performed under the supervision of a trained clinician. Although isokinetic evaluation is not risk free, there is little chance of serious injury given the safety mechanisms engineered into isokinetic devices. Failure of a subject to meet any specified force or torque level will not put the applicant at risk. Isokinetic devices only produce forces or torques that meet the output of the subject. Angular velocity of movement is controlled. Resistance is variable, totally accommodating to the force or torque output of the subject. Therefore, the resistance generated by the isokinetic device is always proportional to the force or torque applied by a subject.

In comparison, risk of injury is higher when a test load in a lift test surpasses the capability of the applicant. Failure in a functional simulation test may occur when trying to determine a subject's maximum lift capacity. Failure during such a lift test, in which the load is not controlled, may injure a subject.

## Isokinetic Testing and Physical Job Demands

Discussion continues regarding the connection between functional capacity evaluations and isokinetic evaluations and the ability of each to demonstrate a worker's ability to perform a specific job task safely. Some scientists believe an FCE is synonymous with work simulation, a set of tasks in which subjects perform actual work tasks. Other scientists believe that an isokinetic evaluation can be used as a physical capacity evaluation to measure function of a specific joint. The main issue of discussion is whether or not function on an isokinetic device demonstrates functional capability. Work simulation evaluation simulates function but in most cases does not measure it in quantitative terms. Isokinetic testing measures muscle performance capabilities—torque generation within a joint's selected range of motion. It is the torque generated at a joint that creates joint motion and thus the capability to perform occupational tasks. Isokinetic testing provides quantified data concerning such capabilities.

A review of relevant peer-reviewed literature indicates a significant body of knowledge concerning isokinetic testing, its validity, reliability, precision, accuracy, and applications. A similar body of knowledge in peer-reviewed literature is not apparent concerning work simulation. The theory and presumed logic of work simulation have been presented but not quantified or investigated. Unlike work simulation, a number of databases of normative data exist for isokinetic measures (8). The benefits of a large-scale database for the application of isokinetic testing and injury prevention are reported for a major United States airline (15). The reduction in injury rates, and the economic impact of such injury reduction rates, presented in these data are reflective of the predictive values, positive and negative, that can be obtained by appropriately designed and applied isokinetic test protocols.

Although movements performed on an isokinetic device may not in themselves be deemed functional for the purpose of performing occupational tasks, the measurements obtained by movements on an isokinetic device can demonstrate the ability to generate torque at specific joints that allows occupational tasks to be performed safely. Measurement of torque generation by an isokinetic device demonstrates the ability to perform functional occupational tasks. Application of specific torque-generating capabilities to functional task performance can be developed by careful ergonomic analysis.

Without measuring the actual function of the body part, a database is desirable to validate that the FCE is measuring the function and that there is a direct correlation between what the person can safely do and the simulated function. A normative database derived from noninjured workers may not exist that will allow the therapist to directly make the connection between the work simulation process and the actual function.

# Applications of Isokinetic Testing

Preplacement physical capability testing has been in widespread use throughout the United States for many years. The National Safety Council (16) makes the following statement:

*Industry spends more than $120 billion on work-related injury costs that include wage and productivity losses, medical costs of $21 billion, and administrative expenses of $23 billion. Also included are employer costs of $10 billion such as the money value of time lost by workers other than those with disabling injuries, who are directly or indirectly involved in injuries, and the cost of time required to investigate injuries, write up injury reports, etc.*

Whatever method of testing is used, the tests should be standardized, objective, defensible, and represent the essential functions of the job.

## Pre- and Post-Offer

Isokinetic evaluation to quantify muscle performance can be administered pre-offer or post-offer. There are significant differences in how a potential employee can be questioned or tested, depending upon whether the muscle performance testing (or any other physical task performance testing) is pre- or post-offer. Isokinetic muscle performance testing may also be used to document ability to return to work.

## Reproducibility

Isokinetic testing is highly reproducible when maximal voluntary effort by the subject is used. Maximal voluntary efforts produce similar curves with respect to amplitude and shape. Attempting to feign injury produces inconsistent curve shapes and abnormally large variance in torque measurements. Differences in maximum ROM, average ROM, and angle at which peak torque is achieved may be indicative of invalid test results if they exceed 5°.

## Muscle Performance

Isokinetic testing permits isolation of individual muscle groups in the performance of their primary function. Work simulation permits compensation for weakness in one joint with strength in another. While such compensation and substitution is possible during occupational tasks, compensation for impaired muscle performance in one joint places other joints at greater risk for injury. For example, when upper extremity muscle performance capability is deficient, changes are made in spinal posture to accommodate a decreased ability to support loads as they are moved away from the axis of the axial skeleton. As spinal posture changes to compensate for deficits in upper extremity muscle performance capability, the spine becomes more susceptible to injury. Another example occurs when there are muscle performance deficits in the lower extremities. A common instruction for lifting technique is for an employee to use his legs when lifting. This instruction is based upon the greater muscle performance capabilities of the quadriceps femoris muscles to lift in comparison to the spinal extensor muscles. If there is a muscle performance deficit in the lower extremities, however, the low back is at greater risk for injury. Unfortunately, during training for lifting, muscle performance of the back extensor musculature is often emphasized, and extremity muscle performance is often overlooked.

Isokinetic testing permits the evaluation of muscle performance capability of joints during isolated testing. Appropriate application and statistical analysis may then lead to the creation of an overall isokinetic testing procedure that integrates muscle performance of upper extremities, lower extremities, and trunk. In this way, isokinetic testing demonstrates quantitatively the ability to perform functional occupational tasks. This method of testing provides data on the ability to generate the minimal torque required and the safety zone of reserve muscle performance capability necessary to avoid musculoskeletal injury during unexpected load movement or in the presence of musculoskeletal fatigue. Work simulation does not provide these quantified data.

# Occupational Laws and Regulations

The role of isokinetic testing in occupational health treads a fine line among different laws and governmental regulations. The Americans with Disabilities Act (ADA) does not permit discrimination against hiring potential employees because of disability in the absence of a demonstrated inability to perform essential job tasks. Employers may not ask disability-related questions or conduct medical examinations until after a conditional job offer is made to the applicant. This ensures that an applicant's possible hidden disability or history of disability is not considered before the employer evaluates an applicant's nonmedical qualifications (23). The Equal Employment Opportunity Commission (EEOC) is responsible for investigating and pursuing claims of discrimination. The Occupational Safety and Health Act does not permit employment conditions that place employees at risk. The Occupational Safety and Health Agency (OSHA) is responsible for investigating and pursuing claims of unsafe occupational tasks. Both the EEOC and OSHA rely on avoiding the imposition of a direct threat to either the employee or those working with the employee. Direct threat means that an individual poses a significant risk of substantial harm to himself or herself or others, and this threat cannot be reduced through reasonable accommodation. The Employment Practices Act does not permit discriminatory hiring practices. The Department of Labor (DOL) and the EEOC are responsible for investigating and pursuing claims of discriminatory hiring practices. Mixed in with all of these laws and regulations is the concept of *business necessity*. Business necessity implies that individuals are capable of carrying out all job tasks without having a negative impact on productivity and that a business must have the ability to earn a profit. In many ways, these laws and regulations may be perceived as contradictory, creating a catch-22 for a company wishing to meet the requirements of all laws and regulations.

## Job Relatedness

The first step in meeting the requirements of laws and regulations in occupational settings is to demonstrate that a test relates to the job. When providing muscle performance testing, it is imperative that the test measures job-related functions and is valid. Individuals may be screened out of a job if they are unable to meet minimum standards related to job skills and to demonstrate the capability to perform essential functions of the job safely (7).

The evaluation method used for preplacement screening must show a direct correlation to the job, matching the physical capability of a worker to the physical demands of a job (8, 10). To determine essential functions of jobs, and the level of muscle performance necessary for performing the essential functions, an in-depth ergonomic analysis of jobs should be performed. Data from the ergonomic analysis provide the basis for determining the level of muscle performance required and for setting a cutoff score necessary for performing essential functions safely.

A number of different methods might be used to test muscle performance. Isokinetic testing is appropriate under the requirements of ADA if the muscle performance capabilities tested can be demonstrated to be related to essential functions. Isokinetic testing isolates major muscle groups involved in performance of physically demanding jobs. The movement patterns are the same movement patterns (at least 80% of the time) used in performing the job. This demonstrates job relatedness. Since the movement patterns assessed are the same movement patterns used in job performance, function is being evaluated. Isokinetic evaluations provide the most objective measure of function in comparison to any other assessment tool currently available.

Although disability-related questions cannot be asked or medical examinations be required at the pre-offer stage, alternatives exist to evaluate whether an applicant is qualified for a job. An employer may state the physical requirements of a job (such as the ability to lift a certain amount of weight, or the ability to climb ladders) and ask if an applicant can satisfy these requirements. Physical agility and muscle performance tests in which an applicant demonstrates the ability to perform actual or simulated job tasks are not a medical examination under ADA (23). A test in which an applicant's performance of physical tasks such as running or lifting is measured is not a medical examination (23, 24), although the criteria of the test must be job related. Measuring an applicant's heart rate or blood pressure (biological or physiological responses) makes the test a medical examination. Using isokinetic equipment as a screening tool for new hires may be considered job related and consistent with business necessity (11, 23). Under these guidelines, isokinetic evaluations may be administered pre-offer (11). When requiring an appropriate isokinetic test, an employer may ask an applicant to assume responsibility and release the employer of liability for injuries incurred in performing the test (23).

Following a bona fide offer of work, employers may ask disability-related questions, and medical examinations may be performed. At the post-offer stage, the questions and examinations need not be job related. If an employer chooses to ask post-offer disability-related questions, all employees entering the same job category must be subjected to the same inquiry or examination. All medical information obtained in this manner must be kept confidential (23).

## Return-to-Work Conditions

Because isokinetic testing is not considered a medical examination under the ADA, its use on current employees to assess readiness to return to work is permitted if all similarly situated individuals are tested. Under ADA return-to-work guidelines, medical examinations are permitted if the medical examination is job related and consistent with business necessity (21). Isokinetic evaluations may be used as a condition of returning to work, even for employees eligible under the Family Medical Leave Act (FMLA), where such evaluation is governed by state law (including workers' compensation law), or the terms of a collective bargaining agreement (6, 21).

It must be noted that not all essential functions of a job are related to muscle performance capability. Therefore, final decisions concerning the suitability of a potential employee should not be based solely on isokinetic testing. Isokinetic testing is only one part of the hiring or return-to-work process.

# Considerations for Testing

There are several issues related to the defensibility of isokinetic testing, with respect to both scientific method and legal constraints. Each issue must be considered when developing such tests.

## Equipment Validity, Accuracy, and Reliability

The intersite, intertester, intratester, interday, and intraday validity, accuracy, and reliability of isokinetic peak torque measurements have been demonstrated (4, 5, 8). A prominent requirement to ensure these parameters is dynamic calibration of equipment throughout the entire range of torque and range of motion. Such calibration requires a method of applying and comparing, in a dynamic mode, known inputs to measured outputs. Calibration verifies that all system components are functioning correctly.

*Validity* is the extent to which an instrument truly measures what is intended to be measured (18). Validity is demonstrated when the test instrument used produces measurements that are indicative of the parameter to be measured. The measurement of force by a strain gauge would be valid. Measurement of force by a goniometer would not be valid. *Accuracy* is freedom from error or conformity of a measure to a true value. Accuracy may be compromised by measurement error (18). Accuracy is demonstrated when a known parameter such as 100 N force is applied to a load cell, and the equipment presents a measurement of 100 N. *Reliability* is the extent to which a test or measurement procedure yields measurements that are consistent and free from error over repeated trials (18). Reliability is demonstrated if a known parameter, such as the 100 N force, is applied to the load cell repeatedly, and the equipment presents the same measurement repeatedly. Equipment is considered reliable and accurate when the repeated measurement is consistently the same as the known parameter being measured.

## Objectivity

To correlate test measurements to essential tasks, objective measurements are necessary. Isokinetic testing avoids subjective human evaluation methods that are likely to affect test results. The result is an objective measure of isolated joint torque-generating capability. These measures of torque-generating capability permit multiple within subject comparisons, including contralateral deficits and within joint muscle imbalances.

## Subject Stabilization

Subject stabilization is an important issue in test accuracy and reliability. In isokinetic testing, stabilization helps ensure that only the desired muscle performance is being tested. A lack of stabilization on an isokinetic device allows a subject to substitute or supplement desired muscle activity using other body segments. When this occurs, inaccurate or unreliable measurements may occur. If accuracy and reliability are not ensured, test validity is not supported.

## Consistency of Effort

A key feature of isokinetic testing is the ability to document consistency of effort. Strict adherence to test procedures and equipment familiarization help ensure consistency of effort. Matching curve shape for multiple repetitions demonstrates consistency of effort. Studies verify this characteristic as a measure of consistency of effort. There is, however, no conclusive evidence in peer-reviewed literature indicating that curve shape can be used to diagnose specific musculoskeletal pathology.

## Standardization of Procedures

For scientific and legal reasons, it is important that each isokinetic test is administered consistently. It is a legal requirement of the ADA and employment law that job applicants or workers be accorded consistent procedures. Scientific integrity requires standardized protocols of measurement and recording. Standardized procedures, including standardized test procedures and protocols, documented equipment calibration, and consistent analysis of data, help ensure valid and reliable data. This helps ensure a high degree of reproducibility and generalizability. Additional advantages of isokinetic testing include maximal voluntary exertion throughout the full range of motion, reciprocal testing, and the ability to standardize evaluation methods and procedures with respect to angular velocity, range of motion, and maintenance of joint alignment during testing.

## Data Interpretation and Analysis

Effective data interpretation and analysis are affected by test administration. Consistency of effort influences the validity of test results. A database can be used to decide how much effort is required to do work at specific levels. The interpretive process allows standard comparisons of specific variables to be made as related to the appropriate normative database. Results can be compared to specific groups, or age and gender, of workers. All persons involved in the interpretive process must follow the same guidelines if valid comparisons are to be made.

# An Isokinetic Testing System: Injury Reduction Technology

A company named INRTEK (**In**jury **R**eduction **Tec**hnology) has developed a system of muscle performance testing using isokinetic technology. The INRTEK system has been available to industry since 1982. Muscle performance of the knees, shoulders, and back is tested to determine if a potential or injured employee can perform the essential functions of his job without creating a direct threat of injury to himself or those in close proximity. During the life of muscle performance testing in this system, a database of over 80,000 subjects and approximately 100,000 tests has been compiled.

The database consists of raw isokinetic data. Raw data from isokinetic testing does not by itself create a useful database with respect to measuring functional lift capability. Statistical analyses and subsequent manipulation of these isokinetic testing data permit recommendations to be made concerning functional ability to perform essential functions of jobs and the likelihood of injury occurring while performing essential functions of jobs. The system has been validated statistically by

1. isokinetic testing of the range of necessary muscle performance characteristics of the knees, shoulders, and back of uninjured incumbent workers;

2. isokinetic testing of new hires and their subsequent record of knee, shoulder, and back injuries, in comparison with hire/do not hire recommendations based on the isokinetic testing system; and

3. retrospective review of injury rates and medical costs for knee, shoulder, and back injuries in client companies that use INRTEK's isokinetic testing system.

The statistical validation has been used to determine a Standard Index Score (SIS). The SIS formula was derived using discriminate function analysis based upon data from injured versus uninjured, tested versus untested, and matched versus mismatched (with respect to matching an individual's physical capabilities and the physical task demands of essential job functions) employees. Key foundation components of this system are

1. matching isokinetic test parameters to actual job functions,
2. matching isokinetic test parameters to physical task demands determined by ergonomic analysis,
3. comparison of measured physical task demands to U.S. Department of Labor guidelines and data in *Selected characteristics of occupations as defined in the revised dictionary of occupational titles* (22),
4. verification of test reliability and validity using statistical methods,
5. maintaining high standards of equipment calibration, and
6. strictly following a specific test protocol.

Building on the key foundation components cited, isokinetic testing of functional lift capacity has been demonstrated to work very well. Isokinetic muscle performance testing has been demonstrated to be appropriately selective when determining the ability of workers to perform safely the physical demands of work (8, 15). Without the key foundation components cited, isokinetic testing of functional lift capacity would lack validity and generalizability and would be in conflict with numerous laws and regulations.

There are two major functions of the INRTEK isokinetic testing system: preplacement evaluation (PP), and return-to-work readiness evaluation (RTW-RE). The objectives of the preplacement evaluation are to

1. evaluate new hires, job transfers, and job bids;
2. match physical capabilities of potential employees to the physical task demands of essential job functions;
3. identify the baseline status of physical capability for each new hire;
4. reduce the incidence rate and severity of injuries in the work place;
5. provide documentation accepted as courtroom testimony; and
6. provide an isokinetic evaluation that can be administered pre- or post-offer.

The preplacement evaluation is designed to aid employers and employees in reducing the incidence rate of injuries in the work place. Preplacement screening permits an employer to use objective measures to place a new hire (or job transfer/job bid employee) in an employment situation in which the physical capabilities of the employee are matched to the physical task demands of the essential job functions.

The return-to-work readiness evaluation is designed to determine if individuals who have been injured have recovered the physical capabilities necessary to meet the physical task demands of essential job functions. The objectives of the RTW-RE are to

1. lower return-to-work costs,

2. prevent overtreatment by providing an accurate record of progress,

3. provide objective and defensible results,

4. verify progress in the enhancement of muscle performance to prevent reinjury if more conditioning is necessary, and

5. provide a cost-effective return-to-work evaluation for injured employees.

When an injured employee does not meet the criteria to return to work based on the RTW-RE, a physical capacity evaluation may provide a more detailed procedure and report mechanism.

## Isokinetic Testing System Protocols

The first step in the testing system is to determine factors of job relatedness. Client company job descriptions are reviewed to determine job classifications in which employees might be at risk. Job descriptions, however, rarely provide objective data describing the actual physical task demands of an employee performing the job. Therefore, an ergonomic analysis is performed to provide measured essential job functions. Data generated by the ergonomic analysis are used for comparison with U.S. Department of Labor guidelines and data (22) and for comparison with the INRTEK database. Subsequently, each job is classified with respect to the database and Department of Labor definitions. A final Standard Index Score is set based upon data from ergonomic analysis of the client company, statistical analyses of the database, and Department of Labor definitions (22).

The test protocol used in the INRTEK isokinetic testing system focuses on the knees, shoulders, and back as individual joints and as an integrated system. Each of the five joints is tested individually, using multiple angular velocities of movement for the knees and shoulders but not the back. The final SIS is a composite score of muscle performance testing for the five areas tested.

The angular velocities chosen for the knees and shoulders cover the spectrum of velocities observed during manual materials handling tasks in industry. The different velocities demonstrate a subject's muscle performance capability under changing conditions. The single angular velocity chosen for testing of the back is a common angular velocity of low back flexion/extension observed in a variety of manual materials handling tasks. Angular velocity of back motion does not seem to demonstrate the variability of angular velocities presented by the knees and shoulders during occupational tasks. The repetition of back testing twice at an angular velocity of 60°/s also provides an opportunity to verify consistency of effort and force reproducibility by each subject tested.

Each test session is performed in the same sequence. Knees are tested first, then shoulders, and then the back. The sequences and parameters of testing are presented sequentially in tables 12.1–12.3.

A training and procedure manual is given to each test provider at the time of training in the specifics of the test protocols. The instructor who wrote the training and procedure manual provides the training, which ensures consistency of training and testing. Strict adherence to the stated protocol is required of test providers. Monthly calibration of each piece of equipment used for testing is also required. Calibration results are faxed to INRTEK for review and comparison with previous calibration results. Each of these steps has been initiated to maintain reliability of test results with respect to the overall database.

## Table 12.1   Knee Test Protocol

| Right knee warm-up | Right knee test |
|---|---|
| 2 light contractions of extension/ flexion at 180°/s | 5 repetitions of extension/flexion at 60°/s |
| | 5–10 repetitions for cool-down |
| 2 medium contractions of extension/ flexion at 180°/s | 30 s rest |
| 1 hard contraction of extension/ flexion at 180°/s | Familiarization at 180°/s by 3–5 repetitions at maximum force |
| Repeat 5-contraction sequence at 120°/s, 90°/s, and 60°/s | 30 s rest |
| | 5 repetitions of extension/flexion at 180°/s |
| Rest 1 min | 30 s rest |
| | Familiarization at 240°/s by 3–5 repetitions at maximum force |
| | 30 s rest |
| | 5 repetitions of extension/flexion at 240°/s |
| | Rest 2 min while changing set-up to test left knee |
| **Left knee warm-up** | **Left knee test** |
| 2 light contractions of extension/ flexion at 180°/s | 5 repetitions of extension/flexion at 60°/s |
| | 5–10 repetitions for cool-down |
| 2 medium contractions of extension/ flexion at 180°/s | 30 s rest |
| 1 hard contraction of extension/ flexion at 180°/s | Familiarization of 180°/s by 3–5 repetitions at maximum force |
| Repeat 5-contraction sequence at 120°/s, 90°/s, and 60°/s | 30 s rest |
| | 5 repetitions of extension/flexion at 180°/s |
| Rest 1 min | 30 s rest |
| | Familiarization at 240°/s by 3–5 repetitions at maximum force |
| | 30 s rest |
| | 5 repetitions of extension/flexion at 240°/s |

## Table 12.2   Shoulder Test Protocol

| Dominant shoulder warm-up | Dominant shoulder test |
|---|---|
| 2 light contractions of extension/ flexion at 60°/s<br><br>2 medium contractions of extension/ flexion at 60°/s<br><br>1 hard contraction of extension/ flexion at 60°/s<br><br>Rest 1 min | 5 repetitions of extension/flexion at 60°/s<br><br>30 s rest<br><br>Familiarization at 180°/s by 3–5 repetitions at maximum force<br><br>30 s rest<br><br>5 repetitions of extension/flexion at 180°/s<br><br>Rest 2 min while changing set-up to test nondominant shoulder |
| **Nondominant shoulder warm-up** | **Nondominant shoulder test** |
| 2 light contractions of extension/ flexion at 60°/s<br><br>2 medium contractions of extension /flexion at 60°/s<br><br>1 hard contraction of extension /flexion at 60°/s<br><br>Rest 1 min | 5 repetitions of extension/flexion at 60°/s<br><br>30 s rest<br><br>Familiarization at 180°/s by 3–5 repetitions at maximum force<br><br>30 s rest<br><br>5 repetitions of extension/flexion at 180°/s |

## Table 12.3   Back Test Protocol

| Back warm-up | Back test | Back retest |
|---|---|---|
| 2 light contractions of flexion/extension at 60°/s<br><br>2 medium contractions of flexion/extension at 60°/s<br><br>1 hard contraction of flexion/ extension at 60°/s<br><br>Additional graded submaximal repetitions may be required if the tester determines further familiarization is required to facilitate motor learning. | 5 repetitions of flexion/ extension at 60°/s<br><br>Rest 30 s<br><br>Refamiliarization at 60°/s by 5 additional repetitions at submaximal levels | 5 repetitions of flexion/ extension at 60°/s |

The INRTEK system uses 32 measures taken directly from raw data generated by the isokinetic testing. More than 50 additional variables (including comparisons of like joints, similar joint motions, and torque/body weight ratios) are derived from the initial 32 isokinetic measures. From these data, a specific SIS score for the potential or injured employee is calculated. The individual's SIS is compared to the baseline SIS derived from ergonomic analysis, database, and Department of Labor data. Potential or injured employees whose individual SIS meets or exceeds the derived SIS are recommended for hire or return to work. Individuals whose SIS are below the derived SIS are not recommended for hire or return to work. The final decision rests with the client company for whom the employee wishes to work. In many cases, individuals who are not recommended for hire or return to work are provided an opportunity to exercise to improve their muscle performance and are then retested.

# A Case for Using the Isokinetic Testing System

A major United States airline company began using the INRTEK isokinetic testing system in December 1995. The primary objective of the client company was to reduce workplace injuries to ramp workers (baggage handlers). This job is rated as "heavy" based on an ergonomic analysis, U.S. Department of Labor (22) guidelines and data, and examination of the INRTEK database. Over the course of seven months, 1,884 applicants were screened, of which 1,428 (76%) met or exceeded the SIS for the essential job functions of a ramp worker. Historically, the injury rate of knees, shoulders, and backs for this group of employees was 14 per 100 workers. Following implementation of the INRTEK program, the actual injury rate dropped to 1.1 per 100 workers. Costs averaged $1,177 per claim following program implementation, compared with historical costs of $17,013 per claim. This change represents a 69-fold decrease in costs of these injuries. The airline realized a net savings of $1 million in claim costs alone during the program's first seven months (15). In a three-year follow-up, the lower injury rate and cost per claim has held steady.

# Practical Outcomes

Several outcomes accrue to the appropriate use of isokinetic technology when testing functional lift capacity. First, carefully designed protocols provide for the scientific necessity of validity, accuracy, and reliability. Second, appropriate statistical analysis demonstrates the job relatedness of isokinetic testing for functional lift capability. Third, the appropriate application of isokinetic technology has been demonstrated to be a significant factor in the reduction of injuries in occupational settings. Reviews of the INRTEK database in comparison with injury statistics from client companies demonstrate that for potential employees tested using the isokinetic testing system, 95% of those recommended for hire remain free of injury during the first year of employment. These are employees who are considered matched (by comparison of the individual's physical capabilities to the physical task demands of essential job functions). The 5% of "matched" employees who do suffer injuries of the knees, shoulders, or back during the first two years incur medical costs at a lower level than employees who are considered "unmatched" by the INRTEK protocol. Of potential employees who were considered unmatched by isokinetic testing (the individual's physical capabilities do not meet the physical task demands of essential job functions) but were hired despite not being recommended for hire, 76% incurred injuries of the knee, shoulder, or back during the first year of employment. The impact of applying isokinetic technology is apparent from either side of the issue.

In light of the business environment in which employment testing is performed, there are additional points to make concerning the use of isokinetic testing. First, the outcomes of the isokinetic testing system are nondiscriminatory with respect to gender or age. In jobs that require extensive torque-generating capability, the difference in numbers of males and females recommended for hire is related to scientifically known differences between genders in the ability to generate torque. Job matching is performed independently of gender or age. The objective test criterion is torque-generating capability and not gender or age. When challenged by a claim of gender bias the INRTEK system of isokinetic testing, when used as designed and applied to all potential employees equally, was determined not to be discriminatory on the basis of gender by the Equal Employment Opportunity Commission.

Second, there are significant economic benefits to preplacement testing. Correctly matching an individual's physical capability to the physical task demands of essential job functions can prevent overexertion injuries to the knees, shoulders, and back. There is also a concomitant decrease in the incidence and severity of initial injuries and in reinjury rates. Reduced worker's compensation costs contribute directly to return on investment. The costs of hiring temporary or replacement employees is also reduced. Employers who have utilized the INRTEK program have realized at least a 7 to 1 return on investment for every $1 invested for preplacement testing, with some reporting a 30 to 1 return on investment.

# Summary

Isokinetic technology, when applied appropriately, is an excellent tool for testing functional lift capacity. Appropriate application requires demonstration of equipment validity, accuracy, and reliability; well-calibrated equipment; strict adherence to a specific testing protocol; and statistical analyses that support the development of scoring levels and formulas. When used appropriately, isokinetic technology provides objective data that are useful in occupational settings and meet the legal and regulatory constraints of employment law.

# References

1. American Physical Therapy Association. 1997. Guide to physical therapist practice. *Physical Therapy* 77(11): 1175–650.

2. American Physical Therapy Association. 1997. Adapted from *Occupational health guidelines: Evaluating functional capacity*. BOD 11-97-16-53. Alexandria, VA: American Physical Therapy Association.

3. American Physical Therapy Association. 1997. Adapted from the Guide to physical therapist practice. *Physical Therapy* 77(11): 1175–650.

4. Byl NN and Sadowsky HS. 1993. Intersite reliability of repeated isokinetic measurements: Cybex back systems including trunk rotation, trunk extension/flexion, and lift task. *Isokinetics and Exercise Science* 3: 139–47.

5. Byl NN, Wells L, Grady D, Friedlander A., and Sadowsky S. 1991. Consistency of repeated isokinetic testing: Effect of different examiners, sites, and protocols. *Isokinetics and Exercise Science* 1: 122–30.

6. Committee on Interstate and Foreign Commerce, U.S. House of Representatives. February 1976. *A discursive dictionary of health care*. Washington, DC: GPO.

7. Edwards FC, McCallum RI, and Taylor PJ, eds. 1988. *Fitness for work: The medical aspects*. Oxford, New York: Oxford University Press.

8. Freedson PS, Gilliam TB, Mahoney T et al. 1993. Industrial torque levels by age group and gender. *Isokinetics and Exercise Science* 3: 34–42.

9. Hazard RG, Reid S, Fenwick J, and Reeves V. 1988. Isokinetic trunk and lifting strength measurements: Variability as an indicator of effort. *Spine* 13: 54–57.

10. Isernhagen SJ. 1988. *Work injury management and prevention*. Rockville, MD: Aspen.

11. Jackson, Lewis, Schnitzler and Krupman (Law Firm). 1995 *An analysis regarding the application of Title I of the Americans With Disabilities Act (ADA) and the Family and Medical Leave Act (FMLA) to INRTEK's Preplacement and Return to Work isokinetic evaluations*.

12. Malone TR, ed. 1988. Evaluation of isokinetic equipment. *Sports Injury Management* 1(1): 1–90.

13. Mayer TG, Gatchel RJ, Kishino N et al. 1985. Objective assessment of spine function following industrial injury. *Spine* 10: 482–93.

14. Mayer TG, Smith SS, Keeley J, and Mooney V. 1985. Quantification of lumbar region: II. Sagittal plane trunk strength in chronic low back pain patients. *Spine* 10: 765–72.

15. McKenas D, Gilliam TB, Green K, and Martin J. 1996. Injury reduction in commercial aviation ramp workers through post-offer screening [abstract]. Dallas-Ft. Worth: American Airlines Corporate Medical Dept.

16. National Safety Council. 1995. *Accident facts*. Itasca, IL: National Safety Council.

17. Porterfield JA, Mostardi RA, King S et al. 1987. Simulated lift testing using computerized isokinetics. *Spine* 12: 683–87.

18. Portney LG and Watkins MP. 1993. *Foundations of clinical research: Applications to practice*, 69. Norwalk, CT: Appleton & Lange.

19. Smith SS, Mayer TG, Gatachel RJ, and Becker TJ. 1985. Quantification of lumbar function: I. Isometric and multispeed isokinetic trunk strength measures in sagittal and axial planes in normal subjects. *Spine* 10: 757–64.

20. Timm KE. 1988. Isokinetic lifting simulation: A normative data study. *Journal of Orthopaedic and Sports Physical Therapy* 10: 156–66.

21. U.S. Code of Federal Regulations. 1990. 29 CFR § 825.310 (b). Washington, DC: GPO.

22. U.S. Department of Labor. 1993. *Selected characteristics of occupations as defined in the revised dictionary of occupational titles.* Washington, DC: U.S. Department of Labor (NTIS No. PB 94-116 282).

23. U.S. Equal Employment Opportunity Commission. 1995. *ADA enforcement guidance: EEOC guidance on preemployment inquiries under Americans with Disabilities Act.* Washington, DC: GPO.

24. U.S. Equal Employment Opportunity Commission. 1995. *ADA enforcement guidance: Preemployment disability related inquiries and medical examinations under the Americans with Disabilities Act of 1990, May 19, 1994.* Notice No. 915.002. Washington, DC: GPO.

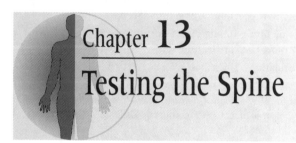

# Chapter 13

# Testing the Spine

Kent E. Timm

This chapter presents a compilation of knowledge regarding the application of isokinetic principles to the lumbar spine. The text reviews the physiological effects that spinal isokinetic activity has on the various systems and certain tissues in the body that require consideration for the development of effective assessment and exercise protocols. Testing is presented in terms of appropriate protocols. The chapter discusses the different methods that are available for the interpretation of spinal isokinetic test results, including the normalization of data. The data interpretation process is applied to the area of lifting analysis, with the presentation of specific methods for the determination of a subject's lifting capacity. This chapter concludes with a description of the concepts that may be used to develop effective spinal isokinetic exercise protocols, using both the traditional approach of the velocity spectrum sequence and the contemporary method of exercise to 50% fatigue. This information should enable the reader to effectively practice spinal isokinetic principles and technology regardless of the setting—athletic, clinical, or research.

## Isokinetic Effects on the Spine

Isokinetic activity for the spine can induce a variety of physiological changes in the different systems of the body. Such changes stem from the principle of specific adaptation to imposed demands (SAID) and reflect the body's response to the conditions that accompany isokinetic training. Spinal isokinetic activity results in changes within the following physiological systems (in alphabetical order): bone, cardiovascular, connective tissue, intervertebral disk, muscle, and neurological. In addition to these physiological adaptations, isokinetic activity also influences changes in spinal kinesiology through effects on postural biomechanics and on kinetic chain states.

# Bone Adaptations

Spinal isokinetic activity induces changes in bone under Wolff's law of tissue remodeling, which states that living tissue will adapt as a direct response to specific external demands (9, 16–18, 24). Adaptation takes place to physically strengthen the bone tissues of the spinal column, making them more resistant to external force loads that may cause injury. Specifically, isokinetic training causes an increase in bone density, bone mass, and bone mineral content through facilitation of osteoblast activity and of calcium and vitamin D metabolism. However, a training period of at least eight-week duration is needed to impart such adaptation (9, 16–18, 24).

# Cardiovascular Adaptations

Spinal isokinetic activity influences the cardiovascular system by promoting changes in the left ventricle of the heart. The left ventricular wall undergoes muscle hypertrophy to increase potential ventricular filling volume during the diastolic phase of the cardiac cycle (9, 11, 16–18, 24). This leads to an increase in stroke volume and, therefore, to a decrease in resting heart rate as the cardiac system becomes more efficient. This adaptation also requires an isokinetic-training period of at least eight weeks (9, 16–18, 24).

# Connective Tissue Adaptations

Isokinetic exercise enhances the process of collagen synthesis, which reinforces the structural integrity of the spinal ligaments and tendons; therefore, the stronger tissues have a greater resistance to injury. Isokinetic activity also facilitates the development of new collagen fibers in an area of connective tissue that has sustained injury (9, 16–18, 24). Once new collagen fibers have formed, the accommodating resistance of isokinetic exercise promotes tissue remodeling along a path of controlled force, which produces a parallel alignment of collagen fibers (16–18, 24). The overall effect is the development of normal, flexible connective tissue, as opposed to an inflexible, dysfunctional scar, in the region of a spinal injury (9, 16–18, 24).

# Intervertebral Disk Adaptations

Spinal isokinetic activity will enhance the physiology of the intervertebral disk. The spinal motion and the increased cardiovascular activity that accompany isokinetic exercise increase the rate of nutrient diffusion across the vertebral endplate from the capillary beds of the vertebral body into the interstitial fluid matrix of the annulus fibrosus and the nucleus pulposus (16–18, 24). In addition, the spinal motion and increased cardiovascular activity help to pump metabolic wastes across the vertebral endplate from the intervertebral disk matrix into the capillary beds of the vertebral body for removal through the circulatory system. The overall effect ensures optimal conditions of disk height and tissue health, so that the intervertebral disk can effectively serve its primary function as a physiological shock absorber of load forces transmitted through the spinal column (9, 16–18, 24).

## Muscle Adaptations

As is the case with other modes of progressive resistance exercise, spinal isokinetic activity promotes muscle hypertrophy. Hypertrophication, which requires a training period of at least eight weeks, occurs at the cellular level through the stimulation of increased protein synthesis in myocytes (9, 16–18, 24). This enables the production of more actin and myosin proteins for the improvement of the muscular contractile apparatus (16–18, 24). Therefore, the spinal muscles increase in both size and ability to produce force output. Also, as a possible short-term, high-intensity mode of muscle training, isokinetic exercise enhances the development of the type II muscle fibers (5, 6, 8–10, 14, 16–18, 24). This particular muscle adaptation is especially important because lumbar disorders are accompanied by type II fiber atrophy in the spinal muscle groups (5, 6, 8–10, 14, 16–18, 24). Conversely, type II muscle fiber development is positively correlated with overall spinal health (10, 16–18, 24).

## Neurological Adaptations

Spinal isokinetic activity influences the alpha motoneuron system to enhance overall muscle performance (5, 6, 9, 16–18, 24). Specifically, isokinetic exercise increases the level of a subject's maximal volitional contraction, as represented by an increase in EMG output during exercise (5, 6, 24). The effect is a composite of separate actions: a more synchronous discharge of motoneurons within a muscle motor unit, the recruitment of additional motor units, lowering of the threshold for the excitation contraction coupling process, and a dampening of inhibitory reflexes. These processes are responsible for the relatively early gains in performance ability after a subject undertakes an isokinetic training regimen; other adaptation processes require a training period of at least eight weeks (9, 16–18, 24).

# Postural Biomechanics

Spinal isokinetic dynamometer systems are constructed in a configuration that duplicates the normal lumbar biomechanical actions during test and exercise movement activities. In the sagittal plane, spinal isokinetic systems permit the natural reversal of the lumbar lordotic curve during flexion, the return to lordosis during extension from a forward-flexed position, and an increased lordosis during hyperextension, which prevents the application of abnormal stresses to the spine during isokinetic activity (5–9, 14–21, 24). This also facilitates a natural degree of contractile activity in the spinal muscle groups. Specifically, flexion recruits the eccentric action of the spinal extensor muscle complex and the concentric actions of the rectus abdominis, internal and external obliques, and the iliopsoas muscle groups, while extension involves the concentric action of the spinal extensor muscle complex and the hamstring and gluteal muscle groups (5–9, 14–21, 24).

In the transverse plane, spinal isokinetic systems allow for left and right rotation in the natural anatomical neutral position of the lumbar lordotic curve (5–9, 14–21, 24). This configuration also facilitates the actions of left and right lumbar lateral flexion, since the motions of segmental rotational and side bending are normally coupled in the lumbar spine (16, 17, 21). The coupled rotation and side bending activity involves the concentric actions of the multifidi, internal oblique, and external oblique muscle groups. The action of these muscle groups also creates an increase in tension within the thoracolumbar fascia, which helps to reduce the chance of lumbar injury through a reinforcement of the normal lordotic curve (5–9, 14–21, 24).

## Kinetic Chain States

The kinetic chain is a fundamental concept in modern biomechanics and orthopedic medicine. The feet are dynamically linked to the lumbar spine by way of the ankle, knee, hip, and sacroiliac joint complexes. Furthermore, the legs are linked to the upper back, shoulders, arms, and neck through the lumbar spine. Influences at one point in the kinetic chain are known to produce a compensatory effect at other points in the chain, either proximal or distal to the point of influence. The compensatory effect may include changes in joint mechanics or muscle responses. In addition, compensatory effects may differ with the relative state of the kinetic chain, which may be open, partially closed, or closed, as a function of the weight-bearing status of the specific joints in the kinetic chain.

The state of the kinetic chain has been found to affect the performance of the lumbar spine muscle groups under isokinetic test and exercise conditions (21). A closed lower extremity kinetic chain results in greater spinal flexor and extensor muscle peak torque output when compared to different forms of an open kinetic chain (21). Also, lumbar muscle torque production decreases as the lower extremity kinetic chain becomes more open (21). These results are summarized in figure 13.1. This information would benefit strength and conditioning professionals in the design of isokinetic exercise protocols to address different lumbar and lower extremity kinetic chain configurations. However, since no data exists for upper spinal and upper extremity influences, information on the effects of different kinetic chain states relative to the lumbar spine under isokinetic conditions is incomplete.

## Spinal Testing Procedures and Protocols

Isokinetic testing of the spine may complement other common procedures that are used to diagnose a spinal problem or to assess performance ability in healthy subjects. Spinal isokinetic testing is somewhat unique in that it collects objective, reliable, and valid data on muscle function during dynamic activity;

**Spinal flexion peak torque (Nm) at 60°/s**

| KCS | Closed | Open 1 | Open 2 | Open 3 |
|------|--------|--------|--------|--------|
| Mean | 268.50 | 166.00 | 162.50 | 49.42 |
| SD | 22.42 | 19.12 | 23.54 | 36.13 |

**Spinal extension peak torque (Nm) at 60°/s**

| KCS | Closed | Open 1 | Open 2 | Open 3 |
|------|--------|--------|--------|--------|
| Mean | 296.90 | 176.75 | 171.60 | 65.30 |
| SD | 34.11 | 50.67 | 47.36 | 29.98 |

Key: Nm = Newton-meters (1 Nm = 0.74 ft-lb); KCS = kinetic chain state; Closed = ankles, knees, and hips weight bearing; Open 1 = knees and hips weight bearing; Open 2 = ankles and hips weight bearing; Open 3 = ankles, knees, and hips nonweight bearing; SD = standard deviation.

**Figure 13.1**   Kinetic chain state performance data.
See Timm (21).

most traditional spinal diagnostic procedures incorporate static methods of testing. The information on dynamic muscle performance may be merged with the information achieved through other traditional methods such as radiographs, EMG procedures, and static strength tests in order to create a comprehensive analysis of overall spinal function (2, 4–9, 12, 14–16, 19–21, 23, 24).

Spinal isokinetic test protocols are based on a series of traditional factors, which include the isokinetic velocity spectrum for the spine, the number of test repetitions at each test speed, the length of the rest interval between test speeds, and the spinal range of motion (ROM) for the test subject. These factors apply to testing in both the sagittal and the transverse planes of spinal motion (16, 19–22, 26).

## Spinal Velocity Spectrum

The traditional isokinetic velocity spectrum for the spine is 30 to 150°/s (2, 4–9, 14–21, 24, 26). Also traditionally, testing occurs across this velocity spectrum in a sequence of speeds that increase by 30°/s: 30, 60, 90, 120, and 150°/s. However, more current findings suggest that, at least for the knee, the specific order of test speeds is not important, since combinations of different speed sequences produce the same overall test outcome (26). Also, other studies suggest that testing across a velocity spectrum is not necessary in the spine, because physiological overflow readily occurs between the spinal test velocities

(22), and no statistically significant difference exists between single and multi-speed test protocols (19, 20).

## Test Repetitions

A traditional test format would incorporate a minimum of four repetitions at each speed of a spinal isokinetic test protocol (2, 4–9, 14–21, 24, 26). The number of test repetitions could expand to a minimum of 20 at the fastest speed of a multispeed protocol for the collection of endurance data. However, current findings suggest that a minimum of five repetitions at a particular test speed is necessary for the collection of accurate data (19, 20).

## Rest Interval

The minimum rest interval used to separate speeds of a multispeed test sequence is 20 s (2, 4–9, 14–21, 24, 26). A shorter rest period between speeds does not provide a sufficient degree of recovery by the test subject, which threatens the accuracy of the data collection process. The maximum rest interval has been found to be 90 s. Longer rest intervals also threaten the accuracy of the test results, since the test subject begins to cool down too much between speeds (2, 4–9, 14–21, 24, 26).

## Test ROM

The traditional approach to spinal isokinetic testing suggested that the test subject move through a particular ROM for either flexion/extension or left/right rotation data collection (2, 4–9, 14–21, 24). However, the prescribed ROM was arbitrary and did not reflect any definitive physiological requirement for an accurate test outcome. Also, the various methods for the interpretation of spinal isokinetic test data, which are described in the following section, are independent of spinal ROM. Therefore, the current thought is to test through a spinal ROM that is comfortable, and preferably functional, for the test subject (16, 17, 19, 20, 24). An example test protocol, which could be useful for flexion/extension, left/right rotation testing, or for both arcs of movement, appears in figure 13.2.

| Speed | 30 | 60 | 90 | 120 | 150 |
|---|---|---|---|---|---|
| Reps | 4 | 4 | 4 | 4 | 20 |
| Rest | Interval of 20–90 s between speeds | | | | |
| ROM | Comfortable, functional for the subject | | | | |

Key: Speed = °/s; reps = minimum number of test repetitions per speed; rest = rest interval between speeds; ROM = spinal range of motion.

**Figure 13.2** Traditional spinal isokinetic test protocol.
See Timm (16).

# Data Interpretation

The interpretation of isokinetic test data for the shoulder and knee has involved the comparison between the injured and the normal muscle groups for both the upper and lower extremities (1, 16, 19, 20). Comparisons between peak torque, total work, average power, and endurance data are used to determine the state of muscle function, which is then extrapolated to overall performance ability (2, 4–9, 14–16, 19–22, 26). However, isokinetic test data interpretation must be different for the spine, since there is no reference limb for the generation of a bilateral comparison. The isokinetic spinal data systems include the average performance deficit, the muscle performance index, and normative data for peak torque percent body weight.

## Average Performance Deficit

The average performance deficit (APD) method of isokinetic spinal data interpretation has demonstrated high levels of intra- and interrater reliability (16, 19, 20). The method incorporates the minimum necessary criteria for accurate isokinetic testing: four maximal repetitions at a test speed and a 20 s rest interval between speeds. The method is also practical because it is based on a reference criterion of 100% as being normal spinal muscle function (16, 19, 20). However, the procedure requires a testing protocol of five different test speeds (30, 60, 90, 120, and 150°/s), which has been found to be inefficient as compared to a single test speed (19, 20). Also, the APD method needs to be employed independently for each spinal movement direction (flexion, extension, left rotation, and right rotation) to achieve a complete result for the overall analysis of a subject's spinal muscle performance. The APD formula and examples for its use in data interpretation appear in figure 13.3.

## Muscle Performance Index

The muscle performance index (MPI) is a robust method for the interpretation of spinal isokinetic data that incorporates parameters of peak torque, average power, and total work (3). The MPI may be adapted to any testing protocol that uses two or more test speeds. A minimum of four maximal test repetitions at each speed and a minimum rest interval of 20 s between speeds are required for accurate results. The procedure is performed separately for the test motions of flexion, extension, left rotation, and right rotation. As opposed to the APD method, which uses a set standard of 100% for normal spinal muscle function, the MPI is a comparative method for data analysis; an increased score from a retest indicates improvement while a decreased score indicates decreased performance as compared to the first test (3). The MPI formula and an example of its application appear in figure 13.4. Figure 13.5 contains a comparison between the APD and MPI methods of isokinetic spinal data interpretation.

## Data collection format

| Speed, °/s | 30 | 60 | 90 | 120 | 150 |
|---|---|---|---|---|---|
| Parameter | PT%BW | PT%BW | AP%BW | AP%BW | AP%BW |
| Parameter | TW%BW | TW%BW | TW%BW | TW%BW | TW%BW |
| Parameter | | | | | ER |

Key: PT%BW = peak torque percent body weight; AP%BW = average power percent body weight; TW%BW = total work percent body weight; ER = endurance ratio.

### Formulas

APD = 100% − average performance ratio (APR)

APR = (PT%BW$_{30}$ + PT%BW$_{60}$ + AP%BW$_{90}$ + AP%BW$_{120}$ + AP%BW$_{150}$ + TW%BW$_{30}$ + TW%BW$_{60}$ + TW%BW$_{90}$ + TW%BW$_{120}$ + TW%BW$_{150}$ + ER$_{150}$)/11

### Example calculation

| Speed, °/s | 30 | 60 | 90 | 120 | 150 |
|---|---|---|---|---|---|
| Data | 110 | 100 | 89 | 94 | 76 |
| Data | 100 | 96 | 65 | 59 | 50 |
| Data | | | | | 66 |

APR = (110 + 100 + 89 + 94 + 76 + 100 + 96 + 65 + 59 + 50 + 66)/11
  = 905/11
  = 82%

APD = 100% − APR
  = 100% − 82%
  = 18%

**Interpretation:** Subject has an 18% deficit in muscle function.

**Figure 13.3** Average performance deficit (APD).
See Timm (16).

# Normative Data—Peak Torque Percent Body Weight

A meta-analysis of the published data (2–9, 14–21, 24) for spinal isokinetic testing reveals several interesting and important results. The results may be grouped into two categories: statistically significant differences and differences that are not statistically significant. The overall analysis is based on a total subject population of 38,740 normal, healthy individuals. The statistically significant findings (19) include the following:

1. Differences in results between genders, with male performance usually exceeding female performance
2. Differences between test motions, with a hierarchy of extension > flexion > rotation

MPI = (peak torque at the slowest test speed + peak torque at the next slowest test speed + average power at the fastest test speed + average power at the next fastest test speed + total work at the slowest test speed + total work at the next slowest test speed + total work at the fastest test speed + total work at the next fastest test speed)/8

**Example calculation**

| Speed, °/s | 30 | 60 | 90 | 120 |
|---|---|---|---|---|
| Peak torque | 235 | 242 | 216 | 144 |
| Average power | 112 | 248 | 334 | 191 |
| Total work | 182 | 204 | 140 | 68 |

MPI = (235 + 242 + 191 + 334 + 182 + 204 + 68 + 140)/8
    = (1596)/8
    = 199.5

---

**Figure 13.4** Muscle performance index (MPI).
See Jerome et al. (3).

---

**Regression equations**

Spinal flexion: MPI – 25.164 = APR

Spinal extension: MPI – 59.641 = APR

---

Key: MPI = muscle performance index; APR = average performance ratio; APD = 100% – APR; APD = average performance deficit.

---

**Figure 13.5** Comparison between APD and MPI data interpretations.

3. Differences between decades, with performance generally decreasing from the 10–19 decade through the 70–79 decade

4. Differences between accuracy of isokinetic data parameters, with peak torque percent body weight (PT%BW) being the single most important measurement of spinal isokinetic muscle function

Similar to a finding for the knee (1), for data on the spine PT%BW also predicts the common isokinetic parameters of average power and total work. Conversely, additional isokinetic parameters do not appear to add any more accuracy or practicality to the overall measurement of spinal muscle performance capacity through isokinetic testing beyond the contribution of PT%BW (1, 19). Therefore, PT%BW alone is both accurate and sufficient for the interpretation of spinal isokinetic data (19). The findings (19) that were not statistically significant include the following:

1. No difference between right rotator and left rotator muscle performance; right and left rotation are equal in normal subjects

2. No difference in overall muscle performance between the common spinal isokinetic test speeds of 30, 60, 90, 120, and 150°/s

3. No difference in overall performance measurement between single speed and multispeed isokinetic test protocols

The latter two findings present two practical implications for spinal isokinetic testing. The first is that testing at multiple speeds is not necessary, since there is no gain to the accuracy, reliability, or validity of the test results. The second is that a subject may be tested accurately at the most comfortable single test speed within the velocity spectrum of 30°/s through 150°/s (19). The normative data for PT%BW and the overall trends for spinal isokinetic data comparisons are summarized in table 13.1 and figure 13.6, respectively.

### Table 13.1   Normative Data— Mean Peak Torque Percent Body Weight

| Decade | Gender | Flexion | Extension | Rotation |
|--------|--------|---------|-----------|----------|
| 10–19 | F | 98.1 | 117.8 | 67.5 |
|       | M | 108.5 | 130.8 | 75.5 |
| 20–29 | F | 93.8 | 111.8 | 65.7 |
|       | M | 103.2 | 122.0 | 71.4 |
| 30–39 | F | 89.7 | 105.4 | 62.1 |
|       | M | 98.5 | 118.2 | 68.9 |
| 40–49 | F | 85.5 | 101.5 | 59.9 |
|       | M | 93.9 | 112.3 | 65.5 |
| 50–59 | F | 81.6 | 96.9 | 56.7 |
|       | M | 89.7 | 108.0 | 61.4 |
| 60–69 | F | 77.8 | 91.8 | 54.5 |
|       | M | 85.6 | 103.1 | 59.9 |
| 70–79 | F | 74.4 | 87.4 | 50.9 |
|       | M | 81.8 | 97.0 | 57.3 |

All data reported in ft-lb (1 ft-lb = 1.3558 Nm). See Timm (19).

# Lifting Capacity Assessment

Isokinetic technology has been effective for the determination of a worker's lifting capacity. Such information is useful as additional data in the overall processes of preplacement screening, functional capacity evaluations, return-to-work evaluations, and disability assessment (2, 4, 12, 13, 16, 23). However, as is the case with all applications of the technology, isokinetic testing is designed to complement other methods of clinical and physiological performance testing and is not meant to exist as a single, or the only, means of worker assessment (4, 12, 13, 23).

Flexion:     PT%BW declines 3.4% per decade in females
             PT%BW declines 3.5% per decade in males
             Female:Male PT%BW ratio = 1.00:1.15

Extension:   PT%BW declines 3.7% per decade in females
             PT%BW declines 3.7% per decade in males
             Female:Male PT%BW ratio = 1.00:1.11

Rotation:    PT%BW declines 3.5% per decade in females
             PT%BW declines 3.4% per decade in males
             Female:Male PT%BW ratio = 1.00:1.11

Females:     Flexion:Extension PT%BW ratio = 1.00:1.19
             Rotation:Flexion PT%BW ratio = 1.00:1.38
             Rotation:Extension PT%BW ratio = 1.00:1.71
             Right:Left rotation PT%BW ratio = 1.00:1.00

Males:       Flexion:Extension PT%BW ratio = 1.00:1.20
             Rotation:Flexion PT%BW ratio = 1.00:1.44
             Rotation:Extension PT%BW ratio - 1.00:1.72
             Right:Left rotation PT%BW ratio = 1.00:1.00

Key: PT%BW = peak torque percent body weight.

**Figure 13.6**   Isokinetic spinal data trends.
See Timm (19).

# Normative Data

The literature reports two different methods for the testing of lifting capacity with isokinetic technology: normative data and ergonomic formulas. Both methods employ an isokinetic lifting dynamometer instead of a freestanding spinal dynamometer or a spinal testing attachment to an extremity system. The existing normative database encompasses 2,688 healthy subjects (1,236 females; 1,452 males) in the age range of 10 to 79 years (23). The subjects were tested across a variety of linear lift speeds using a flexed knees-flexed back lifting posture, which is still the routine method for lifting in many industries (23). The data, which may be generalized to any isokinetic lifting dynamometer, are summarized in tables 13.2 and 13.3.

# Ergonomic Formulas

The other method for isokinetic lift testing uses a set of two ergonomic formulas. The formulas require the collection of isokinetic average force data over a minimum of five maximal lift efforts at the linear speed of 30 in/s (13). The formulas, which appear in figure 13.7, generate two pieces of data: MDL and MAL. MDL is the acronym for maximum dynamic lift, which is the amount of weight that a worker may lift safely only once per hour for each hour of a standard eight-hour workday (13). The MDL may be thought of as the one hour repetition maximum (1 HRM) or as the eight repetition maximum per day (8 RM/D). However, the MDL has limited application to contemporary

## Table 13.2    Normative Data—Female Lifting Performance

| Speed | Decade | PF | | PF%BW | |
|-------|--------|------|------|------|------|
|       |        | Mean | SD | Mean | SD |
| 60  | 10–19 | 130.8 | 27.6 | 74.9 | 13.1 |
|     | 20–29 | 138.3 | 29.2 | 79.2 | 13.9 |
|     | 30–39 | 120.9 | 25.5 | 69.2 | 12.1 |
|     | 40–49 | 115.9 | 24.4 | 66.4 | 11.6 |
|     | 50–59 | 105.9 | 22.4 | 60.7 | 10.6 |
|     | 60–69 | 99.7 | 21.0 | 57.1 | 10.0 |
|     | 70–79 | 83.5 | 17.6 | 47.8 | 8.4 |
| 120 | 10–19 | 118.8 | 39.5 | 64.9 | 22.2 |
|     | 20–29 | 129.0 | 42.9 | 70.5 | 24.2 |
|     | 30–39 | 111.9 | 37.2 | 61.2 | 21.0 |
|     | 40–49 | 103.9 | 34.6 | 56.8 | 19.5 |
|     | 50–59 | 93.6 | 31.2 | 51.2 | 17.5 |
|     | 60–69 | 89.1 | 29.6 | 48.7 | 16.7 |
|     | 70–79 | 74.2 | 24.7 | 40.6 | 13.9 |
| 180 | 10–19 | 111.8 | 33.8 | 64.6 | 18.9 |
|     | 20–29 | 126.0 | 38.1 | 72.8 | 21.4 |
|     | 30–39 | 105.2 | 31.8 | 60.8 | 17.8 |
|     | 40–49 | 100.8 | 30.4 | 58.2 | 17.1 |
|     | 50–59 | 89.9 | 27.1 | 51.9 | 15.2 |
|     | 60–69 | 86.6 | 26.1 | 50.0 | 14.7 |
|     | 70-79 | 72.3 | 21.8 | 41.8 | 12.3 |
| 240 | 10–19 | 115.5 | 51.2 | 55.9 | 22.2 |
|     | 20–29 | 125.6 | 55.7 | 60.8 | 24.2 |
|     | 30–39 | 106.5 | 47.2 | 51.6 | 20.5 |
|     | 40–49 | 100.9 | 44.7 | 48.9 | 19.4 |
|     | 50–59 | 90.8 | 40.2 | 43.9 | 17.5 |
|     | 60–69 | 86.3 | 38.3 | 41.8 | 16.6 |
|     | 70–79 | 71.7 | 31.8 | 34.8 | 13.8 |
| 300 | 10–19 | 84.7 | 50.6 | 60.6 | 28.0 |
|     | 20–29 | 91.3 | 54.6 | 65.3 | 30.2 |
|     | 30–39 | 77.2 | 46.1 | 55.2 | 25.6 |
|     | 40–49 | 73.0 | 43.6 | 52.3 | 24.2 |
|     | 50–59 | 64.7 | 38.7 | 46.3 | 21.4 |
|     | 60–69 | 61.4 | 36.7 | 43.9 | 20.4 |
|     | 70–79 | 51.5 | 30.8 | 36.8 | 17.0 |
| 360 | 10–19 | 74.8 | 39.0 | 51.9 | 19.2 |
|     | 20–29 | 81.3 | 42.4 | 56.4 | 20.8 |
|     | 30–39 | 69.7 | 36.4 | 48.4 | 17.8 |
|     | 40–49 | 66.1 | 34.5 | 45.9 | 16.9 |
|     | 50–59 | 59.5 | 31.1 | 41.3 | 15.2 |
|     | 60–69 | 56.6 | 29.6 | 39.3 | 14.5 |
|     | 70–79 | 47.2 | 24.6 | 32.8 | 12.1 |

Key: Speed = in/s; PF = peak force (lb; 1kg = 2.2 lb); PF%BW = peak force percent body weight (bw in lb); SD = standard deviation. Data from Timm (23).

## Table 13.3 Normative Data—Male Lifting Performance

| Speed | Decade | PF Mean | PF SD | PF%BW Mean | PF%BW SD |
|-------|--------|---------|-------|------------|----------|
| 60  | 10–19 | 257.5 | 21.2 | 141.1 | 27.7 |
|     | 20–29 | 272.2 | 22.4 | 149.2 | 29.3 |
|     | 30–39 | 237.8 | 19.6 | 130.4 | 25.6 |
|     | 40–49 | 228.0 | 18.8 | 125.0 | 24.6 |
|     | 50–59 | 208.4 | 17.2 | 114.2 | 22.4 |
|     | 60–69 | 196.2 | 16.2 | 107.5 | 21.1 |
|     | 70–79 | 164.3 | 13.5 | 90.0 | 17.7 |
| 120 | 10–19 | 235.1 | 36.7 | 129.1 | 20.2 |
|     | 20–29 | 255.5 | 39.9 | 140.2 | 21.9 |
|     | 30–39 | 221.6 | 34.6 | 121.6 | 19.0 |
|     | 40–49 | 205.8 | 32.1 | 112.9 | 17.6 |
|     | 50–59 | 185.4 | 28.9 | 101.8 | 15.9 |
|     | 60–69 | 176.4 | 27.5 | 96.8 | 15.1 |
|     | 70–79 | 146.9 | 22.9 | 80.7 | 12.6 |
| 180 | 10–19 | 211.5 | 47.5 | 113.6 | 30.4 |
|     | 20–29 | 238.5 | 53.6 | 128.1 | 34.3 |
|     | 30–39 | 199.1 | 44.7 | 106.9 | 28.6 |
|     | 40–49 | 190.8 | 42.9 | 102.5 | 27.4 |
|     | 50–59 | 170.1 | 38.2 | 91.3 | 24.4 |
|     | 60–69 | 163.8 | 36.8 | 88.0 | 23.5 |
|     | 70-79 | 136.9 | 30.8 | 73.5 | 19.7 |
| 240 | 10–19 | 183.5 | 66.5 | 105.5 | 72.4 |
|     | 20–29 | 199.6 | 72.4 | 114.7 | 35.0 |
|     | 30–39 | 169.3 | 61.4 | 97.3 | 29.7 |
|     | 40–49 | 160.4 | 58.1 | 92.2 | 28.2 |
|     | 50–59 | 144.3 | 52.3 | 82.9 | 25.4 |
|     | 60–69 | 137.2 | 49.7 | 78.7 | 24.1 |
|     | 70–79 | 114.0 | 41.3 | 65.5 | 20.0 |
| 300 | 10–19 | 191.4 | 49.4 | 95.1 | 41.3 |
|     | 20–29 | 206.5 | 53.2 | 102.5 | 44.6 |
|     | 30–39 | 174.6 | 45.0 | 86.7 | 37.7 |
|     | 40–49 | 165.2 | 42.6 | 82.0 | 35.6 |
|     | 50–59 | 146.4 | 37.8 | 72.7 | 31.6 |
|     | 60–69 | 138.9 | 35.8 | 68.9 | 29.9 |
|     | 70–79 | 116.4 | 30.0 | 57.8 | 25.1 |
| 360 | 10–19 | 173.6 | 65.4 | 85.4 | 34.5 |
|     | 20–29 | 188.8 | 71.1 | 92.8 | 37.5 |
|     | 30–39 | 161.8 | 61.0 | 79.6 | 32.2 |
|     | 40–49 | 153.4 | 57.8 | 75.4 | 30.5 |
|     | 50–59 | 138.2 | 52.1 | 67.9 | 27.5 |
|     | 60–69 | 131.5 | 49.5 | 64.7 | 26.1 |
|     | 70–79 | 109.6 | 41.3 | 53.9 | 21.8 |

Key: Speed = in/s; PF = peak force (lb; 1kg = 2.2 lb); PF%BW = peak force percent body weight (bw in lb); SD = standard deviation.

MDL = 295 + 0.66 (AF) – 148 (S)

MAL = 0.22 (MDL)

Key: MDL = maximum dynamic lift (lb; 1 kg = 2.2 lb); MAL = maximum acceptable load (lb;); AF = average isokinetic force (at 30 in/s); S = gender factor (for females = 2, for males = 1)

**Figure 13.7**  Ergonomic lifting formulas.
See Pytel and Kamon (13).

worker testing and conditioning practices and is not recognized by state workers' compensation systems.

In contrast, the formula for MAL is quite usable for industrial applications. MAL is the acronym for maximum acceptable load, which is the amount of weight that a worker may lift frequently, or continuously, up to a maximum frequency of six lifts per minute (13). The maximum frequency of six lifts per minute is the upper legal limit for safe material handling and lifting as established by the National Institute for Occupational Safety and Health (NIOSH). Therefore, isokinetic testing can fulfill the practical expectation of determining a worker's safe lifting capacity. Normative data for the ergonomic lifting formulas appear in table 13.4, *a* and *b*.

# Training Principles

Isokinetic technology may be used as a means of exercise directed toward the goal of facilitating the physiological adaptations that have been described previously. The enhancement of the cardiovascular, connective tissue, intervertebral disk, muscle, neurological, and biomechanical systems would be a

### Table 13.4a  Normative Data for Ergonomic Lifting Formulas (Means) for Females

| Decade | AF | MDL | MAL |
|--------|------|------|-----|
| 10–19 | 46.7 | 29.8 | 6.6 |
| 20–29 | 50.4 | 32.3 | 7.1 |
| 30–39 | 42.6 | 27.1 | 6.0 |
| 40–49 | 40.3 | 25.6 | 5.6 |
| 50–59 | 35.7 | 22.6 | 5.0 |
| 60–69 | 33.9 | 21.4 | 4.7 |
| 70–79 | 28.4 | 17.7 | 3.9 |

Key: AF = average force at a speed of 30 in/s; MDL = maximal dynamic lift (lb; 1 kg = 2.2 lb); MAL = maximum acceptable load (lb)

**Table 13.4b Normative Data
for Ergonomic Lifting Formulas (Means) for Males**

| Decade | AF | MDL | MAL |
|--------|-------|-------|------|
| 10–19 | 105.5 | 216.6 | 47.6 |
| 20–29 | 113.7 | 222.0 | 48.8 |
| 30–39 | 96.2 | 210.5 | 46.3 |
| 40–49 | 90.9 | 206.9 | 45.5 |
| 50–59 | 80.6 | 200.2 | 44.0 |
| 60–69 | 76.5 | 197.5 | 43.4 |
| 70–79 | 64.1 | 189.3 | 41.6 |

Key: AF = average force at a speed of 30 in/s; MDL = maximal dynamic lift (lb; 1 kg = 2.2 lb); MAL = maximum acceptable load (lb)

desired outcome for a wide variety of athletes or clients. The two guiding principles for the construction of isokinetic training protocols have been the traditional—the velocity spectrum—and the contemporary—exercise to 50% fatigue.

## Velocity Spectrum

The traditional velocity spectrum approach to isokinetic exercise involves a pyramid sequence of increasing and then decreasing training speeds (5, 6, 8, 9, 14–16, 19, 20). The subject starts exercising at a relatively slow speed, progresses at distinct increments toward a faster speed, and then returns in set increments to the starting, slower speed. As is the case with traditional testing methods, the usual velocity spectrum for spinal isokinetic activity is 30°/s through 150°/s. This spectrum, which may be used for both flexion/extension and left/right rotation training, appears in table 13.5.

**Table 13.5 Velocity Spectrum Training Protocol**

| Speed (°/s) | 30 | 60 | 90 | 120 | 150 | 150 | 120 | 90 | 60 | 30 |
|-------------|----|----|----|-----|-----|-----|-----|----|----|----|
| Reps | 10 | 10 | 10 | 10 | 10 | 10 | 10 | 10 | 10 | 10 |

Rest    20–90 s between speeds

ROM    Subject comfort or functional range

Possibilities for progression:

1. Increase the number of repetitions per speed.

2. Decrease the rest interval between speeds.

3. Increase the number of sequences (sets).

See Timm (16).

The basic speed pyramid for the spine begins at a velocity of 30°/s and progresses in speed increments of 30°/s up to the top velocity of 150°/s. The subject performs 10 repetitions of flexion/extension or left/right rotation exercise at each speed, with a rest interval of 20–90 s between each training speed (5, 6, 8, 9, 14–16). As is also the case with spinal isokinetic testing, the subject exercises through a ROM that is comfortable or, preferably, functional for the individual (16, 17, 24).

The velocity spectrum format of training may be progressed in several ways. The usual methods include increasing the number of repetitions performed at each speed from the base unit of 10, decreasing the rest interval between training speeds, or performing multiple sets of the speed pyramid sequence (16, 17, 24). Any, or a combination of several, of these methods may be used to adjust the intensity and volume of exercise for the conditioning of the spinal muscle groups. As is the case with many programs of progressive resistance exercise, the velocity spectrum is best performed under the guidelines ·three sessions per week, with at least 48 h rest in between training sessions , 17, 24).

# Exercise to 50% Fatigue

Instead of a distinct number of repetitions performed in increments of speed across a velocity spectrum, exercise to 50% fatigue involves training at a single isokinetic speed (16, 25). Training at a single exercise velocity is reinforced by the findings that a statistically significant difference does not exist for performance outcomes between different spinal isokinetic test speeds (19) and a sufficient physiological overflow effect occurs between all speeds across the isokinetic velocity spectrum for the spine (16, 22). These factors enable the practical guideline of having training occur at a single exercise velocity that is most comfortable for the subject (18, 19, 24).

Exercise to 50% fatigue is based on the physiological concept that the most efficient way to train a muscle system is to exercise until force production drops to one-half of the initial output (16, 25). Peak torque is the isokinetic parameter most commonly used to monitor a subject's muscle force production (1, 16, 19, 20, 25). Thus, unlike the velocity spectrum approach to spinal isokinetic training, exercise occurs independent of a distinct number of repetitions, since the number of repetitions needed to achieve a level of 50% fatigue varies with each individual subject during exercise. Also unlike the velocity spectrum method, exercise encompasses a single set of repetitions because additional sets would promote muscle fatigue below a level of 50%, which increases the risk of muscle overuse injury (16, 25).

The concept of isokinetic exercise to 50% fatigue may be clarified through the following example sequence. First, the subject would complete a preparatory warm-up activity, similar to the pretest warm-up used for spinal isokinetic testing. Second, the subject would be positioned for exercise in a spinal isokinetic dynamometer system. Third, a single, comfortable exercise speed would be selected from the spinal isokinetic velocity spectrum of 30°/s through 150°/s. Fourth, the subject would begin exercising and would be coached to provide maximal efforts of either flexion/extension or left/right rotation through the desired plane of motion. Fifth, the initial level of peak torque output for the first repetition in the first direction of motion would be recorded for use in monitoring the subject's progress toward 50% fatigue. Sixth, the subject would be coached to continue maximal exercise efforts as the peak torque level is monitored during each repetition. Seventh, the subject would be instructed to stop the training bout once the level of peak torque output dropped to 50% of the peak torque output recorded from the initial exercise repetition. Eighth and lastly, the exercise process would continue in a format of two to three sessions per week, with a break period of at least 48 h rest in between sessions. This regimen should produce an effective training response, since the spinal muscles are exercised efficiently to a physiological level of fatigue that simultaneously promotes the enhancement of overall muscle performance and protects against muscle overuse injury (16, 25).

# Summary

This chapter has presented current information on the aspects of isokinetic technology as applied to the lumbar spine. It has examined the effects that isokinetic activity has on different systems of the body to produce physiological adaptations in bone, the cardiovascular system, connective tissue, the intervertebral disk, muscle, and the neurological system. Biomechanical effects have also been examined relative to the influence that isokinetic activity has on the posture of the lumbar lordotic curve and during different kinetic chain states.

The process of spinal isokinetic testing has also been examined. Testing may be used to determine muscle function in the sagittal and transverse planes of motion or to determine a subject's lifting ability for functional applications. Testing protocols have evolved from a multispeed approach across the velocity spectrum requiring a distinct ROM to the current format of data collection from a single test speed within the spectrum of 30 to 150°/s over a test ROM established as comfortable for each subject.

This chapter has also discussed data interpretation. In parallel to testing, the processes for interpreting spinal isokinetic test data have advanced from the formula method of APD and MPI to the use of normative data for PT%BW. Conversely, normative data for lifting ability are not as practical as the MDL and MAL ergonomic formulas to predict a subject's functional capacity.

Lastly, the chapter presented material on the use of isokinetic procedures for spinal muscle training. The velocity spectrum approach was described as the traditional method of spinal isokinetic exercise. This involves 10 repetitions performed at each speed as the subject progresses up and then down the pyramid of 30 through 150°/s. However, the format of isokinetic exercise to 50% fatigue at a single velocity was suggested as a more physiologically efficient method of spinal muscle training. A working knowledge of all of these concepts should enable the appropriate use of spinal isokinetic technology by the practitioner for the collection of accurate data and the design of effective exercise prescriptions.

# References

1. Bandy, W.D., and K.E. Timm. 1992. Relationship between peak torque, work, and power for knee flexion and extension in clients with grade I medical compartment sprains of the knee. *Journal of Orthopaedic and Sports Physical Therapy* 16: 288–92.

2. Hazard, R.G., S. Reid, and J. Fenwick. 1988. Isokinetic trunk and lifting strength measurements. *Spine* 13: 54–57.

3. Jerome, J.A., K. Hunter, P. Gordon, and N. McKay. 1991. A new robust index for measuring trunk flexion and extension. *Spine* 16: 804–8.

4. Kishino, N.D., T.G. Mayer, and R.J. Gatchel. 1985. Quantification of lumbar function, part 4: Isometric and isokinetic lifting simulation in normal subjects and low back dysfunction patients. *Spine* 10: 921–27.

5. Langrana, N.A., and C.K. Lee. 1984. Isokinetic evaluation of trunk muscles. *Spine* 9: 171–75.

6. Langrana, N.A., C.K. Lee, and H. Alexander. 1984. Quantitative assessment of back strength using isokinetic testing. *Spine* 9: 287–90.

7. Marras, W.S., and A.I. King. 1984. Measurement of loads on the lumbar spine under isometric and isokinetic conditions. *Spine* 9: 176–87.

8. Mayer, T.G., S.S. Smith, and J. Keeley. 1985. Quantification of lumbar function, part 2: Sagittal plane trunk strength in chronic low back pain patients. *Spine* 10: 765–72.

9. Newton, M., M. Thow, D. Somerville, I. Henderson, and G. Waddell. 1993. Trunk strength testing with iso-machines. *Spine* 18: 812–24.

10. Ng, J.K., C.A. Richardson, V. Kippers, and M. Parnianpour. 1998. Relationship between muscle fiber composition and functional capacity of back muscles in healthy subjects and patients with back pain. *Journal of Orthopaedic and Sports Physical Therapy* 27: 389–402.

11. Peel, C., and M.J. Alland. 1990. Cardiovascular responses to isokinetic trunk exercise. *Physical Therapy* 70: 503–10.

12. Porterfield, J.A., R.A. Mostardi, and S. King. 1987. Simulated lift testing using computerized isokinetics. *Spine* 12: 683–87.

13. Pytel, J.L., and E. Kamon. 1981. Dynamic strength tests as a predictor for maximal acceptable lifting. *Ergonomics* 24: 663–72.

14. Smith, S.S., T.G. Mayer, and R.J. Gatchel. 1985. Quantification of lumbar function, part 1: Isometric and multispeed isokinetic trunk strength measures in sagittal and axial planes in normal subjects. *Spine* 10: 757–64.

15. Thompson, N.N., J.A. Gould, and G.J. Davies. 1985. Descriptive measures of isokinetic trunk testing. *Journal of Orthopaedic and Sports Physical Therapy* 7: 43–49.

16. Timm, K.E. 1989. *Back injuries and rehabilitation*. Baltimore, MD: Williams & Wilkins.

17. Timm, K.E. 1994. A randomized-control study of active and passive treatments for chronic low back pain following L5 laminectomy. *Journal of Orthopaedic and Sports Physical Therapy* 20: 276–86.

18. Timm, K.E. 1987. Case studies: Use of the Cybex trunk extension flexion unit in the rehabilitation of back patients. *Journal of Orthopaedic and Sports Physical Therapy* 8: 578–81.

19. Timm, K.E. 1995. Clinical applications of a normative database for the Cybex TEF and TORSO spinal isokinetic dynamometers. *Isokinetics and Exercise Science* 5: 43–49.

20. Timm, K.E. 1994. Comparison of test data from the Cybex TEF and 6000-TMC isokinetic spinal dynamometers. *Isokinetics and Exercise Science* 4: 112–15.

21. Timm, K.E. 1991. Effect of different kinetic chain states on the isokinetic performance of the lumbar muscles. *Isokinetics and Exercise Science* 1: 153–60.

22. Timm, K.E. 1987. Investigation of the physiological overflow effect from speed-specific isokinetic activity. *Journal of Orthopaedic and Sports Physical Therapy* 9: 106–10.

23. Timm, K.E. 1988. Isokinetic lifting simulation: A normative data study. *Journal of Orthopaedic and Sports Physical Therapy* 10: 156–66.

24. Timm, K.E. 1991. Management of the chronic low back pain patient: A retrospective analysis of different treatment approaches. *Isokinetics and Exercise Science* 1: 44–48.

25. Timm, K.E. 1987. Suggestion from the field: Isokinetic exercise to 50% fatigue. *Journal of Orthopaedic and Sports Physical Therapy* 8: 505–6.

26. Timm, K.E. and D. Fyke. 1993. The effect of test speed sequence on the concentric isokinetic performance of the knee extensor muscle group. *Isokinetics and Exercise Science* 3: 123–28.

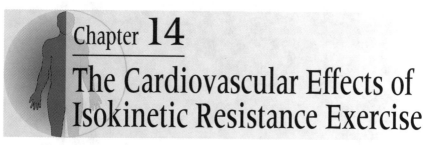

# Chapter 14
# The Cardiovascular Effects of Isokinetic Resistance Exercise

Douglas M. Kleiner

**R**esistance exercise has become a very popular form of exercise for enhancing one's performance. The effects of resistance exercise on the development of skeletal muscle are becoming more widely known; however, far less is known about its effects on more central parameters such as the cardiovascular system. Isokinetic resistance was introduced in 1967 (27, 57) and today remains a very popular form of exercise for strength gains; it is becoming more widely accepted as a mode of resistance exercise for performance enhancement. Much of what we know about the cardiovascular effects of resistance exercise has been learned by studying forms of resistance other than isokinetics (i.e., isometric or constant load). It is reasonable to assume that many of the cardiovascular responses or adaptations that can be encountered or stimulated by constant load resistance exercises (fixed or variable resistance) can also be encountered or stimulated by isokinetic resistance. It is far less reasonable to make inferences between static (isometric) and dynamic (constant load or isokinetic) resistance exercises (47).

The literature reveals few publications addressing the chronic cardiovascular effects (adaptations) of resistance exercises and even fewer for the acute cardiovascular effects (responses). Perhaps one reason that such little information exists on this topic is because of the difficulty in obtaining accurate cardiovascular measurements, particularly blood pressure measurements. The only way to truly "measure" blood pressure is to obtain it directly from within the artery (see figures 14.1 and 14.2). This procedure, called intraarterial blood pressure monitoring, is an invasive technique that requires the involvement of a physician. All other indirect methods (such as auscultation) are only estimates of arterial blood pressure. Although these indirect methods are generally accepted as valid during rest, they are not considered valid during exercise and especially during resistance exercise. One problem with auscultation during resistance exercise is the occurrence of a potent pressor response that is

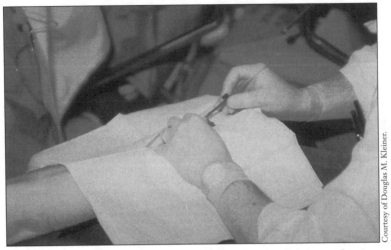

Courtesy of Douglas M. Kleiner.

**Figure 14.1** The introduction of the arterial catheter by a guide wire.

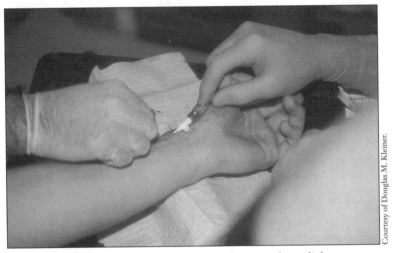

Courtesy of Douglas M. Kleiner.

**Figure 14.2** Placement of the arterial catheter in the radial artery.

known to dramatically elevate blood pressure during resistance exercises. These sudden elevations can remain undetected by measurements obtained postexercise or by discontinuous, indirect methods of measurement such as by auscultation (5, 17, 24, 60). Furthermore, it has been shown that indirect measures of blood pressure underestimate actual arterial pressures. This inaccuracy is even greater during exercise and particularly with resistance exercises (25, 51, 52, 60).

Knowing the cardiovascular response to a specific resistance exercise is important because of the stress that is placed on the heart and vasculature as a result of the exercise. In a number of instances, and in a number of populations, it might be prudent to avoid those resistance exercises or protocols that may excessively stress the cardiovascular system.

# Chronic Cardiovascular Adaptations

The effects of resistance exercise on strength and muscular function have been investigated by many prominent researchers (2, 3, 6, 8, 20, 49, 56). While a number of investigators have compared the effects of using different forms of resistance, or methods of training, on strength (7, 10, 19, 48, 55), limited information is available regarding the cardiovascular adaptation.

Although few studies have used isokinetics as the form of resistance, there is no reason to think that cardiovascular adaptations would not take place with isokinetic resistance training. The one study that did use isokinetic resistance as the means of training did not evaluate the typical cardiovascular parameters such as heart rate and blood pressure. The chronic adaptation study by Haennel and others (22) used hydraulic circuit training as the form of resistance to examine maximal oxygen consumption, stroke volume, and cardiac output. The experimental design for that study had two groups of subjects performing circuit weight training (each with different protocols), while a third group of subjects (the control group) trained by cycling. The results showed an increase in maximal oxygen consumption for all three groups. The authors attributed the increases in oxygen consumption to the increases in stroke volume and cardiac output (22). In a follow-up study, the researchers trained 16 individuals immediately after coronary artery bypass surgery (23). Subjects were divided into an aerobic exercise group (cycle ergometer) and an isokinetic resistance training group. The results from that study demonstrated significant increases in oxygen consumption, stroke volume, and cardiac output in both groups. However, strength gains were observed only in the resistance training group (23).

# Acute Cardiovascular Responses

The acute cardiovascular responses to resistance exercises are equally, if not more, important than the chronic adaptations that may take place. That is because the chronic adaptations occur as a result of many "acute stresses" that are repeatedly placed on the system over time. However, it is this "acute stress" that can by more dangerous, particularly when an individual is unable to tolerate the physiological stress. Although this can be an important consideration when dealing with healthy individuals, it can become critical when dealing with individuals who have a pathology, such as athletes who are hypertensive.

## Heart Rates

In 1990, Kleiner (31) reported a study in which heart rate was measured directly and continuously by electrocardiogram in response to isokinetic resistance exercises at four different speeds. Subjects performed single-leg flexion and extension exercises at the knee until exhaustion at 12°/s, 46°/s, 96°/s, and 192°/s on a Cybex II isokinetic dynamometer (see figure 14.3). The results showed that both the mean peak heart rates and the mean increase in heart rate from resting values increased with each increase in isokinetic velocity.

Past acute cardiovascular studies have examined heart rate as the only cardiovascular parameter, even though heart rate is not the only contributor to cardiovascular stress. As one author states,

> *"the use of heart rate alone as a measure of circulatory load has a rather restricted value. It is shown that the intrinsic value of each heartbeat as a measure of circulatory load differs greatly in different types of work-load since apart from heart rate, stroke-volume and mean blood pressure show various patterns of reaction in these conditions"* (4: p. 857).

Hence, many of the studies that examined heart rate alone have been dismissed for being rather incomplete. Still, the process of obtaining accurate blood pressure measurements during an acute bout of resistance exercise remains a challenge.

Some acute cardiovascular response studies investigated blood pressure in addition to heart rate. However, many of these studies have used indirect methods of obtaining blood pressure (by auscultation via a sphygmomanometer), despite the known inaccuracy of these methods during exercise (see figure 14.4). In an acute response study with isokinetics being used as the form of resistance, indirect measurements of blood pressure and heart rate were evalu-

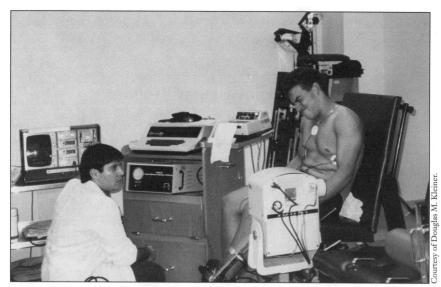

Courtesy of Douglas M. Kleiner.

**Figure 14.3** Heart rate being monitored by electrocardiogram in response to exhaustive exercises with the Cybex II dynamometer.

ated in response to velocity-specific exercises. In this study, subjects performed as many repetitions as possible during a one-minute exercise session. Heart rates and systolic and diastolic blood pressures were observed, although blood pressures were taken by auscultation (9). This study found that during exercise heart rate increased with increases in velocity. The findings from this study were similar to the previously reported study by Kleiner, which did not attempt to take blood pressure because of the known limitations of indirect measurement (31). It is interesting to note the similar findings with these two studies, even though their methods were different. In the Douris (9) study the subjects only performed for one minute, whereas in the Kleiner (31) study, the subjects were instructed to complete as many repetitions as they could, until failure (30).

## Limitation of Indirect Measures of Blood Pressure

While indirect methods may be accurate during rest, it has been reported that blood pressure measurements taken after exercise, even immediately after exercise, are grossly inaccurate (17). This inaccuracy is exaggerated even more when the form of exercise is resistance exercise. Specifically, blood pressure is known to become dramatically elevated during resistance exercise due to a potent pressor response. These sudden elevations are not detectable by measurements obtained postexercise or by noncontinuous, indirect methods of measurement such as auscultation (5, 17, 24, 60).

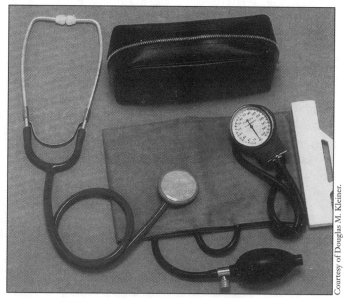

Courtesy of Douglas M. Kleiner.

**Figure 14.4** A sphygmomanometer and stethoscope as an example of an indirect method used to estimate blood pressure.

In each case when compared with indirect measurements, the direct measurements were higher than the indirect measurements. That is to say, the estimates given by indirect methods such as auscultation underestimate the actual blood pressure (both systolic and diastolic blood pressure) during rest, exercise, and recovery (52). This has been supported by other reports as well (25, 32, 45, 51, 52, 60).

Lastly, automated measurements of blood pressure correlate poorly with auscultation measures and are thought to be less accurate, especially during exercise and with resistance exercise in particular (28, 36).

The problem with indirect measurement, even automated measurement, is that the pressor response can go undetected. The pressor response, although not yet completely understood, is an immediate increase in blood pressure that occurs during muscular actions. It is largely the result of an increased cardiac output and to a lesser extent a reflex vasoconstriction of the vascular beds in nonexercising muscles (21, 41). Its purpose is to maintain perfusion pressure in an exercising muscle, which may become partially occluded with the increased intramuscular pressure (muscle pump) that is experienced during the actions of resistance exercise. In addition to creating very sudden and short-lived spikes in blood pressure, the pressor response can also produce a rapid drop in blood pressure immediately after exercise as large vasodilated muscles that were occluded are suddenly perfused, all of which would go undetected by indirect methods of measurement.

The pressor response has been shown by Fleck and Dean (13, 14) to be lessened with resistance training experience. Fleck and Dean also went on to hypothesize as to why the pressor response is attenuated with resistance exercises. Their hypotheses include the resetting of the peripheral barroreceptor threshold and the desensitization of the sympathetic nervous system (13, 14). In another study, Fleck and coworkers (15) reported that a linear relationship does indeed exist between intrathoracic pressure (caused by the Valsalva maneuver) and systolic blood pressure, diastolic blood pressure, cardiac output, and stroke volume during resistance exercises. However, a nonlinear relationship exists between heart rate and blood pressure, and active muscle mass involvement. In addition, it was reported that the cardiovascular response varied between exercises (leg press and leg extension) and varied with manipulations made in the exercise protocol (resistance and number of repetitions) (15).

Maximal oxygen uptake, changes in range of motion, and high-intensity exercises have all been evaluated with regard to the pressor response, although none of these variables was found to be strongly correlated to the response (1, 29, 46). However, a lower pressor response has been correlated to muscles composed predominantly of slow twitch muscle fibers (12).

MacDougall and colleagues (39) have examined the effects of the Valsalva maneuver (along with joint angle, muscle size, and strength) on the blood pressure response to resistance exercises. Many important findings were reported in this study, including their conclusion that the greatest rise in blood pressure occurred at the weakest point in the strength curve (39). That conclusion may be an important factor when discussing isokinetic resistance, since isokinetics were developed, in part, to compensate for the different points in the strength curve (57).

Other researchers have reported values of blood pressure and mouth pressure (estimating intrathoracic pressure in response to the Valsalva maneuver) during resistance exercises. MacDougall and coworkers (41, 42) reported perhaps a more important finding that pressures were substantially higher during the concentric phase of the exercise as opposed to the eccentric phase, with the highest numbers in blood pressure and heart rate occurring during the last several repetitions in the set (mean blood pressure value for the group was 320/250 mm Hg; one subject had a value of 480/350 mm Hg). Again, because many isokinetic devices allow for dual concentric exercise (during flexion and extension, with no eccentric component) (59), this finding could have important implications in the acute cardiovascular response to isokinetic resistance exercise. The MacDougall group concluded that when subjects perform heavy weight-lifting exercises, the mechanical compression of blood vessels with each contraction combines with a potent pressor response and a Valsalva response to produce extreme elevations in systolic and diastolic pressures. These elevations are extreme even when exercise is performed with a relatively small muscle mass (41, 42).

A later study by MacDougall and colleagues (40) was designed to examine the contributions of the Valsalva maneuver, muscle size and strength, force of muscle action, type of muscle action, changes in the joint angle, and the effects of muscle fatigue on the blood pressure response to resistance exercises. Data revealed no effect from muscle size or strength or type of action. However, joint angle (weakest point of the strength curve) and the Valsalva maneuver were again found to be contributors to increases in blood pressure. MacDougall and colleagues have stated that the Valsalva maneuver is an unavoidable consequence of high resistance exercise with repeated muscle actions to failure (40).

However, Kleiner and colleagues (32) discouraged subjects from performing the Valsalva maneuver and took precautions to avoid any occurrence of the Valsalva maneuver. The subjects were instructed and prompted to inhale and exhale continuously during both the concentric and eccentric portion of each repetition. In addition, the subjects' respiratory pattern was observed by impedance pneumography and the very sensitive intraarterial blood pressure waveform was printed (see figure 14.5). Thus, any occurrence of the Valsalva maneuver should have been evident in the pressure tracings. The authors state that they were confident that little or no breath holding occurred (32). They concluded, like those before them, that extremely high intraarterial blood pressures could occur even in the absence of a Valsalva maneuver (11, 38).

# Direct Measurement of Blood Pressure During Isokinetic Resistance Exercise

Several forms of resistance exercise equipment are commercially available, and some forms vary the resistance throughout the range of motion in order to

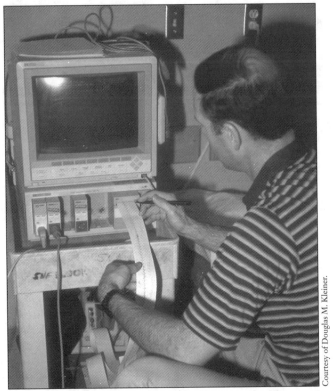

**Figure 14.5** Impedance pneumography and intraarterial blood pressure wave forms being continuously monitored and printed.

more closely match the strength curve of the subject. This is done, in part, to lessen the biomechanical "sticking region," which may introduce an isometric component into the maneuver. These isometric components are believed to further contribute to the elevated cardiovascular response associated with resistance exercises (26). However, few studies have investigated the acute cardiovascular effects of resistance exercise, and those that have did not consider the form of resistance as a variable. Kleiner and coworkers have stated that the form or mode of resistance selected is as important a contributor to the cardiovascular response of the exercise as the exercise itself (32).

## Isokinetic Resistance Versus Other Forms of Resistance

There have only been a few intraarterial studies to compare the blood pressure response during resistance exercise from different forms of resistance. In one study, the investigators compared 10 repetitions of free weight bench press at 25% and 50% of maximum isometric strength versus isokinetic (hydraulic) resistance at fast and slow speeds. The slow isokinetic speed produced the greatest mean systolic and diastolic blood pressure values, followed by the 50% constant load fixed resistance, the 25% constant load fixed resistance, and the fast isokinetic speed producing the least values (18).

Kleiner and coworkers (32) also conducted an intraarterial study that evaluated the acute cardiovascular responses to resistance exercises with different forms of resistance. In that study, six normotensive males performed a cycle ergometer test and one set of resistance exercises to failure with constant load fixed resistance, variable resistance, and isokinetic resistance. The resistance exercises used were single-leg, concentric leg extension and eccentric leg flexion exercises at the knee. These exercises were performed on the Kin-Com 125E+ isokinetic testing and exercise device, on the David leg extension machine for variable resistance, and on the Universal leg extension machine for constant load resistance. Every subject performed one continuous set of exercises until they reached momentary muscular failure or were unable to continue (32).

Significant differences ($p < .05$) were reported for heart rate, systolic blood pressure, diastolic blood pressure, and rate pressure product, among the conditions. However, most of the differences were between the aerobic exercise and the three resistance exercises. Mean peak values for heart rate, systolic blood pressure/diastolic blood pressure, and rate pressure product were 189 bpm, 330 mm Hg/184 mm Hg, and 545, respectively (see table 14.1). Heart rates were higher during the aerobic exercise than during any of the resistance exercises. Post hoc analysis for heart rate response data revealed

### Table 14.1 Mean Cardiovascular values (± *SD*) at Rest and During Exercise

| Variable | Rest | Bike | Peak Acc | Var | Fix |
|----------|--------|--------|----------|--------|--------|
| HR | 57.8 | 189.0 | 166.0 | 157.2 | 156.8 |
| | (10.3) | (6.6) | (12.8) | (23.7) | (11.5) |
| SBP | 142.0 | 244.7 | 329.5 | 282.5 | 296.0 |
| | (6.0) | (31.1) | (28.2) | (31.0) | (29.7) |
| DBP | 61.8 | 74.0 | 184.3 | 162.5 | 164.3 |
| | (8.0) | (17.6) | (25.5) | (39.2) | (14.2) |
| RPP | 82.2 | 461.7 | 545.3 | 445.7 | 463.6 |
| | (15.8) | (53.6) | (56.0) | (93.5) | (49.7) |

Note: Values during exercise obtained at peak HR. HR = heart rate, bpm; SBP = systolic blood pressure, mm/Hg; DBP = diastolic blood pressure, mm/Hg; RPP = rate pressure product; Rest = resting values; Bike = values obtained during cycle ergometry; Acc = isokinetic (accommodating) resistance; Var = isotonic variable resistance; Fix = isotonic fixed resistance. From *Journal of Strength and Conditioning Research* 1996.

significant differences between the cycle ergometer and all resistance exercises. There were no significant differences between the resistance exercises. Conversely, both systolic blood pressure and diastolic blood pressure were higher during the resistance exercises than during the aerobic exercise (see figure 14.6). Post hoc analysis revealed significant pairwise comparisons for systolic blood pressure between the cycle ergometer and all other exercises, and between the isokinetic exercise and all other exercises. Post hoc analysis for diastolic blood pressure revealed significant differences only between the cycle ergometer and the resistance exercises. The rate pressure product was highest during isokinetic exercise, followed by constant load fixed resistance exercise, aerobic (cycle ergometer) exercise, and finally variable resistance exercise. The rate pressure product, which is a noninvasive indicator of myocardial oxygen consumption and incorporates both heart rate and systolic blood pressure, was significantly different between isokinetic resistance and the other two forms of resistance (variable resistance and constant load fixed resistance) (32).

One possible explanation for these results is that isokinetic resistance had more "aerobic" qualities than the other resistance exercises. The higher heart rate and increase in systolic blood pressure that were observed with the isokinetic

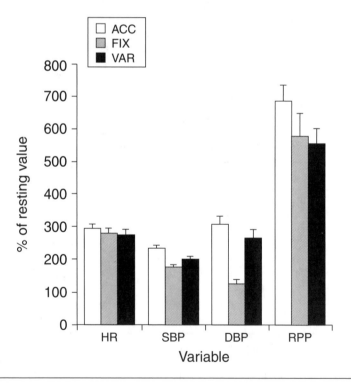

**Figure 14.6** Mean cardiovascular responses for all exercises, reported as % of resting value (peak/resting).

From *Journal of Strength and Conditioning Research* 1996.

resistance is similar to what we would observe in response to aerobic exercise and would be consistent with the greater duration of exercise (less resistance and more repetitions). Fleck and Dean (14) have shown a higher arterial blood pressure response in longer duration sets (70–80% 1 RM) than in shorter duration sets with near maximal resistance (90–100% 1 RM). It is possible that rate pressure product was highest during the isokinetic condition because of the increase in systolic blood pressure. This may be a result of more straining by the subject as a result of providing maximal resistance throughout the full range of motion by more closely matching the subject's strength curve. The increase in systolic blood pressure and rate pressure product may also be the result of stimulating the pressor response.

# Velocity-Specific Effects of Isokinetic Resistance Exercise

Most velocity-specific research conducted with isokinetic resistance has addressed the effects of exercise on peak torque or power (35), and very little information is available regarding the cardiovascular effects of manipulating the velocity of isokinetic resistance exercise.

Although several investigators have previously reported increases in heart rate while utilizing different speeds of isokinetic exercise (9, 31), they usually assessed changes in systolic blood pressure, diastolic blood pressure, and the rate pressure product with indirect methods (9). Freedson and associates (18), however, did report intraarterial blood pressures with isokinetic resistance at unidentified slow and fast speeds. They reported significant differences in peak systolic blood pressure and diastolic blood pressure for slow versus fast isokinetic speeds, with the slower speed producing the greater value (18).

In a more recent study, Kleiner and colleagues (33) evaluated the acute cardiovascular responses, including intraarterial blood pressure, to isokinetic resistance exercises and compared the response to aerobic exercise. The resistance exercises were single-leg, dual concentric flexion and extension isokinetic exercises at the knee. These exercises were performed on the Kin-Com 125E+ isokinetic testing and exercise device (see figure 14.7). All subjects executed one continuous set of isokinetic exercise to failure at each of three isokinetic speeds (50°/s, 100°/s, and 200°/s). Subjects were instructed to provide maximal effort during each repetition until they could no longer continue (see figure 14.8). The use of an isokinetic device enabled the investigators to (a) preset a minimum force requirement to ensure that subjects continued to produce sufficient torque, (b) limit the subjects' range of motion to exactly 90° (from 90° to 0° of flexion) for each repetition, (c) standardize the speed of the exercise, (d) isolate the joint being used (34), (e) count each repetition completed, and (f) measure the torque produced (16, 33).

Changes were observed in the cardiovascular data from resting to peak values (see table 14.2). Systolic blood pressures, diastolic blood pressures, and the

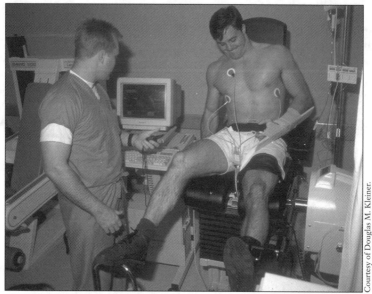

**Figure 14.7** Intraarterial blood pressure monitoring system used during isokinetic testing with the Kin-Com 125E+.

Courtesy of Douglas M. Kleiner.

## Table 14.2 Mean Cardiovascular Values (± *SD*) at Rest and During Exercise

| Peak variable | Rest | Bike | 50°/s | 100°/s | 200°/s |
|---|---|---|---|---|---|
| HR | 70.3 | 192.8 | 163.3 | 174.7 | 183.5 |
| | (10.9) | (13.1) | (28.4) | (20.3) | (16.8) |
| SBP | 154.3 | 212.0 | 348.2 | 337.2 | 335.5 |
| | (10.1) | (28.2) | (18.1) | (23.7) | (27.4) |
| DBP | 77.0 | 91.4 | 157.3 | 47.2 | 135.0 |
| | (11.9) | (16.3) | (34.0) | (25.3) | (31.1) |
| RPP | 108.8 | 404.5 | 569.2 | 589.1 | 616.7 |
| | (19.6) | (49.6) | (104.8) | (79.9) | (84.1) |

Note: Values during exercise obtained at peak HR. HR = heart rate, bpm; SBP = systolic blood pressure, mm/Hg; DBP = diastolic blood pressure, mm/Hg; RPP = rate pressure product; Rest = resting values; Bike = values obtained during cycle ergometry. From *Journal of Strength and Conditioning Research* 1999.

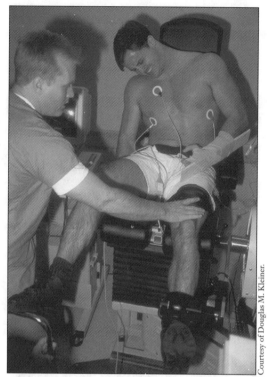

**Figure 14.8** A subject completing maximal isokinetic exercise to exhaustion during the 100°/s trial.

rate pressure product were all higher during the isokinetic resistance exercises, while heart rate was highest during the cycle ergometer. The response data are presented in figure 14.9. The analysis of variance revealed significant differences ($p < .05$) among the treatments regarding heart rate, systolic blood pressure, diastolic blood pressure, and rate pressure product.

Much of the early research involving the acute cardiovascular response to resistance exercise has been conducted with isometric resistance. These studies have shown that cardiovascular responses increase with changes in the duration, intensity (% of maximum voluntary contraction), and muscle mass involved (37, 44, 53, 54, 58). As a result, many researchers believe that a slower isokinetic velocity, which allows the subject to produce greater torque, may also produce a greater cardiovascular response. In the study by Kleiner and associates (33), increases in blood pressure were related to decreases in isokinetic velocity or exercises that enabled the subject to produce more force. Heart rate increased with increases in isokinetic velocity. At 200°/s the mean heart rate response was almost as great as it was during the cycle ergometer test, with values of 184 and 193 bpm, respectively. The authors attributed this trend

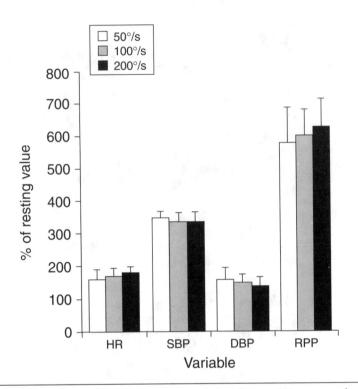

**Figure 14.9**  Mean cardiovascular responses for all exercises, reported as % of resting value (peak/resting).

From *Journal of Strength and Conditioning Research* 1999.

to the higher isokinetic speeds producing less resistance and more closely resembling "aerobic" activity than the lower velocity, less aerobic resistance exercises that often produce straining (33).

The peak systolic pressures reported by Kleiner and coworkers (33) were similar to the pressures reported by MacDougall and colleagues (41) (group mean of 320 mm Hg/250 mm Hg and a peak pressure of 480 mm Hg/350 mm Hg in one subject). It had been hypothesized that the extremely high pressures reported by MacDougall were due to the location of the catheter. However, other resistance exercise studies, which also used intrabrachial pressures, failed to produce similar extreme values. The radial artery was cannulated in the Kleiner group's studies and mean systolic blood pressure and diastolic blood pressure values were considerably higher than in other reported intraradial studies (13–15, 43), though still not as high as the MacDougall group has reported (41).

The great systolic blood pressure and diastolic blood pressure observed in the study by Kleiner and associates (group mean of 348 mm Hg/157 mm Hg and a peak in one subject of 380 mm Hg/185 mm Hg at 50°/s) may be because isokinetics was the form of resistance used (32). Earlier, Kleiner and colleagues reported a greater response in all cardiovascular parameters (heart rate, systolic blood pressure, diastolic blood pressure, and rate pressure product) with isokinetic resistance than with constant load (fixed or variable) resistance (32).

## Practical Considerations

The cardiovascular response to resistance exercises is significantly different than during aerobic exercise. Great elevations in heart rate, systolic blood pressure, diastolic blood pressure, and the rate pressure product have been documented with isokinetic resistance exercises. These increases occur even in the absence of a Valsalva maneuver. Although these extreme values during isokinetic resistance exercise do not appear to pose problems in healthy subjects, they are a stress to the cardiovascular system nonetheless. This information should not discourage anyone from using isokinetic resistance, but instead particular attention should be paid to the form and speed of resistance chosen when prescribing resistance exercises to special populations such as hypertensive athletes. The strength and conditioning professional must consider the cardiovascular consequences from the form and speed of resistance selected.

## Summary

Resistance exercises have become a very popular form of exercise. The effects of these exercises on skeletal muscle are known. However, less is known about what effects these exercises have on the cardiovascular system. Chronic isokinetic training is thought to have the same positive effects on resting heart and resting blood pressure as other types of exercise and other forms of resistance. However, each acute bout of isokinetic resistance exercise can temporarily elevate cardiovascular parameters such as blood pressure to dangerous levels. Proper instruction of exercise technique, including the avoidance of the Valsalva maneuver, may lessen the effects of the pressor response that are observed with resistance exercises. While the Valsalva maneuver may have orthopedic benefits, and while its occurrence may be unavoidable, it is a stress to the cardiovascular system.

We currently know very little about the cardiovascular responses or adaptations to isokinetic resistance exercise; however, we do know enough to form some general conclusions and to make some general recommendations. The rate pressure product is a noninvasive indicator of myocardial oxygen demand and should be of particular interest to populations whose myocardial workloads should be minimized during exercise. Studies that utilized appropriate methods, including direct and continuous monitoring of intraarterial blood pressure, have shown that the rate pressure product is lower during exercises at lower isokinetic speeds. However, it is important to recall that these are the same exercises that produce the greatest response in systolic blood pressure and diastolic blood pressure. It is more likely that a strength and conditioning professional will encounter an athlete who is hypertensive (whether she is aware of the athlete's condition or not) than an individual with ischemia. Thus, to minimize the blood pressure response to isokinetic resistance the following factors should be considered. A pressor response does occur with isokinetic resistance exercise; however, proper breathing patterns can minimize any affects that the Valsalva maneuver may have on the pressor response. Systolic blood pressure and diastolic blood pressure values are known to increase as the isokinetic velocity decreases (which is an inverse relationship to that of heart rates and velocity).

Finally, consider other forms of resistance for individuals who may be compromised by the acute cardiovascular response to isokinetic resistance. Cardiovascular response values are higher with isokinetic resistance than they are with constant load fixed resistance or variable resistance. Resistance exercises of any mode are an important part of overall body development and conditioning. However, it must be remembered that the effects of these exercises are not limited to the skeletal muscle. While more research may be needed into the cardiovascular effects of these various exercises, currently, there are no known contraindications to isokinetic resistance exercise in healthy individuals.

# References

1. Becque, M.D., D. Mistry, F.I. Katch, and T. Hortobagyi. 1991. Effect of $\dot{V}O_2$max on the pressor response to static and dynamic exercise. *Med. Sci. Sports Exerc.* 23(4): S162.

2. Berger, R. 1962. Effect of varied weight training programs on strength. *Res. Q. Exerc. Sport* 33(2): 168–81.

3. Berger, R.A. 1963. Comparative effects of three weight training programs. *Res. Q.* 24: 334–38.

4. Burger, G.C.E. 1969. Heart rate and the concept of circulatory load. *Ergonomics* 12(6): 857–64.

5. Butler, R.M., W.H. Beierwaltes, and F.J. Rogers. 1987. The cardiovascular response to circuit weight training in patients with cardiac disease. *J. Cardiopulmonary Rehabil.* 7: 402–9.

6. Clarke, D.H., and G. A. Stull. 1970. Endurance training as a determinant of strength and fatigability. *Res. Q.* 41: 19–26.

7. Coleman, A.E. 1977. Nautilus vs. Universal gym strength training in adult males. *Am. Corrective Therapy J.* 31(4): 103–7.

8. DeLateur, B.J., J.F. Lehmann, and W.E. Fordyce. 1968. A test of the DeLorme axiom. *Arch. Phys. Med. Rehabil.* 49: 245–48.

9. Douris, P.C. 1991. Cardiovascular response to velocity-specific isokinetic exercise. *J. Ortho. Sports Phys. Ther.* 13(1): 28–32.

10. Duncan, P.W., J.M. Chandler, D.K. Cavanaugh, K.R. Johnson, and A.G. Buehler. 1989. Mode and speed specificity of eccentric and concentric exercise training. *J. Orthop. Sports Phys. Ther.* 11(2): 70–75.

11. Falkel, J.E., S.J. Fleck, and T.F. Murray. 1992. Comparison of central hemodynamics between power lifters and bodybuilders during resistance exercise. *J. Appl. Sport Sci. Res.* 6(11): 24–35.

12. Fleck, S.J. 1988. Cardiovascular adaptations to resistance training. *Med. Sci. Sports Exerc.* 20(5): S146–51.

13. Fleck, S.J., and L.S. Dean. 1985. Influence of weight training experience on blood pressure response to exercise. *Med. Sci. Sports Exerc.* 17(2): 185.

14. Fleck, S.J., and L.S. Dean. 1987. Resistance training experience and the pressor response during resistance exercise. *J. Appl. Physiol.* 63(1): 116–20.

15. Fleck, S.J., J. Falkel, E. Harman, W.J. Kraemer, P. Frykman, C.M. Maresh, K.L. Goetz, D. Campbell, M. Rosenstein, and R. Rosenstein. 1989. Cardiovascular responses during resistance training. *Med. Sci. Sports Exerc.* 21(2): S114.

16. Foran, B. 1985. Advantages and disadvantages of isokinetics, variable resistance, and free weights. *NSCA J.* Feb-Mar: 24–25.

17. Franklin, B.A., S. McClintock, P. Bendick, D. Bakalyar, S. Gordon, and G.C. Timmis. 1990. Inaccuracy of blood pressure measurements taken immediately after weightlifting. *Med. Sci. Sports Exerc.* 22(2): S37.

18. Freedson, P., B. Chang, F. Katch, W. Kroll, J. Rippe, J. Alpert, and W. Byrnes. 1984. Intraarterial blood pressure during free weight and hydraulic resistive exercise. *Med. Sci. Sports Exerc.* 16(2): 131.

19. Gettman, L.R., L.A. Culter, and T.A. Strathman. 1980. Physiological changes after 20 weeks of isotonic vs. isokinetic circuit training. *J. Sports Med.* 20: 265–74.

20. Gillespie, J., and C. Gabbard. 1984. A test of three theories of strength and muscular endurance development. *J. Hum. Movement Studies* 10: 213–23.

21. Guyton, A.C., B.H. Douglas, J.B. Langston, and T.Q. Richardson. 1962. Instantaneous increase in mean circulatory pressure and cardiac output at onset of muscular activity. *Circ. Res.* XI: 431–41.

22. Haennel, R., K.-K. Teo, A. Quinney, and C.T. Kappagoda. 1989. Effects of hydraulic circuit training on cardiovascular function. *Med. Sci. Sports Exerc.* 21(5): 605–12.

23. Haennel, R.G., H.A. Quinney, and C.T. Kappagoda. 1991. Effects of hydraulic circuit training following coronary artery bypass surgery. *Med. Sci. Sports Exerc.* 23(2): 158–65.

24. Haslam, D.R.S., N. McCartney, R.S. McKelvie, and J.D. MacDougall. 1988. Direct measurements of arterial blood pressure during formal weightlifting in cardiac patients. *J. Cardiopul. Rehab.* 8: 213–25.

25. Henschel, A., F. DeLaVega, and H.L. Taylor. 1954. Simultaneous direct and indirect blood pressure measurements in man at rest and work. *J. Appl. Physiol.* 6: 506–8.

26. Hill, D.W., and S.D. Butler. 1991. Hemodynamic responses to weightlifting exercise. *Sports Med.* 12(1): 1–7.

27. Hislop, H., and J.J. Perrine. 1967. The isokinetic concept of exercise. *Phys. Ther.* 47: 114–17.

28. Hossack, K.F., B.W. Gross, J.B. Ritterman, F. Kusumi, and R.A. Bruce. 1982. Evaluation of automated blood pressure measurements during exercise testing. *Am. Heart J.* 104(5): 1032–38.

29. Hunter, G., and J.P. McCarthy. 1983. Pressor response associated with high-intensity anaerobic training. *Phys. Sports Med.* 11(4): 151–62.

30. Katch, F.I., P.S. Freedson, and C.A. Jones. 1985. Evaluation of acute cardiorespiratory responses to hydraulic resistance exercise. *Med. Sci. Sports Exerc.* 17(1): 168–73.

31. Kleiner, D.M. 1990. The effects of manipulating the speed of maximal isokinetic resistance training on heart rate. *Med. Sci. Sports Exerc.* 22(2): S45.

32. Kleiner, D.M., D.L. Blessing, W.R. Davis, and J.W. Mitchell. 1996. Acute cardiovascular responses to various forms of resistance exercise. *J. Strength and Cond. Res.* 10(1): 56–61.

33. Kleiner, D.M., D.L. Blessing, J.W. Mitchell, and W.R. Davis. 1999. A description of the acute cardiovascular responses to isokinetic resistance at three different speeds. *J. Strength and Cond. Res.*

34. Lander, J.E., B.T. Bates, J.A. Sawhill, and J. Hamill. 1985. A comparison between free weight and isokinetic bench pressing. *Med. Sci. Sports Exerc.* 17(3): 344–53.

35. Lesmes, G.R., D.L. Costill, E.F. Coyle, and W.J. Fink. 1978. Muscle strength and power changes during maximal isokinetic training. *Med. Sci. Sports* 10(4): 266–69.

36. Lightfoot, J.T., C. Tankersley, S.A. Rowe, A.N. Freed, and S.M. Fortney. 1989. Automated blood pressure measurements during exercise. *Med. Sci. Sports Exerc.* 21(6): 698–707.

37. Lind, A.R., S.H. Taylor, P.W. Humphreys, B.M. Kennelly, and K.W. Donald. 1964. The circulatory effects of sustained voluntary muscle contraction. *Clin. Sci.* 27: 229–44.

38. Linsenbardt, S.T., T.R. Thomas, and R.W. Madsen. 1992. Effect of breathing techniques on blood pressure response to resistance exercise. *Br. J. Sports Med.* 26: 97–100.

39. MacDougall, D., R. McKelvie, D. Moroz, D. Sale, and N. McCartney. 1989. Effects of the Valsalva maneuver, joint angle, muscle size and strength on the blood pressure response to weightlifting. *Med. Sci. Sports Exerc.* 21(2): S2.

40. MacDougall, J.D., R.S. McKelvie, D.E. Moroz, D.G. Sale, N. McCartney, and F. Buick. 1992. Factors affecting blood pressure during heavy weightlifting and static contractions. *J. Appl. Physiol.* 73: 1590–97.

41. MacDougall, J.D., D. Tuxen, D.G. Sale, J.R. Moroz, and J.R. Sutton. 1985. Arterial blood pressure response to heavy resistance exercise. *J. Appl. Physiol.* 58(3): 785–90.

42. MacDougall, D., D. Tuxen, D. Sale, A. Sexton, J. Moroz, and J. Sutton. 1983. Direct measurement of arterial blood pressure during heavy resistance training. *Med. Sci. Sports Exerc.* 15(2): 158.

43. Maresh, C.M., W.J. Kraemer, S.J. Fleck, K.L. Goetz, E. Harman, P. Frykman, and J. Falkel. 1989. Effects of heavy resistance exercise on hemodynamic, stress hormone, and fluid regulatory factors. *Med. Sci. Sports Exerc.* 21(2): S37.

44. Misner, J.E., S.B. Going, B.H. Massey, T.E. Ball, M.G. Bemben, and L.K. Essandoh. 1990. Cardiovascular response to sustained maximal voluntary static muscle contraction. *Med. Sci. Sports Exerc.* 22(2): 194–99.

45. Nagle, F.J., J. Naughton, and B. Balke. 1966. Comparisons of direct and indirect blood pressure with pressure-flow dynamics during exercise. *J. Appl. Physiol.* 21(1): 317–20.

46. Ng, A.V., J.C. Agre, M.S. Harrington, and F.J. Nagle. 1989. Pressor and endurance response of isometric knee extension to changes in knee angle. *Med. Sci. Sports Exerc.* 21(2): S3.

47. Pipes, T.V. 1977. Strength-training modes: What's the difference? *Scholastic Coach* 46(10): 96, 120–24.

48. Pipes, T.V. 1978. Variable resistance versus constant resistance strength training in adult males. *Eur. J. Appl. Physiol.* 39(1): 27–35.

49. Pipes, T.V., and J.H. Wilmore. 1975. Isokinetic vs. isotonic strength training in adult men. *Med. Sci. Sports* 7(4): 262–74.

50. Pollock, M.L., J.H. Wilmore, and S.M. Fox. 1978. *Health and fitness through physical activity.* New York: Wiley.

51. Rasmussen, P.H., B.A. Staats, D.J. Driscoll, K.C. Beck, H.W. Bonekat, and W.D. Wilcox. 1985. Direct and indirect blood pressure during exercise. *Chest* 87(6): 743–48.

52. Robinson, T.E., D.Y. Sue, A. Huszczuk, D. Weiler-Ravell, and J.E. Hansen. 1988. Intraarterial and cuff blood pressure responses during incremental cycle ergometery. *Med. Sci. Sports Exerc.* 20(2): 142–49.

53. Sagiv, M., P. Hanson, M. Besozzi, and F. Nagle. 1985. Left ventricular responses to upright isometric handgrip and dead lift in men with coronary artery disease. *Am. J. Cardiol.* 55(1): 1298–302.

54. Sharkey, B.J. 1966. A physiological comparison of static and phasic exercise. *Res. Q.* 37(4): 520–31.

55. Smith, M.J., and P. Melton. 1981. Isokinetic versus isotonic variable resistance training. *Am. J. Sports Med.* 9(4): 275–79.

56. Stull, G.A., and D.H. Clarke. 1970. High-resistance, low-repetition training as a determiner of strength and fatigability. *Res. Q.* 41: 189–93.

57. Thistle, H.G., H.J. Hislop, M. Moffroid, and E.W. Lowman. 1967. Isokinetic contraction: A new concept of resistance exercise. *Arch. Phys. Med. Rehabil.* 48: 279–82.

58. Tuttle, W.W., and S.M. Horvath. 1957. Comparison of effects of static and dynamic work on blood pressure and heart rate. *J. Appl. Physiol.* 10(2): 294–96.

59. Westing, S.H., J.Y. Seger, and A. Thorstensson. 1991. Isoacceleration: A new concept of resistive exercise. *Med. Sci. Sports Exerc.* 23(5): 631–35.

60. Wiecek, E.M., N. McCartney, and R.S. McKelvie. 1990. Comparison of direct and indirect measures of systemic arterial pressure during weightlifting in coronary artery disease. *Am. J. Cardiol.* 66: 1065–106.

# Part IV
## Unique Populations

Part IV collectively presents a review of the relevant literature as it relates to special populations. Chapter 15 is dedicated to testing and training in youth with emphasis placed on maturation and strength gains. Chapter 16 explores an aging population and the ramifications of assessment within this, the fastest growing population in the world. Chapter 17 describes the singular adaptations and manifestations of females within an isokinetic paradigm. Chapter 18 delves deeper into the upper extremity design by investigating how athletes who participate in overhead sports exhibit unusual force couplings. Chapter 19 inquires into another group of athletes (baseball players), who, like tennis players, are predominantly unilateral in their athletic endeavors. Chapter 20 analyzes football from a new perspective of comparing and contrasting the different codes of football as displayed in American, Australian Rules, and soccer. Chapter 21 examines an area often overlooked by the average practitioner, space flight. The exclusive maladaptations associated with zero gravity are explored through attempts to ameliorate muscular atrophy.

Every attempt has been made in this section to cover unique populations the reader may not be completely familiar with. This reading should further promote research in these areas and foster new understanding in these and other insufficiently researched topics. The shortage of research into human performance related to isokinetics and sports as well as industrial environments such as space is one reason this book was written.

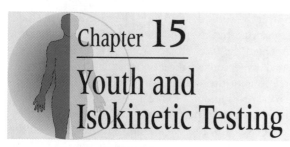

# Chapter 15

# Youth and Isokinetic Testing

Joseph P. Weir

Isokinetic testing of muscle strength provides an objective approach to examining and easily quantifying muscle strength and endurance in children and adolescents. Isokinetic testing, specifically the ability to examine strength at different contraction velocities, has the potential to further our understanding of muscle mechanics during growth and development. However, there are many gaps in the literature regarding isokinetic responses in youths. This chapter provides an overview of the available research literature regarding a variety of issues surrounding isokinetic testing in youths. Specific attention is given to issues such as unique aspects of youth data, isokinetic strength development across age, and associations with athletics. In addition, areas of inquiry related to neuromuscular function in youths that lend themselves to isokinetic assessment are examined and holes in our current knowledge are discussed.

## Testing and Analysis Issues

In general, one must consider the same issues when testing a younger or an older population. When testing youths, however, especially on equipment designed primarily for adults, the examiner often must correct for differences in body size.

### Reliability

To date, surprisingly little research has been performed examining the reliability of isokinetic test parameters in youths, and many studies did not employ the preferred data analysis approach of the intraclass correlation coefficient (ICC). Alexander and Molnar (2) were the first to report reliability data on isokinetic strength in youths; however, the small sample size in their analysis (n = 3) was insufficient for adequate evaluation. A subsequent study by Molnar, Alexander, and Gutfeld (56) examined 7- to 15-year-old boys and girls both with (n = 30 per gender) and without (n = 50 per gender) mental retardation. The motions examined were flexion and extension at the hip, shoulder, elbow, and knee as well as abduction at the shoulder and hip. The specific test velocity was not reported in the manuscript, but the procedures were noted to be similar to previous work (2) in which the test velocity was 30°/s. The researchers reported high reliability, based on percentage deviation calculations, for intratest reliability (repeated contractions in the same session; mean deviation scores ranged from 5.4 to 5.9% in controls and 4.9 to 6.2% in children with mental retardation), intertest reliability (testing performed 7 to 10 days apart; mean deviation scores varied between 7.9% and 9.8%), and intertester reliability (subjects tested by two different operators; mean deviation scores ranged from 8.7 to 10.0%). They noted that similar reliability scores were obtained from both groups of children, and the authors argued that these relatively low deviation scores indicate that isokinetic testing can be reliably performed in children of this age.

More recent studies have also reported high reliability for youth isokinetic testing. For example, Burnett and coworkers (14) found ICCs ranging from .63 to .84 for hip flexion and extension at 30°/s and 90°/s, but they found low values (.49–.59) for hip abduction and adduction in 29 boys aged 6 to 10 years old. For the thigh muscles, Merlini, Dell'Accio, and Granata (53) found high reliability for the knee extensors (ICC = .95; 95% CI = .91–.97) and flexors (ICC = .85; 95% CI = .77–.91) in 12 boys aged 6 to 8 years. Similarly, Van den Berg-Emons and coworkers (76) found high intraday test-retest reliability in isokinetic knee extension and flexion peak torque at 30, 60, and 120°/s in 38 healthy children (Spearman rank correlation coefficients ranged from .88 to .95). However, in 12 children with cerebral palsy, the correlations tended to be lower with extension peak torque at 60 and 120°/s, being .55 and .42, respectively.

In general, the available literature indicates that the reliability of isokinetic testing in youths is acceptable. However, more research needs to be performed. Specifically, most studies have examined the knee extensors and flexors and fewer studies have examined other muscles, especially in the upper extremities. No studies have reported reliability for eccentric torque measures in youths. In addition, use of the ICC and associated standard error of measurement needs to be incorporated into the analyses.

## Positioning and Stabilization

Positioning and stabilization have been shown to significantly affect torque output in adults (31, 32, 78). Because of obvious differences in body dimensions between children and adults, modification of the testing apparatus is needed. However, relatively little information has been reported regarding specific modifications required for youth testing. Upper body testing may require raising the subject to a level that physically permits testing to occur (83). For the leg extensors and flexors, the primary modification appears to be to provide added support behind the back of the subject (83). This allows the subject to maintain proper knee position relative to the dynamometer axis of rotation while still maintaining adequate support for the back. In addition, Henderson and associates (33) reported the use of the upper extremity dynamometer input arm for leg extension and flexion testing in small children on a Cybex II dynamometer.

## Scaling for Differences in Body Size

A complicating factor in the analysis of isokinetic strength in children and adolescents is the effect of body size on the isokinetic torque. Because of differences in body size across age and gender, examination of strength differences in subjects of different ages and between boys and girls requires accounting for body size differences. There are two issues that need to be addressed when scaling for body size differences. First is the choice of body size variable with which to scale. Authors have often used body mass (see, e.g., 30, 40) and height (see, e.g., 2–5, 44) as these are easily measured, and it is intuitively appealing that bigger individuals, on average, are stronger than smaller individuals. However, because of differences in body composition, use of body mass or height alone may result in misleading results, especially when comparing across gender. Indeed, use of different scaling variables can result in different outcomes. Gilliam and colleagues (30) found no knee extension or flexion strength differences between boys and girls (ages 7–13 years) at 120°/s when using height as a covariate, while use of body weight did show gender differences. Similarly, Docherty and Gaul (23) found no gender differences between preteen boys and girls when correcting for lean body weight (from skinfolds), but some gender differences were found following corrections for body mass. Use of fat free weight (FFW) and muscle cross-sectional area (CSA) can improve the partitioning of body size but requires the ability to determine body composition (for FFW) or CSA. Body composition assessment in children and adolescents can be problematic because of the differences in densities of fat free weight components of children versus adults (51). Similarly, direct measures of CSA require technology such as ultrasound, computed tomography, and magnetic resonance imaging.

The second issue concerns the choice of how to "correct" for body size differences. A common approach is to simply divide the strength score by the body size variable. So-called ratio scaling is intuitively appealing and results in a strength per unit of body size variable. Indeed, this approach is common for a variety of variables in the exercise science literature; for example, maximal oxygen consumption expressed as $ml \cdot kg^{-1} \cdot min^{-1}$ is a ratio scale score. However, as early as 1949, Tanner (70) pointed out the potential pitfalls in ratio scaling. Most notably, the use of ratio scaling only removes the effect of the body size variable under very limited conditions. That is, ratio scaling can result in a body size-adjusted strength score that is still correlated with the body size variable. An alternate approach involves the use of regression analysis, or the equivalent LY analysis of covariance (ANCOVA), to remove the effects of the body size variable. This approach is more likely than ratio scaling to effectively remove the effects of body size. However, a traditional regression approach can result in a nonzero $y$ intercept, which is physiologically unreasonable. The fit to the data is required to be linear, which does not always result in the best-fitting model. In addition, the assumption of homoscedasticity is often not met.

An alternative approach is the use of allometric scaling. In the 1950s, Asmussen and Heeboll-Nielsen (4, 5) used an allometric approach to examine body size and strength relationships in boys. Only recently, however, has allometric scaling been increasingly used in exercise science research to remove the effects of body size. With allometric scaling, the relationship between body size and strength is modeled as a power function of the form

$$strength = a \cdot size^b$$

where a is a constant multiplier, and b is the scaling exponent. The size of the scaling exponent can be predicted based on dimensionality theory. For example, the scaling exponent for muscle force is suggested to be $b = 2/3$, while the scaling exponent for torque should theoretically approximate $b = 1.0$ (6). Allometric scaling has advantages over traditional regression in that the resulting equation goes through the origin, the curve can be nonlinear, and the statistical assumptions are more likely to be met. However, to date there is little data in the literature (44, 80) in which allometric scaling was used in assessing isokinetic strength in youths. Future research should more completely examine this approach to body size scaling in youth isokinetic data. Nonetheless, in subsequent sections where authors have employed body size adjustments, the approach (e.g., ratio scaling, ANCOVA) used by the authors will be noted.

## Load Range

Because isokinetic contractions involve acceleration and deceleration phases in addition to periods of constant angular velocity (load range), recent attention has focused on load range, which is the range of motion where the actual velocity equals the selected isokinetic velocity. In adults, load range has been shown to vary inversely with contraction velocity (60, 71). Examination of load range in conjunction with torque data may provide unique insights into neuromuscular function. For example, it has recently been reported in adults that there are gender differences in load range, indicating that the periods of acceleration and deceleration differ between sexes (12). Furthermore, because resistance from an isokinetic dynamometer is provided only during load range, additional load range data may affect recommendations for isokinetic training protocols. To date, only one study has examined load range in youths. Brown and coworkers (11) examined load range during internal and external rotation of the shoulder in elite junior tennis players (n = 12 males, mean age = 16.2 years). At high contraction velocities (> 240°/s), less than 75% of the range of motion occurred at the preset velocity. At the highest velocity (450°/s), no subject was able to achieve load range for external rotation, and only a small portion ($< 25\%$) of the internal rotation range of motion was load range. It was suggested that high velocity isokinetic training, and therefore low load range training, might not provide sufficient overload for optimal strength gains. Further research needs to be performed to examine load range issues in youths of different ages.

# Torque-Velocity Relationships

Numerous studies have examined various aspects of isokinetic torque-velocity curves in adults (see, e.g., 17, 64, 74, 79). Less work has been performed with children, but some evidence presented below indicates that the shape of the torque-velocity curve in youths may be different than that of adults. In addition, no studies have reported torque-velocity curve data in youths in which the data were recorded at a constant joint angle (and therefore constant muscle length) as opposed to peak torque. These studies may provide insight into the extent of neuromuscular inhibition present in youths across age.

## Concentric

Studies using isokinetic dynamometry in adults have shown that less peak torque is produced at higher concentric contraction velocities (17, 64, 74, 79). This general relationship has also been shown in youths (16, 34, 35, 82). For example, Burnie and Brodie (16) found lower leg extension peak torque values at 240 versus 60°/s in 18 preadolescent (mean age = 11.4 years) boys. Weltman and associates (83) showed higher torque outputs at 30 than at 90°/s for flexion and extension at the knee, elbow, and shoulder in 29 prepubescent boys (mean age = $8.2 \pm 1.3$ years). In contrast, Calmels and coworkers (18) did not find significant differences in knee extension and flexion peak torque at 60 versus 120°/s in 9 elite female gymnasts (mean age = $11.3 \pm 1.2$ years). However, low statistical power associated with their small sample size may have led to their results, as an examination of their table 2 shows a trend for smaller scores at the faster speed. Interestingly, Hill and colleagues (34) found a significant interaction effect between muscle group (knee extensors versus flexors) and contraction velocity (velocities = 60, 120, and 180°/s) in 7 girls and 8 boys between 9 and 11 years of age. Their follow-up procedures indicated that increases in contraction velocity were associated with decreased torque, however the nature of the interaction effect was not fully explained. That is, the interaction suggests that the pattern of torque change across velocities differed as a function of muscle group. Further, examination of their figure 1 shows a low velocity torque plateau for the extension but not the flexion data. Specifically, extension peak torque at 0°/s was lower than that at 60°/s while the opposite was true for the flexion data. Similar low velocity torque plateaus in the knee extensors have been reported for adults (16, 64, 79).

In children, there are indications that the pattern of decline in torque with increases in contraction velocity may vary across age and may differ between muscle groups. Data from Backman and Oberg (7) show that decreases in dorsiflexion torque with increased velocity are more pronounced in older subjects. That is, differences in torque between age groups were larger at slow contraction velocities. They hypothesized that these age-related torque-velocity differences were due to increased muscle stiffness with age. However, their analyses were based on absolute torque values, and because absolute torque values are generally higher at low speeds, it follows that the absolute differences between age groups will be larger at low speeds, giving the appearance of steeper torque decay at higher velocities in older subjects. Future studies examining this issue using both absolute as well as relative analyses are warranted.

## Eccentric

The development of eccentric measurement capabilities with isokinetic dynamometers is new relative to concentric measurements, and therefore fewer studies have examined eccentric torque in children and adolescents. Consistent with adult data, several studies have shown that eccentric torque at a given speed is higher than concentric torque in youths (18, 46, 55). Mohtadi and associates (55) have shown that young males (ages 10–12) produce more quadriceps torque under eccentric than concentric testing (60°/s). Similar results were reported by Calmels and colleagues (18) for both knee flexion and extension. Kawakami and coworkers (46) also found that elbow flexor peak torque was higher under eccentric versus isometric and concentric testing (speeds = 12, 30, and 60°/s in 13-year-old boys). However, there were no differences in eccentric peak torque across velocities. These results were reported to differ from low velocity eccentric elbow flexor data in adults (47), which indicated an increase in eccentric torque with increases in eccentric velocity. It was suggested that the lack of velocity dependence of eccentric torque was similar to the data from "weak" adult subjects reported by Hortobagyi and Katch (36) and suggests that weak adults and boys are inhibited from recruiting all available motor units during high force eccentric contractions.

# Antagonist Strength Ratios

Numerous studies have examined the strength ratios of agonist versus antagonist muscles in adults with the belief that large strength imbalances are associated with increased risk of injury. These analyses are complicated by several factors (1). Specifically, the strength ratios at a joint tend to be speed specific, and the magnitude of the ratios can be affected by gravity (the weight of the leg, for example, inflates hamstring strength scores and decreases quadriceps strength scores). Nonetheless, data do exist supporting the notion that agonist/antagonist strength ratios predict injury risk. Notably, Knapik and coworkers (49) found that a knee flexor/extensor ratio at 180°/s of 75% or less was associated with increased lower extremity injury risk in collegiate female athletes. Similarly, knee flexor strength differences between limbs (15%) were also associated with increased risk.

To date, several studies have examined isokinetic strength ratios in youths. However, those that have been published are inconsistent in their use of gravity corrections, and no data are available examining associations with injury risk. In high school football players (n = 115, ages 15–17 years), Gilliam and associates (29) found that the knee flexion/extension ratio at a slow speed (30°/s) varies by player position. Specifically, linemen had significantly higher knee flexion/extension ratios (65%) than receivers and backs (59%) while position differences were not significant at a faster speed (180°/s). However, these results were not corrected for gravity. In pre- and postpubescent boys (n = 30) and girls (n = 30) between 10 and 15 years of age, Tabin, Gregg, and Bonci (69) found mean knee flexion/extension ratios between 58.5% and 65.8% at 60°/s (scores were not corrected for gravity). They found mean dorsiflexor/plantar-flexor ratios between 27.6% and 32.1% in these groups.

Similar to results from adults (1, 57), several studies have reported that the knee flexion/extension ratio in youths varies with contraction velocity (15, 16, 18, 35, 59). For example, Burnie and Brodie (16), based on their own as well as other published data, showed an increased concentric knee flexion/extension ratio at higher contraction velocities (n = 18, mean age = 11.4 years). Similarly, Calmels and coworkers (18) found a higher knee flexion/extension ratio at 120°/s than at 60°/s in nine elite female gymnasts (mean age = 11.3 ± 1.2 years). (Interestingly, the ratios were not different for eccentric versus concentric contractions.) In addition, Burnie (15) examined knee flexion/extension ratios in untrained prepubescent males (n = 14, mean age = 11.4 ± 0.6 years) and preadolescent female gymnasts (n = 12, mean age = 10.6 ± 0.5 years). For both groups, increases in contraction velocity resulted in increases in the knee flexion/extension ratio. Together, these results indicate that the decline in hamstring torque with increases in contraction velocity is less than for the quadriceps and suggest that the slope of the torque-velocity curve is different for the hamstrings versus the quadriceps in youths (1). These results are similar to data from adults and suggest that recommendations for knee flexion/extension ratios should be speed specific.

Some data exist in the literature to suggest that strength ratios may vary with age and body size. Kanehisa and associates (44) found differential results in flexion/extension peak torque ratios (60°/s) for the elbow and knee across ages (n = 130 boys, ages 7–13). Specifically, the elbow ratio increased with age while there was no age effect for the knee ratio. Interestingly, the flexor/extensor CSA (via ultrasound) ratios were not related to age for the elbow but increased across age at the knee. These disparate results suggest dissociation between strength and CSA development in youths. Similarly, the trunk flexion/extension ratio was shown to differ across age in boys versus girls (8). At 30°/s, the ratio decreased with age in girls but increased with age in boys. In addition, the relationships between age, body size, and strength ratios may vary with contraction velocity. Gilliam and coworkers (30) found that the elbow and knee flexion/extension ratios in 7- to 13-year-old boys and girls were affected by body size and age at 120°/s but not at 30°/s. Specifically, at 120°/s the ratios decrease with increases in body size (height and mass) and age.

With respect to differences between limbs, Burnie (15) found no side-to-side differences in knee flexion/extension ratios in preadolescent males and females. In addition, several papers have also reported data examining possible gender differences in antagonist strength ratios. In most studies, gender differences have not been found (30, 35, 58).

## Muscle Endurance

Thorstensson and Karlsson (75) developed an isokinetic protocol to assess muscle fatigue in which the percentage decline across 50 repeated maximal isokinetic contractions was correlated with muscle fiber composition. Kanehisa and coworkers (45) have shown that 14-year-old boys (n = 26) have a smaller percentage decline in knee extension torque across 50 maximal contractions at 180°/s than 18- to 25-year-old men (n = 26). The authors noted that while the literature indicates that the percentage of fast twitch fibers is determined early in life (9), there also are data in the literature to suggest that there is lower utilization of glycolytic metabolism in youths (27, 42). They suggested, then, that the smaller percentage decline of the young subjects might have been due to relatively smaller reliance on glycolysis in these subjects.

Kawakami and coworkers (46) examined fatigue responses over 50 consecutive reciprocal concentric and eccentric contractions of the elbow flexors at 30°/s in 13-year-old boys. Their results showed similar force losses for the concentric and eccentric contractions. They noted that the pattern of force loss with eccentric versus concentric contractions differed from adult data (48), which showed greater eccentric fatigue with similar testing. They suggested that the differences might have been due to the young subjects' inability to maximally recruit motor units during eccentric contractions. However, since no direct comparisons with adults were made in the study, these observations should be viewed as preliminary.

There is little data regarding isokinetic muscle endurance between genders; however, one study by Holmes and Alderink (35) found no differences between genders in high school age subjects (n = 17 males and 32 females, ages 15–18 years).

Collectively, these results suggest that responses during isokinetic endurance testing may differ in youths versus adults. The differences may reflect developmental processes in glycolytic metabolism and possibly neuromuscular inhibition, but further research is necessary to establish more clearly developmental differences and to examine possible mechanisms.

## Age Effects

Many studies have shown that, even after adjusting for differences in body size, older subjects are stronger than younger subjects (8, 37–40, 44, 67, 69,

72, 81). For example, Kanehisa and coworkers have shown that for both females (43) and males (43, 44), young subjects exhibit lower strength per unit of the product of muscle cross-sectional area (from ultrasound scans) times thigh length (product is an estimate of thigh muscle volume), indicating an age effect in which increases in body size are insufficient to account for age-related increases in strength. Similarly, several studies (37–40, 72, 81) have shown (using procedures such as partial correlation analysis, ratio scaling, and ANCOVA) that significant age effects persist even after removing the effects of body weight and fat free weight (FFW).

In addition, the age effect appears to be specific for both muscle group and contraction speed. For example, Housh and coworkers (40) tested knee and elbow extension and flexion peak torque in 195 high school wrestlers (ages 14–19 years) at 30, 180, and 300°/s. After covarying for FFW, significant age differences were still found for leg extension at 30°/s and forearm flexion at 30 and 180°/s. No FFW-adjusted age differences were found for forearm extension or knee flexion. Similarly, differences in the age effect have been reported for motions at the shoulder (38). Flexion and extension of the arm did not show a relationship between age and peak torque (speeds = 30, 180, and 300°/s) after separately covarying for body weight and FFW and anthropometrically estimated muscle mass (n = 40, ages 14–19 years). In contrast, horizontal abduction (30°/s) and adduction (30 and 180°/s) of the arm (n = 60) did result in significant correlation between age and peak torque after separately covarying for body weight, FFW, and muscle mass. Collectively, these results suggest that both contraction speed and motion influence the age effect. It should be noted, however, that the authors suspected that the lack of significant age effect for arm flexion and extension may have been due to relatively low statistical power (n = 40).

We have recently used allometric scaling to examine age-related increases in isokinetic strength across age using data from the Nebraska wrestling study (80). The results showed not only an age effect as described above (statistically a main effect for age), indicating greater strength in older (high school, ages 14–18 years) versus younger (elementary school, ages 8–13) wrestlers, but a significant interaction between age and fat free weight. The interaction effect indicated that the relationship between FFW and isokinetic strength changes across age, with FFW being a stronger determinant of strength differences in elementary school age subjects than high school age subjects. In addition, the leg flexion data indicated that while age was a significant determinant of peak torque in the elementary school age wrestlers, age was not significant in the high school wrestlers, indicating that the age effect can be muscle group dependent. Similarly, Leatt, Shephard, and Plyley (50) did not find significant leg flexion strength differences between Canadian national soccer team players under age 18 (mean age = 16.7 years) versus those under age 16 (mean age = 15.4 years). However, significant differences were noted between the age group teams for the leg extension data at 300°/s (data ratio scaled for body mass and lean body mass).

A variety of hypotheses have been proposed to explain the age effect for strength. At least some of the body size-independent increase in strength across age is likely due to neurological maturation. Specifically, the ability to maximally recruit all motor units during a maximal contraction may increase across age (10). It has been suggested that the percentage of FFW that is composed of muscle tissue may increase with age (40), implying that scaling for differences in FFW may not fully account for differences in muscle mass. In addition, there may be qualitative changes that occur in skeletal muscle across age (22). Clearly, the causes for age-related strength differences require further study. Furthermore, to date no studies have examined age-related differences in eccentric strength. Differences in the age effect between concentric and eccentric contractions may provide insight into skeletal muscle development in youths.

# Gender Effects

Examination of gender differences in isokinetic strength in youths is complicated by two factors. First, because of potential differences in body size and body composition, body size adjustments typically need to be performed as part of the data analysis. Procedures for body size adjustments have been noted previously. In addition, the relationship between gender and isokinetic strength likely changes across age. In this section, where adolescent versus preadolescent distinctions are possible, the studies have been segregated accordingly. The outcomes of the various studies also have been summarized in table 15.1.

Gilliam and colleagues (30) reported one of the first studies of gender differences in isokinetic peak torque in youths. Boys (n = 28) and girls (n = 28) between the ages of 7 and 13 were tested for knee and elbow flexion and extension at 30 and 120°/s. Gender differences were examined statistically using ANCOVA, with separate analyses using height and body mass as covariates. For knee extension and flexion, no differences were found between genders with height as the covariate while gender differences were noted with body mass as the covariate at 120°/s only. There are two points worth noting. First, as pointed out previously, the choice of scaling variable (height versus mass) can significantly affect the outcome of the analyses. Second, gender differences may be affected by the contraction velocity (30 versus 120°/s). For the elbow data, the authors reported that their ANCOVA results indicated violation of the homogeneity of regression assumption for both speeds with height as the covariate and at 30°/s with body mass as the covariate. This assumption violation indicates that the regression slopes between genders for both height and body mass were not parallel. Because violation of this assumption makes examination of ANCOVA adjusted means invalid, the authors did not interpret these analyses. However, the assumption violation is equivalent to a gender by body size interaction effect. That is, their results indicate that for elbow flexion and extension, the fundamental relationship between body size and strength differs between boys and girls. Unfortunately, this interaction was not examined by the authors and is worthy of further study.

## Table 15.1 Gender Differences

| Study | Motion | Speeds (°/s) | Ages and sample size | Body size correction | Outcome |
|---|---|---|---|---|---|
| Gilliam et al. (1979b) | Knee flexion/ extension | 30, 120 | 7–13, n = 28 per gender | ANCOVA for height and body mass | 1. Height: M = F 2. Body mass: M > F at 120°/s |
| Miyashita and Kanehisa (1979) | Knee extension | 210 | 13–17, total n = 569 | None | Increased gender differences across ages 13–17 |
| Sunnegardh et al. (1988) | Elbow flexion, knee flexion/ extension | 12, 90, 150 | 8, 13, total n = 131 | Ratio scaling for body mass, (height)$^2$, estimated CSA | 1. age 8: M = F 2. age 13: M > F for elbow and knee extension |
| Backman and Oberg (1989) | Dorsiflexion | 15, 30, 60, 120, 180, & 240 | 6–15, total n = 137 | Ratio scaling for body mass | M > F at age 15 |
| Docherty and Gaul (1991) | Knee flexion/ extension | 30, 180 | Mean = 11.0, 23 boys, 29 girls | Ratio scaling for lean body mass (skinfolds) | M = F |
| Balague et al. (1993) | Trunk flexion/ extension | 30, 150 | 10–16, total n = 117 | Ratio scaling for body mass index | M > F at age 15 |
| Kanehisa et al. (1994) | Knee extension | 60, 180, 300 | 6–9, n = 30 per gender | Ratio scaling for muscle CSA × thigh length | M > F |
| Cioni et al. (1994) | Knee extension | 30 | 10–18, n = 34 | Unclear | Late childhood: M = F Adolescence: M > F |
| Nyland et al. (1997) | Knee extension | 60, 450 | Mean = 16.1 | Ratio scaling for lean body mass | M = F |

# Preadolescents

There are several reports in the literature concerning differences in isokinetic strength between boys and girls prior to puberty. The data generally show few strength differences between sexes prior to puberty, but strength differences tend to show up after puberty. Kanehisa and coworkers (43) have shown that young boys (ages 6–9 years) have higher isokinetic knee extension strength (speed = 60, 180, and 300°/s), relative to the product of muscle cross-sectional area (ultrasound scans) times thigh length, than young girls of the same age. In contrast, Cioni and associates (20) found no differences between boys and girls (mean age = 12.5 years; n = 9) in isokinetic knee extension peak torque at 30°/s (scores not adjusted for body mass). Similarly, Docherty and Gaul (23) found no gender differences between elementary school boys (n = 23, mean age = 10.8 years) and girls (n = 29, mean age = 11.1) for knee extension and flexion at 30 and 180°/s. This was true for both absolute as well as ratio-scaled data (denominator = lean body mass from skinfolds). For trunk flexion and extension, Balague and coworkers (8) found increases in peak torque across age in 117 boys and girls at both 30 and 150°/s (age range = 10–16 years) after ratio scaling for body mass index. Further, examination of their figures 8 and 9 indicated that by age 15 males exhibited higher strength than females at 150°/s, however these comparisons were not addressed in the paper. In the dorsiflexors (test speeds = 15, 30, 60, 120, 180, and 240°/s), Backman and Oberg (7) found no significant gender differences in 6, 9, and 12 year age groups, however significant gender differences were found for the 15 year age group (see discussion on "Adolescents" below). Similarly, Sunnegardh and coworkers (68) found that in general, 8-year-old boys and girls (total n = 131) showed similar elbow flexion (12 and 90°/s) and knee extension and flexion (12, 90, and 150°/s) strength. However, 13-year-old boys were significantly stronger than girls for elbow and knee extension while knee flexion values were similar between sexes. These results were found using both absolute as well as a variety of ratio-scaled (for body weight, lean body mass, height$^2$, and estimated muscle cross-sectional area) scores.

# Adolescents

In contrast to data from preadolescents, gender differences are apparent during adolescence. For the leg extensors, Cioni and coworkers (20) found significant gender differences for isokinetic peak torque at 30°/s in adolescent subjects (mean age = 15.3 years), and Miyashita and Kanehisa (54) found an increase in peak torque from ages 13 to 17 in males and no differences in females from ages 14 to 17 (total n = 569, test speed = 210°/s). Therefore, while not analyzed in their study, their results suggest a widening of the differences in strength between boys and girls through the teenage years. Similarly, as noted previously, Backman and Oberg (7) found significant gender differences in dorsiflexion torque in 15-year-old subjects. In contrast, Nyland and coworkers (59) reported no gender difference for knee extension peak torque (speeds = 60 and 450°/s) in male (mean age = 15.7 ± 0.7 years; n = 16) versus female (mean age = 16.4 ± 1.1 years) high school soccer players after ratio scaling for lean body weight (skinfolds). These latter results suggest that athletic conditioning may eliminate gender differences in strength.

## Side Dominance

Strength differences between limbs can have important functional implications. Evaluation of rehabilitation progress in an injured limb is often assessed by comparing the injured limb to the uninjured limb (33). Clearly, an understanding of expected side-to-side differences will aid in interpretation of such data. Functionally, gross strength imbalances may affect motor performance, perhaps leading to a preferred side in certain athletic tasks. In addition, in adults a bilateral deficit has been observed in which the bilateral expression of strength is less than the sum of the individual limb strengths used unilaterally (13, 77). To date however, this effect has not been studied in children.

While a variety of studies have reported comparisons of strength between limbs, the available literature presents no clear consensus as to whether such differences are present. The results of these studies are addressed below and summarized in table 15.2. Alexander and Molnar (2) were the first to examine interlimb strength differences in youths. They reported statistically significant strength differences between the dominant and nondominant limbs for elbow and knee flexion and extension in 36 boys and 34 girls between the ages of 7 and 15 years. However, the magnitude of the limb differences was not reported. More recently, Sunnegardh and coworkers (68) found that right-handed children (n = 112, ages 8 and 13) were significantly stronger on the right side for elbow flexion and knee extension and flexion. The left-handed subjects (n = 12) were stronger in elbow flexion on the left side but were generally stronger at the knee on the right side. Backman and Oberg (7) indicated that in adults, lower limb strength is greater in the side opposite to the dominant arm. Their data for dorsiflexion strength, however, shows that in young children (age groups = 6 and 9 years) there is greater strength on the same side as the dominant hand at the faster contraction velocities (speeds = 120, 180, and 240°/s). Older children (age groups = 12 and 15 years) exhibited the adult pattern of handedness at slow contraction velocities (15 and 30°/s), indicating that the adult pattern of lower limb side dominance for strength develops between ages 9 and 12 years.

Rochcongar and associates (66) found no differences between limbs in knee extension and flexion strength (speeds = 30 and 180°/s) in youth soccer players ages 12 to 18. However, Chin and coworkers (19) showed a 36.4% difference in knee extension peak torque between the dominant versus nondominant limb at 60°/s in elite junior soccer players (mean age = 17.3 years) at 240°/s. Additionally, the knee flexors on the dominant side were significantly stronger than the nondominant flexors at both speeds; however, the differences were more modest (4.5% at 60°/s and 10% at 240°/s). These results suggest that intense soccer training may induce interlimb strength imbalances.

## Table 15.2  Side Dominance

| Study | Motion | Speeds (°/s) | Ages and sample size | Outcome |
|---|---|---|---|---|
| Alexander and Molnar (1973) | Elbow flexion/ extension Knee flexion/ extension | 30 | 7–15, n = 70 | D > ND |
| Gilliam et al. (1979a) | Knee flexion/ extension | 30, 180 | 15–17, n = 115 | 2–3% right to left differences |
| Holmes and Alderink (1984) | Knee flexion/ extension | 60, 180 | 15–18, n = 49 | D = ND |
| Burnie and Brody (1986) | Knee flexion/ extension | 60, 240 | Mean = 11.4, n = 18 | D = ND |
| Rochcongar et al. (1988) | Knee flexion/ extension | 30, 180 | 12–18, n = 136 | D = ND |
| Sunnegardh et al. (1988) | Elbow flexion Knee flexion/ extension | 12, 90 12, 90, 150 | 8 and 13, n = 131 | Right handed: R > L for all motions Left handed: L > R for elbow flexion, R > L for knee flexion/extension |
| Weltman et al. (1988) | Knee flexion/ extension Shoulder flexion /extension Elbow flexion/ extension | 30, 90 | 6–11, n = 29 | Knee: ND > D |
| Backman and Oberg (1989) | Dorsiflexion | 15, 30, 60, 120, 180, 240 | 6–15, n = 137 | Ages 6 and 9: D > ND at high speeds (120–240) Age 12: D < ND at 15 Age 15: D < ND at 15, 30 |
| Chin et al. (1994) | Knee flexion/ extension | 60, 240 | Mean = 17.3, n = 21 | Flexion: 60: D > ND; 240: D > ND Extension: 60: D > ND; 240: D = ND |
| Calmels et al. (1995) | Knee flexion/ extension (concentric and eccentric) | 60, 120 | Mean = 11.3, n = 9 | D = ND |

In contrast, several studies have reported no interlimb strength differences in youth athletic groups. Gilliam and colleagues (29) reported only minimal (2–3%) side-to-side differences for knee flexion and extension in high school football players (speeds = 30 and 180°/s). It should be noted, however, that their comparisons were made between right and left limbs and therefore dominant versus nondominant differences may have been obscured. Calmels and associates (18) found no significant knee strength differences between the dominant versus nondominant limbs in female gymnasts (mean age = 11.3 ±1.2 years). This was true for both flexion and extension at both 60 and 120°/s as well as for both concentric and eccentric strength. Similarly, Holmes and Alderink (35) found no strength differences between the dominant versus nondominant limbs for knee extension and flexion peak torque at 60 and 180°/s. No side differences were found by Weltman and coworkers (83) for the elbow and shoulder, but a small difference was reported for the knee flexors and extensors (nondominant > dominant side; speeds = 30 and 90°/s; mean differences ranged from 5.4 to 10.9%). However, it is unclear if the effects were significantly different. Similarly, Burnie and Brody (16) did not find a stronger side for leg extension in preadolescent boys (mean age = 11.4 years) at 60 and 240°/s.

## Isokinetic Assessment of Training Effects

A variety of studies have examined strength increases consequent to training in youths, with many studies specifically examining prepubertal children (26). In prepubescent subjects, most studies show significant increases in strength with little evidence of hypertrophy; the lack of hypertrophy has been suggested to be due to relatively low androgen levels prior to puberty, and the strength increases have been attributed to neurological adaptations (26). Regarding neurological adaptations, Ozmun, Mikesky, and Surburg (61) have shown increases in maximal electromyographic amplitude following training, suggesting an increase in maximal motor unit recruitment or firing rate. It may also be the case that improved lifting technique (i.e., learning) has occurred, which may at least partially explain improvements in strength scores. Surprisingly, few studies have examined isokinetic training in youths. However, isokinetic testing has been frequently used to monitor strength changes following other types of resistance training.

With respect to isokinetic testing of training effects, Fukunaga, Funato, and Ikegawa (28) examined 12 weeks of isometric strength training of the elbow flexors and extensors in elementary school children (first, third, and fifth grades). The training resulted in significant increases in isometric strength and muscle cross-sectional area (ultrasound) but no significant increases in isokinetic strength (60, 180, and 300°/s), indicating that, as with adults, responses to strength training are specific to the mode of training.

However, Ozmun, Mikesky, and Surburg (61) did show significant increases in isokinetic elbow flexor strength at 90°/s following 8 weeks of dumbbell curl strength training (3 sets × 7–10 repetitions, 3 times a week) in 9- to 12-year-old boys and girls. The isokinetic strength increases in the training group (27.8% over pretraining values) were comparable to the relative increases in 1 RM strength (22.6%) over pretraining. Significant increases in EMG amplitude were also shown and, coupled with the lack of increase in arm circumference, suggest that the strength increases were primarily due to neural factors. The similarity of strength increases between isokinetic and "isotonic" measures is puzzling in light of the data of Fukunaga, Funato, and Ikegawa (28) in children and data from adults showing much greater increases in isotonic strength following isotonic training than increases in isokinetic strength (79). However, Ramsey and associates (65) also found quite large increases in isokinetic elbow flexion (25.8%) and knee extension (21.3%) peak torque (values are collapsed across contraction velocities of 30, 60, 120, and 180°/s) following 20 weeks of isotonic strength training (preacher curls, leg extensions, leg press, bench press, lat pull-downs, and sit/curl-ups). The increases in 1 RM strength were 34.6% for the bench press and 22.1% for the double leg press. Both the experimental (n = 13) and control subjects (n = 13) were boys classified as Tanner stage 1. Interestingly, these strength increases were not associated with significant increases in muscle cross-sectional area (computed tomography) of the biceps brachii or quadriceps or motor unit activation (twitch interpolation). The authors suggested that the strength gains without hypertrophy were suggestive of improvements in "motor skill coordination" and other "undetermined" neural factors.

Two studies have examined isokinetic adaptations following the effects of hydraulic resistance training. Docherty and coworkers (24) did not show significant increases in isokinetic peak torque (arm adduction, arm abduction, leg extension, and leg flexion) following four weeks (3 sessions/week) of strength training on a hydraulic resistance device (Hydragym) in prepubertal boys (mean age = 12.6 years). The lack of training response was likely due to the training status of the subjects (immediately postseason of either ice hockey or elite soccer), which, coupled with the short training period (4 weeks), minimized the possible training effect. In contrast, Weltman and colleagues (82) showed that a longer training program (14 weeks) using a similar training protocol on similar equipment did result in significant increases in concentric isokinetic elbow flexion (30 and 90°/s), knee flexion (30 and 90°/s), and knee extension (30°/s) mean torque (relative increases ranged from 18.5 to 36.6%).

Isokinetic strength training (concentric and eccentric) of the knee extensors and flexors has been shown by MacPhail and Kramer (52) to significantly increase both concentric and eccentric peak torque and work in 17 adolescents (n = 10 females) with mild cerebral palsy (mean age = 16 ± 3 years; six were classified as preadolescent). All strength training was performed at 90°/s. Increases in strength over the eight-week training period (3 sessions/week) averaged 25% for peak torque and 21% for work. In addition, there were significant increases in gross motor ability and the amount of improvement was positively correlated with the magnitude of strength increase. Significant increases in strength relative to pretraining were still present following three months of detraining.

The studies reported here indicate that, in general, isokinetic testing is sensitive to changes in strength induced by other forms of resistance training. Notably, the data of Ozmun, Mikesky, and Surburg (61) and Ramsey and coworkers (65) show over 20% increases in isokinetic torque following isotonic training. Indeed, these relative increases were comparable to the relative increases in isotonic strength, suggesting that test mode specificity is not as powerful as that in adults. The data of Fukunaga, Funato, and Ikegawa (28), however, do provide evidence of specificity, in that isotonic training did not result in transfer to isokinetic scores. Further research is warranted to examine test specificity issues in youths.

## Associations With Athletics

Surprisingly little research has been conducted examining isokinetic measures and aspects of athletics in youths. Some papers have reported descriptive data on isokinetic strength in various youth athletic groups in an attempt to establish normative data (29, 62). However, the utility of these studies is open to debate, especially considering the differences in the literature concerning scaling for variations in body size and inconsistency in corrections for gravity.

With respect to correlations with athletic performance, limited data exist in the literature. However, several studies have examined isokinetic strength in adolescent wrestlers. Cisar and coworkers (21) used discriminant function analysis to examine predictors of success in high school wrestling. They found two discriminant functions that correlated with wrestling success classification (novice = ≤ 33% winning percentage, average = 34–60%, and highly skilled = ≥ 67%). One of the discriminant functions was highly associated with measures of isokinetic strength (leg and elbow flexion and extension at 30, 180, and 300°/s) ratio scaled to body weight. This discriminant function was more effective at discriminating between the average and novice wrestlers versus comparisons with the highly skilled wrestlers. Their results suggest that isokinetic strength may differentiate between relatively unsuccessful wrestlers but other factors separate more successful wrestlers.

Eckerson and coworkers (25) examined changes in isokinetic strength, anaerobic power, and body composition in varsity high school wrestlers (n = 34, mean age ± $SD$ = 16.6 ± 1.0 years at preseason) across a competitive season. The subjects were tested for elbow and knee flexion and extension peak torque at 30, 180, and 300°/s during preseason training and again just prior to a postseason tournament. Most subjects (n = 26) showed significant reductions in body weight, fat weight, and relative fat. These subjects showed concomitant reductions in leg flexion torque at 180°/s at all speeds. Nine subjects who gained body weight across the season showed no increases in strength and significantly decreased leg extension peak torque at 30°/s and leg flexion at 180°/s. In addition, data for the entire sample, covaried for body weight, showed significant reductions in leg extension torque at 30°/s and leg and forearm flexion at 180°/s, indicating that the strength decreases were not completely explained by changes in body weight. The authors suggested that the strength declines might have been due to overtraining. These results indicate that a competitive wrestling season results in lower isokinetic peak torque. Furthermore, these data suggest that measurement of isokinetic torque may allow for monitoring of overtraining in high school athletes.

In a similar study, Roemmich and Sinning (67) compared changes in a variety of measures, including isokinetic strength and power (elbow and knee flexion and extension at 60 and 180°/s) between nine adolescent wrestlers (mean age = 15.4 years) and seven controls (mean age = 15.7 years). As with the data of Eckerson and coworkers (25), strength scores were significantly lower at the end of the season relative to the preseason, along with simultaneous reductions in body weight. After covarying for fat free weight, elbow flexion peak torques at both speeds were still reduced; however, the knee strength values were no longer significant. During the postseason, significant increases in isokinetic strength, body weight, and fat free weight occurred. The results indicate that much of the strength loss during the season was due to loss of lean tissue; however, loss of elbow flexion peak torque was more than could be attributed simply to loss of fat free weight.

Some evidence suggests that isokinetic testing can discriminate between youth subjects who excel in sports requiring different contractile and metabolic characteristics. Thorland and coworkers (72) reported that in female athletes (ages = 10–18), sprinters (n = 12) were significantly stronger than distance runners (n = 19) in knee extension at high contraction velocities (240–300°/s) but not at lower contraction velocities (30–180°/s). These effects were present in both younger subjects (ages 10–12 years) and older subjects (ages 12–18) and after covarying for differences in FFW. Another report by the same group (73) found comparable results in competitive male runners (n = 24 sprinters and n = 24 middle distance runners, ages 10–17 years). In this study, leg extension peak torque (speeds = 30, 60, 120, 180, 240, and 300°/s), covaried for body weight, was significantly higher in sprinters versus the middle distance runners. Similarly, Housh and coworkers (41) examined knee extension and flexion (speed = 180°/s) isokinetic strength differences among elite (Olympic development camp participants) adolescent female track and field athletes (mean age = 16.4 ± 1.6 years, n = 16 throwers, 11 long and high jumpers, 12 distance runners, and 23 sprinters). Absolute strength scores were significantly greater in the throwers than the other groups. However, when ratio scaled for body weight or lean body weight (from hydrostatic weighing), few differences were evident. Specifically, the extensor strength/body weight ratio was significantly greater in the sprinters than distance runners while the extension strength/lean body weight ratio was significantly greater in the throwers than the distance runners. Collectively, the results indicate that the distance runners were significantly weaker for extension than the other athletes. However, ratio-scaled differences were not present for flexion. Unfortunately, speed-specific strength differences were not examined. Of note, other than the distance runners, the athletes tested were from events that require brief, high force contractions.

Thus, anaerobic training (or alternatively, a genetic predisposition for success in anaerobic activities) may result in disproportionate strength development in adolescents. This effect does not appear to be present for the leg flexors. Muscle group-specific strength differences between athletes require further study. In addition, these results suggest that isokinetic testing might be used to screen and categorize youth athletes.

Miyashita and Kanehisa (54) found significant correlations between knee extension peak torque at 210°/s and 50-meter running speed in boys ($r = .69$, n = 275) and girls ($r = .37$, n = 298) ages 13 to 17 years. In addition, free style swimming speed (100 meters, n = 35 competitive swimmers, ages 11–21 years) was significantly correlated with isokinetic shoulder strength (210°/s; the specific shoulder motion appears to have been internal and external rotation) in both boys ($r = .73$, n = 19) and girls ($r = .52$, n = 16). Unfortunately, comparisons with other speeds were not performed, so no speed-specific relationships were reported (54).

Similarly, data from isokinetic testing may provide insight into age-related developmental aspects of athletic conditioning. Nemoto, Kanehisa, and Miyashita (58) studied isokinetic knee extension peak torque (dynamic speeds = 30, 180 and 300°/s) in competitive junior speedskaters (n = 132 males and 71 females, ages = 10–18 years) versus controls (n = 236 males and 265 females). They found that at age 16 and above, both male and female speed skaters exhibited significantly higher peak torque at 60°/s than controls; however, there were no differences between younger subjects. At 180°/s, male skaters were stronger than controls only at age 18 while female skaters were stronger than controls at ages 17 and 18. These age-specific strength differences were paralleled by differences in body weight and skinfold-estimated lean body mass. These data suggest that speedskating training results in hypertrophic adaptations that are manifested in increased muscle force at slow contraction speeds but not at a fast speed (300°/s). In addition, these differences were apparent only in older subjects (16+ years). The age- and speed-specific differences between skaters and controls may be due to differences in skating training across age or to underlying differences in biological development across age and require further study with other athletic groups.

# Summary

A variety of studies have examined isokinetic strength in youths. The data suggest that isokinetic testing is reliable, although more detailed analysis is required. Isokinetic testing has been valuable in studying issues such as age and gender effects on strength, side dominance, antagonist strength ratios, and relationships between athletic participation and strength. The available research also suggests several potentially important differences from adult responses. For example, there are hints in the literature that the shapes of the torque-velocity curves are different in youths versus adults. Such differences, including eccentric differences, are particularly suited to examination with isokinetic testing. Similarly, muscle fatigue testing on isokinetic dynamometers suggests possible youth-adult differences. Both of these issues require further study and may provide insight into muscle development across age. In addition, while several studies have employed isokinetic testing to assess the effects of resistance training on strength in youths, there is little data regarding youth responses to isokinetic resistance training. Overall, it is fair to say that our understanding of youth isokinetic responses is not yet well developed, and that future isokinetic research will expand our understanding of neuromuscular function in youths.

# References

1. Aagaard, P., E.B. Simonsen, M. Trolle, J. Bangsbo, and K. Klausen. 1995. Isokinetic hamstring/quadriceps strength ratio: Influence from joint angular velocity, gravity correction, and contraction mode. *Acta Physiologica Scandinavica* 154: 421–27.

2. Alexander, J., and G.E. Molnar. 1973. Muscular strength in children: Preliminary report on objective standards. *Archives of Physical Medicine and Rehabilitation* 54: 424–27.

3. Asmussen, E. 1973. Growth in muscular strength and power. In *Human growth and development*, ed. G.L. Rarick. New York: Academic Press.

4. Asmussen, E., and K.R. Heeboll-Nielsen. 1955. A dimensional analysis of physical performance and growth in boys. *Journal of Applied Physiology* 7: 593–603.

5. Asmussen, E., and K.R. Heeboll-Nielsen. 1955. Physical performance and growth in children: Influence of sex, age, and intelligence. *Journal of Applied Physiology* 8: 371–80.

6. Astrand, P.O., and K. Rodahl. 1986. *Textbook of work physiology*. 3d ed. 393. New York: McGraw Hill.

7. Backman, E., and B. Oberg. 1989. Isokinetic muscle torque in the dorsiflexors of the ankle in children 6 to 15 years of age. *Scandinavian Journal of Rehabilitation Medicine* 21: 97–103.

8. Balague, F., P. Damidot, M. Nordin, M. Parnianpour, and M. Waldburger. 1993. Cross-sectional study of the isokinetic muscle trunk strength among school children. *Spine* 18: 1199–205.

9. Bell, R.D., J.D. MacDougall, R.B. Billeter, and H. Howald. 1980. Muscle fiber types and morphometric analysis of skeletal muscle in six-year-old children. *Medicine and Science in Sports and Exercise* 12: 28–31.

10. Blimkie, C.J.R. 1989. Age- and sex-associated variation in strength during childhood: Anthropometric, morphologic, neurologic, biomechanical, endocrinologic, genetic, and physical activity correlates. In *Perspectives in exercise science and sports medicine*, Vol. 2: *Youth, exercise, and sport*, ed. C.V. Gisolfi and D.R. Lamb, 99–161. Indianapolis: Benchmark Press.

11. Brown, L.E., M. Whitehurst, B.W. Findley, R. Gilbert, and D.N. Buchalter. 1995. Isokinetic load range during shoulder rotation exercise in elite male junior tennis players. *Journal of Strength and Conditioning Research* 9: 160–64.

12. Brown, L.E., M. Whitehurst, R. Gilbert, and D.N. Buchalter. 1995. The effect of velocity and gender on load range during knee extension and flexion exercise on an isokinetic device. *Journal of Orthopaedic and Sports Physical Therapy* 21: 107–12.

13. Brown, L.E., M. Whitehurst, R. Gilbert, B.W. Findley, and D. N. Buchalter. 1994. Bilateral deficit during knee extension and flexion exercise in females. *Isokinetics and Exercise Science* 4: 153–56.

14. Burnett, C.N., E.F. Betts, and W.M. King. 1990. Reliability of isokinetic measurements of hip muscle torque in young boys. *Physical Therapy* 70: 244–49.

15. Burnie, J. 1987. Factors affecting selected reciprocal muscle group ratios in preadolescents. *International Journal of Sports Medicine* 8: 40–45.

16. Burnie, J., and D.A. Brodie. 1986. Isokinetic measurement in preadolescent males. *International Journal of Sports Medicine* 7: 205–9.

17. Caiozzo, V.J., J.J. Perrine, and V.R. Edgerton. 1981. Training-induced alterations of the in vivo force-velocity relationship of human muscle. *Journal of Applied Physiology* 51: 750–54.

18. Calmels, P., I. Van Den Borne, M. Nellen, M. Domenach, P. Minaire, and M. Drost. 1995. A pilot study of knee isokinetic strength in young, highly trained, female gymnasts. *Isokinetics and Exercise Science* 5: 69–74.

19. Chin, M., R.C.H. Raymond, Y.W.Y. Yuan, R.C.T. Li, and A.S.K. Wong. 1994. Cardiorespiratory fitness and isokinetic muscle strength of elite Asian junior soccer players. *Journal of Sports Medicine and Physical Fitness* 34: 250–57.

20. Cioni, M., A. Cocilovo, F. Di Pasquale, M.B. Rillo Araujo, C. Rodrigues Siqueira, and M. Bianco. 1994. Strength deficit of knee extensor muscles of individuals with Down's syndrome from childhood to adolescence. *American Journal of Mental Retardation* 99: 166–74.

21. Cisar, C.J., G.O. Johnson, A.C. Fry, T.J. Housh, R.A. Hughes, A.J. Ryan, and W.G. Thorland. 1987. Preseason body composition, build, and strength as predictors of high school wrestling success. *Journal of Applied Sport Science Research* 1: 66–70.

22. Cooper, D.M., D. Weiler-Ravell, B.J. Whipp, and K. Wasserman. 1984. Aerobic parameters of exercise as a function of body size during growth in children. *Journal of Applied Physiology* 56: 628–34.

23. Docherty, D., and C.A. Gaul. 1991. Relationship of physical size, physique, and composition to physical performance in young boys and girls. *International Journal of Sports Medicine* 12: 525–32.

24. Docherty, D., H.A. Wenger, M.L. Collins, and H.A. Quinney. 1987. The effects of variable speed resistance training on strength development in prepubertal boys. *Journal of Human Movement Studies* 13: 377–82.

25. Eckerson, J.M., D.J. Housh, T.J. Housh, and G.O. Johnson. 1994. Seasonal changes in body composition, strength, and muscular power in high school wrestlers. *Pediatric Exercise Science* 6: 39–52.

26. Faigenbaum, A.D., W.J. Kraemer, B. Cahill, J. Chandler, J. Dziados, L.D. Elfrink, E. Forman, M. Gaudiose, L. Micheli, M. Nitka, and S. Roberts. 1996. Youth resistance training: Position statement paper and literature review. *Strength and Conditioning* 18: 62–75.

27. Fournier, M., J. Ricci, A.W. Taylor, R.J. Ferguson, R.R. Montretit, and B.R. Chaitman. 1982. Skeletal muscle adaptation in adolescent boys: Sprint and endurance training and detraining. *Medicine and Science in Sports and Exercise* 14: 453–56.

28. Fukunaga, T., K. Funato, and S. Ikegawa. 1992. The effects of resistance training on muscle area and strength in prepubescent age. *Annals of Physiological Anthropology* 11: 357–64.

29. Gilliam, T.B., S.P. Sady, P.S. Freedson, and J. Villanacci. 1979a. Isokinetic torque levels for high school football players. *Archives of Physical Medicine and Rehabilitation* 60: 110–14.

30. Gilliam, T.B., J.F. Villanacci, P.S. Freedson, and S.P. Sady. 1979b. Isokinetic torque in boys and girls ages 7 to 13: Effect of age, height, and weight. *Research Quarterly for Exercise and Sport* 50: 599–609.

31. Hanten, W.P., and C.L. Ramberg. 1988. Effect of stabilization on maximal isokinetic torque of the quadriceps femoris muscle group during concentric and eccentric contractions. *Physical Therapy* 68: 219–22.

32. Hart, D.L., T.J. Stobbe, W.W. Till, and R.W. Plummer. 1984. Effect of trunk stabilization on quadriceps femoris muscle torque. *Physical Therapy* 64: 1375–80.

33. Henderson, R.C., C.L. Howes, K.L. Erickson, L.M. Heese, and R.A. DeMasi. 1993. Knee flexor-extensor strength in children. *Journal of Orthopaedic and Sports Physical Therapy* 18: 559–63.

34. Hill, C., R. Croce, J. Miller, and F. Cleland. 1996. Muscle torque relationships between hand-held dynamometry and isokinetic measurements in children ages 9 to 11. *Journal of Strength and Conditioning Research* 10: 77–82.

35. Holmes, J.R., and G.J. Alderink. 1984. Isokinetic strength characteristics of the quadriceps femoris and hamstring muscles in high school students. *Physical Therapy* 64: 914–18.

36. Hortobagyi, T., and F.I Katch. 1990. Eccentric and concentric torque-velocity relationships during arm flexion and extension: Influence of strength level. *European Journal of Applied Physiology* 30: 395–405.

37. Housh, T.J., R.J. Hughes, G.O. Johnson, D.J. Housh, L.L. Wagner, J.P. Weir, and S.A. Evans. 1990. Age-related increases in the shoulder strength of high school wrestlers. *Pediatric Exercise Science* 2: 65–72.

38. Housh, T.J., J.R. Stout, J.P. Weir, L.L. Weir, D.J. Housh, G.O. Johnson, and S.A. Evans. 1995. Relationships of age and muscle mass to peak torque in high school wrestlers. *Research Quarterly for Exercise and Sport* 66: 256–61.

39. Housh, T.J., G.O. Johnson, D.J. Housh, J.R. Stout, D.B. Smith, and K.T. Ebersole. 1997. Isokinetic peak torque and estimated muscle cross-sectional area in high school wrestlers. *Journal of Strength and Conditioning Research* 11: 45–49.

40. Housh, T.J., G.O. Johnson, R.A. Hughes, D.J. Housh, R.J. Hughes, A.S. Fry, K.B. Kenney, and C.J. Cisar. 1989. Isokinetic strength and body composition of high school wrestlers across age. *Medicine and Science in Sports and Exercise* 21: 105–9.

41. Housh, T.J., W.G. Thorland, G.D. Tharp, G.O. Johnson, and C.J. Cisar. 1984. Isokinetic leg flexion and extension strength of elite adolescent female track and field athletes. *Research Quarterly for Exercise and Sport* 55: 347–50.

42. Inbar, O., and O. Bar-Or. 1986. Anaerobic characteristics in male children and adolescents. *Medicine and Science in Sports and Exercise* 18: 264–69.

43. Kanehisa, H., S. Ikegawa, N. Tsunoda, and T. Fukunaga. 1994. Strength and cross-sectional area of knee extensor muscles in children. *European Journal of Applied Physiology* 68: 402–5.

44. Kanehisa, H., S. Ikegawa, N. Tsunoda, and T. Fukunaga. 1995. Strength and cross-sectional areas of reciprocal muscle groups in the upper arm and thigh during adolescence. *International Journal of Sports Medicine* 16: 54–60.

45. Kanehisa, H., H. Okuyama, S. Ikegawa, and T. Fukunaga. 1995. Fatigability during repetitive maximal knee extensions in 14-year-old boys. *European Journal of Applied Physiology* 72: 170–74.

46. Kawakami, Y., H. Kanehisa, S. Ikegawa, and T. Fukunaga. 1993. Concentric and eccentric muscle strength before, during, and after fatigue in 13-year-old boys. *European Journal of Applied Physiology* 67: 121–24.

47. Komi, PV. 1973. Measurement of the force-velocity relationship in human muscle under concentric and eccentric contractions. *Medicine and Sport* 8: 224–29.

48. Komi, P.V., and J.T. Viitasalo. 1977. Changes in motor unit activity and metabolism in human skeletal muscle during and after repeated eccentric and concentric actions. *Acta Physiologica Scandinavica* 100: 246–54.

49. Knapik, J.J., C.L. Bauman, B.H. Jones, J.M. Harris, and L. Vaughan. 1991. Preseason strength and flexibility imbalances associated with athletic injuries in female collegiate athletes. *American Journal of Sports Medicine* 19: 76–81.

50. Leatt, P., R.J. Shephard, and M.J. Plyley. 1987. Specific muscular development in under 18 soccer players. *Journal of Sports Sciences* 5: 165–75.

51. Lohman, T.G. 1986. Applicability of body composition techniques and constants for children and youths. In *Exercise and sport sciences reviews*, ed. K.B. Pandolf, 325–57. New York: MacMillan.

52. MacPhail, H.E.A., and J.F. Kramer. 1995. Effect of isokinetic strength training on functional ability and walking efficiency in adolescents with cerebral palsy. *Developmental Medicine and Child Neurology* 37: 763–75.

53. Merlini, L., D. Dell'Accio, and C. Granata. 1995. Reliability of dynamic strength knee muscle testing in children. *Journal of Orthopaedic and Sports Physical Therapy* 22: 73–76.

54. Miyashita, M., and H. Kanehisa. 1979. Dynamic peak torque related to age, sex, and performance. *Research Quarterly* 50: 249–55.

55. Mohtadi, N.G.H., G.N. Kiefer, K. Tedford, and S. Watters. 1990. Concentric and eccentric quadriceps torque in preadolescent males. *Canadian Journal of Sports Sciences* 15: 240–43.

56. Molnar, G.E., J. Alexander, and N. Gutfeld. 1979. Reliability of quantitative strength measurements in children. *Archives of Physical Medicine and Rehabilitation* 60: 218–21.

57. Morris, A., L. Lussier, G. Bell, and J. Dooley. 1983. Hamstring/quadriceps strength ratios in collegiate middle distance and distance runners. *Physician and Sportsmedicine* 11: 71–77.

58. Nemoto, I., H. Kanehisa, and M. Miyashita. 1990. The effect of sports training on the age-related changes of body composition and isokinetic peak torque in knee extensors of junior speed skaters. *Journal of Sports Medicine and Physical Fitness* 30: 83–88.

59. Nyland, J.A., D.N.M. Caborn, J.A. Brosky, C.L. Kneller, and G. Freidhoff. 1997. Anthropometric, muscular fitness, and injury history comparisons by gender of youth soccer teams. *Journal of Strength and Conditioning Research* 11: 92–97.

60. Osternig, L.R., J.A. Sawhill, B.T. Bates, and J. Hamill. 1983. Function of limb speed on torque patterns of antagonist muscles. In *Biomechanics* VIII-A, Vol. 4A, ed. H. Matsui and K. Kobayashi, 251–57. Champaign, IL: Human Kinetics.

61. Ozmun, J.C., A.E. Mikesky, and P.R. Surburg. 1994. Neuromuscular adaptations following prepubescent strength training. *Medicine and Science in Sports and Exercise* 26: 510–14.

62. Parker, M.G., R.O. Ruhling, D. Holt, E. Bauman, and M. Drayna. 1983. Descriptive analysis of quadriceps and hamstrings muscle torque in high school football players. *Journal of Orthopaedic and Sports Physical Therapy* 5: 2–6.

63. Payne, V.G., J.R. Morrow, L. Johnson, and S.N. Dalton. 1997. Resistance training in children and youth: A meta-analysis. *Research Quarterly for Exercise and Sport* 68: 80–88.

64. Perrine, J.J., and V.R. Edgerton. 1978. Muscle force-velocity and power-velocity relationships under isokinetic loading. *Medicine and Science in Sports and Exercise* 10: 159–66.

65. Ramsey, J.A., C.J.R. Blimkie, K. Smith, S. Garner, J.D. MacDougall, and D.G. Sale. 1990. Strength training effects in prepubescent boys. *Medicine and Science in Sports and Exercise* 22: 605–14.

66. Rochcongar, P., R. Morvan, J. Jan, J. Dassonville, and J. Beillot. 1988. Isokinetic investigation of knee extensors and knee flexors in young French soccer players. *International Journal of Sports Medicine* 9: 448–50.

67. Roemmich, J.N., and W.E. Sinning. 1997. Weight loss and wrestling training: effects on nutrition, growth, maturation, body composition, and strength. *Journal of Applied Physiology* 82: 1751–59.

68. Sunnegardh, J., L.E. Bratteby, L.O. Nordesjo, and B. Nordgren. 1988. Isometric and isokinetic muscle strength, anthropometry and physical activity in 8- and 13-year-old children. *European Journal of Applied Physiology* 58: 291–97.

69. Tabin, G.C., J.R. Gregg, and T. Bonci. 1985. Predictive leg strength values in immediately prepubescent and postpubescent athletes. *American Journal of Sports Medicine* 13: 387–89.

70. Tanner, J.M. 1949. Fallacy of per-weight and per-surface area standards and their relation to spurious correlation. *Journal of Applied Physiology* 2: 1–15.

71. Taylor, N.A.S., R.H. Sanders, E.I. Howick, and S.N. Stanley. 1991. Static and dynamic assessment of the Biodex dynamometer. *European Journal of Applied Physiology* 62: 180–88.

72. Thorland, W.G., G.O. Johnson, C.J. Cisar, T.J. Housh, and G.D. Tharp. 1987. Strength and anaerobic responses of elite young female sprint and distance runners. *Medicine and Science in Sports and Exercise* 19: 56–61.

73. Thorland, W.G., G.O. Johnson, C.J. Cisar, T.J. Housh, and G.D. Tharp. 1990. Muscular strength and power in elite young male runners. *Pediatric Exercise Science* 2: 73–82.

74. Thorstennsson, A., G. Grimby, and J. Karlsson. 1976. Force-velocity relations and fiber composition in human knee extensor muscles. *Journal of Applied Physiology* 40: 12–16.

75. Thorstensson, A., and J. Karlsson. 1976. Fatigability and fiber composition of human skeletal muscle. *Acta Physiologica Scandinavica* 98: 318–22.

76. Van den Berg-Emons, R.J.G., M.A. van Baak, D.C. de Barbanson, L. Speth, and W.H.M. Saris. 1996. Reliability of tests to determine peak aerobic power, anaerobic power, and isokinetic muscle strength in children with spastic cerebral palsy. *Developmental Medicine and Child Neurology* 38: 1117–25.

77. Vandervoort, A.A., D.G. Sale, and J. Moroz. 1984. Comparison of motor unit activation during unilateral and bilateral leg extension. *Journal of Applied Physiology* 56: 46–51.

78. Weir, J.P., S.A. Evans, and M.L. Housh. 1996. The effect of extraneous movements on peak torque and constant joint angle torque-velocity curves. *Journal of Orthopaedic and Sports Physical Therapy* 23: 302–8.

79. Weir, J.P., T.J. Housh, S.A. Evans, and G.O. Johnson. 1993. The effect of dynamic constant external resistance training on the isokinetic torque-velocity curve. *International Journal of Sports Medicine* 14: 124–28.

80. Weir, J.P., T.J. Housh, G.O. Johnson, D.J. Housh, and K.T. Ebersole. 1999. Allometric scaling of isokinetic peak torque: The Nebraska wrestling study. *European Journal of Applied Physiology* 80: 240–48.

81. Weir, J.P., L.L. Wagner, T.J. Housh, and G.O. Johnson. 1992. Horizontal abduction and adduction strength at the shoulder of high school wrestlers across age. *Journal of Orthopaedic and Sports Physical Therapy* 15: 183–86.

82. Weltman, A., C. Janney, C.B. Rians, K. Strand, B. Berg, S. Tippett, J. Wise, B.R. Cahill, and F.I. Katch. 1986. The effects of hydraulic resistance training in prepubertal males. *Medicine and Science in Sports and Exercise* 18: 629–38.

83. Weltman, A., S. Tippett, C. Janney, K. Strand, C. Rians, B.R. Cahill, and F.I. Katch. 1988. Measurement of isokinetic strength in prepubertal males. *Journal of Orthopaedic and Sports Physical Therapy* 9: 345–51.

# Chapter 16
# Aging and Isokinetic Strength

James W. Bellew and Terry R. Malone

Isokinetic testing of muscular strength can provide valuable information about the functional ability or capacity of an individual. The aging individual warrants special attention when assessing muscular strength because of the physiological course of aging. The natural process of aging is accompanied by numerous nonpathological alterations in the muscular system. A general awareness of these physiological changes is prerequisite to working with older people when strength, performance, and conditioning are of specific concern.

The importance of understanding the special considerations of aged individuals with regard to strength is evidenced by the continuous increase in the portion of the population termed "elderly". The twentieth century has been witness to a tremendous demographic development in the United States—the rise in the number of older people in our society. In 1900, only 4% of the population was 65 years of age or older, but by 1986 the Census Bureau reported that the percentage had increased to 12.1% (48). It is projected that by the year 2040, 22% of the population will be 65 or older (42). Additionally, those over the age of 85 years, often called "oldest old," will become the most rapidly growing segment of our society. As the size of an integral component of the population steadily increases, the impending need for more knowledge and better understanding of muscle function in advanced age becomes evident.

The intent of this chapter is to present information regarding the physiological effects of aging on skeletal muscle and the implications specific to isokinetics. Previous investigative findings are presented that address age, skeletal muscle, and isokinetics. Upon conclusion, the reader will have a better understanding of the past and present research in the area of aging and skeletal muscle function as well as the use of isokinetics in the older population.

# Physiological Changes of Aging Skeletal Muscle

The natural physiological process of aging systemically affects all organ systems of the human body (21). The muscular system is no exception, which is of great interest when one considers that skeletal muscle comprises one of the largest organ systems, accounting for approximately 40% of total body weight (21). Investigative interest in the effects of aging on this organ system is diverse.

Research of age-related changes in skeletal muscle strength can be traced to 1836 when Quetelet's seminal work revealed a linear relationship between age and strength. As quoted by Hopp, Quetelet observed that strength declines proportionately as age increases past 25 years (19). The influence of aging on the muscular system has been studied and reported on by many, with varying results (7, 8, 13, 15, 19, 26, 27, 30, 32–34, 50). The changes observed with aging have generally been accepted as a natural part of the aging process and not of a more pathological condition (11, 26, 50), despite being characterized as deleterious.

Investigation into the physiological effects of aging on skeletal muscle has been performed on the microscopic, macroscopic, and functional levels. Numerous investigations have yielded findings at the fiber level, specifically regarding the effects of age on fiber number, ratio, and size (13, 19, 23–26). Much of the original investigative information was attained from the use of rodent and human cadaver muscle (30), because of the technical constraints unique to the study of fiber type distribution in humans. The difficulty of attaining data on age-related fiber changes lies in the procurement of living tissue samples and the statistical errors found in inferences drawn from data taken from very small muscle samples obtained via biopsy.

Driven by the desire to understand the rather ubiquitous declines of physical performance in older individuals, researchers began to investigate the relationship between physiological events and their observations. This led to the identification of certain selective changes in the constituent components of muscle tissue unique to aged samples. With human subjects, the vastus lateralis (VL) became the muscle of preference for biopsy study. This was in direct response to the findings of Serratrice, Raux, and Aquaron (41), who reported that the quadriceps exhibit a decrease in size and strength at an early age. The selection of the quadriceps muscle group for age-related changes has also been supported by Lexell, Taylor, and Sjöström (29), who identified age-induced atrophy in the VL that begins at approximately 25 years of age. The VL was a preferred muscle for studying fiber changes as this muscle has been shown to have a type II/I fiber ratio of approximately 1:1 in younger samples; therefore any effects of age on fiber ratio could be easily compared to older samples.

A vast amount of information exists in the literature on age-induced muscle changes at the microscopic level. In particular, histological and biochemical examinations have revealed significant findings of age-related changes in muscle morphology. Atrophy and absolute loss of fast twitch (type II) fibers have been described. Specifically, aging seemed to impose a preferential loss of type II fibers (13, 19, 23–26). Larsson and colleagues (23–26) reported much of the early information on this still unsettled issue of type II fiber loss as a result of age. They used tissue samples from rats, human cadavers, and living human subjects of various age groups in multiple, cross-sectional investigations. In one investigation, Larsson studied biopsy samples from living vastus lateralis muscles in 55 subjects aged 22 to 65 years. Histochemical and biochemical evaluations revealed a linear decrease in the proportion of type II fiber with increasing age equating to a 14% decline from the third to seventh decade (26).

In a similar study, Larsson and Karlsson (25) biopsied the VL muscles of 50 men, 22 to 65 years of age. A decrease in the proportion of FT fiber was noted with increasing age in the 60- to 65-year-old group. The ratio of FT to ST declined to .99 from 1.3 between the 60- to 69-year-olds and the 20- to 29-year-olds, indicating a greater rate of loss in FT muscle fiber. Lexell, Downham, and Sjöström (30) confirmed the findings of decreased proportions of FT fiber when subjects from three age groups, taken from a population 15 to 83 years of age, revealed significantly less size and total fiber number in the oldest group when compared to a middle (mean 52 years) and young (mean 24 years) group. They asserted that until the age of fifty, fiber loss is minimal, but the ratio of loss steadily increases until nearly 50% has been lost by the age of 80. Further investigation by Lexell, Taylor, and Sjöström (29) showed an average decrease in total fiber number of 39% from 20 to 80 years.

Larsson, Grimby, and Karlsson (24) identified further age-related declines in type II fiber percentages in older subjects. They evaluated biopsy samples and reported that the fiber type distribution reflected a lower percentage of type II fibers (42% decline) with a corresponding increase in type I fibers (23% increase) with increasing age. In a follow-up to his earlier investigative findings, Larsson (23) reviewed the data from his prior studies. His primary findings reflected an alteration in fiber type ratio that was characterized by a decline in the percentage of type II fibers from approximately 60% to 45% between the third and seventh decade of life.

Decreases in type II fiber size and cross-sectional area have likewise been observed by many, and results have shown that aging is correlated with a preferential atrophy of type II fibers (29, 47). Lexell, Taylor, and Sjöström (29), reported that age-related fiber atrophy begins as early as 25 years of age and that by age 50 nearly 10% of the muscle cross-sectional area is lost. Thereafter, the rate of atrophy increases until almost 50% of the area is lost by the age of 80. Most notably, no significance was found to exist between type I fiber size and age, whereas a highly significant correlation was found between type II fiber size decrease and increasing age.

Additional investigations have observed a preferential atrophy of type II fibers. Larsson's (26) study of subjects aged 22 to 65 revealed a decline in the average cross-sectional area of type II muscle fibers with increased age while no such relationship was identified among type I fibers. Larsson also reported a resultant decrease in type II/I fiber area ratio from 1.24, in the 22- to 29-year-old group, to .96, in the 60- to 65-year-old group.

Larsson and Karlsson (25) submitted further evidence of type II atrophy in subjects aged 22 to 65 years. Study results revealed a reduction in type II fiber area while no such reduction was noted in type I area. The fiber area ratio of II/I decreased from 61% to 44% between the group aged 22 to 29 and the group aged 60 to 65. Several additional investigations have confirmed the observation of an age-attenuated atrophy in type II fibers and contend that there is a strong correlation with the decline in skeletal muscle mass and increasing age. Moreover, this reduction is asserted to be chiefly due to a selective atrophy of type II fiber (15, 30).

In a histochemical and biochemical analysis of VL biopsies, Larsson, Sjödin, and Karlsson (27) assessed males up to 65 years of age. They found a linear relationship between increasing age and the decreasing proportion of FT muscle fiber. In the study, they demonstrated that the ST fiber distribution in the 20- to 29-year-old subjects comprised 41% of the total area whereas a 55% distribution was noted in the 60- to 65-year-old subjects. A significant correlation was observed between increasing age and reduced FT fiber size; however, no such relationship existed for ST fibers.

Specific distribution of fiber changes has been reported also. Two separate investigations have revealed progressive FT fiber changes particular to the proximal muscles of the lower extremity in advanced age. Grimby and co-workers (15) biopsied biceps brachii and VL muscles in subjects 78 to 81 years of age and reported that upper extremity skeletal muscle does not display the same age-related changes seen in samples taken from the lower extremity. Marked decreases in total fiber area were noted in FT fiber of the VL musculature, whereas no significant change was noted in the upper extremity musculature. These findings are in agreement with Tomonaga (47), who reported greater atrophy of FT fiber in the proximal muscles of the lower extremity in subjects 60 to 90+ years of age when compared to upper extremity samples.

# General Performance Changes in Aging Muscle

As observations of age-related changes in muscle morphology mounted, research emphasis emerged related to assessment of the functional implications of these changes. Decreases of 10% per year after the age of 60 in endurance, velocity, and maximal voluntary contraction (MVC) of the quadriceps have been reported (36). In reports on age and skeletal muscle function, Graves, Pollock, and Carroll (14) and Birren, Woods, and Williams (6) contend that motor performances of aging skeletal muscle decreased as well as strength and gross muscle mass. Aging skeletal muscle displayed significantly delayed reaction times and prolonged speed of movement during testing of motor performance (6, 14).

More functional assessments of muscle performance in various age groups have been completed. Israel (21) reported that the linear decrease in strength observed with increasing age is different in males and females. According to Israel, the baseline level of strength at age 30 is considerably lower for females.

Therefore, the decline of strength over the ensuing years is less precipitous in females than in males. Brooks and Faulkner (10) presented a review of the functional performance changes of skeletal muscle in advanced age and reported typical decreases of 35% in maximum force, 30% in maximum power, and 20% in normalized force and power.

In his 1978 classic monograph on morphology and function of aging skeletal muscle, Larsson (26) aimed to identify correlations between observed changes in muscle function and muscle morphology. Muscle samples were drawn from the VL of males up to 65 years of age. Muscle performance was assessed with isometric and isokinetic (concentric) actions. A 14% decline in FT fiber distribution was identified between the 20- to 29-year-old subjects and the 60- to 65-year-old subjects whereas no such decline was noted in ST fiber distribution. Dynamic muscle testing also displayed a similar age-related decrease in maximum knee extension velocity. The deficits observed by Larsson were significant and yet each was identified prior to any overt changes in anthropometric measures as traditionally measured. These results suggest that traditional measures of atrophy may be insensitive to the underlying process of atrophy, yet the deficits were detected with the use of isokinetics.

In further study, Larsson, Grimby, and Karlsson (24) investigated relationships between changes in the VL and functional performances using isometric and isokinetic (concentric) actions. Histochemical alterations identified a decreased proportion and selective atrophy of FT fibers, yet no significant anthropometric changes were evident. Both the isometric and concentric strength values demonstrated declining values after the fifth decade. The authors concluded that the decrease in muscle performance in advanced age correlated significantly with the decrease in FT fiber area and size.

Endurance as a function of aging muscle has been significantly less investigated than maximal strength. The findings of early investigations conflicted, some studies suggesting that endurance was not correlated with increasing age yet other investigations suggesting that age was indeed related to declining endurance (4, 28, 37). Nakao, Inoue, and Murakami (34) evaluated knee extensor endurance in 7,412 males and females aged 6 to 79 years as the ability to maintain a half-squat position. Peak values were attained at 13 years of age in males and 12 years of age in females. Thereafter, precipitous decreases in extensor muscle endurance ensued until, by the age of 70 to 79, only 34% of peak knee extensor endurance was achievable.

Further studies of endurance in older subjects have provided information regarding the correlation between age and muscle endurance. Skeletal muscle endurance in the upper and lower extremities was measured by Bemben and coworkers (5) in males 20 to 74 years of age. Maximal endurance of isometric efforts was assessed and results showed that the largest decreases in absolute endurance were noted in muscles of the lower extremity. When normalized to the entire endurance task, no age group differences were observed for endurance. The authors concluded that increasing age was negatively correlated with absolute endurance but relative measures were sustained across all age groups, yielding no differences between age groups.

The findings of Lindstrom and coworkers (31) supported those of Bemben and associates (5) when younger and older males and females with mean ages of 28 and 73 years were assessed for endurance during 100 repetitive maximal knee extension movements at 90°/s. Data showed that endurance in older men and women was significantly less than in the younger subjects; however, no difference was noted in relative force reduction and fatigue rate between older and younger subjects. The authors concluded that the endurance of the older subjects was similar in properties to that of the younger subjects.

# Isokinetic Muscle Performance with Age: "Concentric" and "Isometric"

Following identification of age-related morphological changes and more generalized decreases in the functional performance of human skeletal muscle, several investigators sought more standardized assessment of muscle performance. Isokinetic dynamometry has been the most common method of measuring skeletal muscle performance in age-related studies of skeletal muscle. Investigators have traditionally used isokinetic dynamometers for measuring and recording peak torque (PT). However, measurements of maximal voluntary isometric action have also been used for assessing skeletal muscle strength.

Data have revealed that all muscular actions are affected by aging; however, the magnitude of the age-related effects are not equivalent for all types of muscle action. To date, the majority of isokinetic investigations assessing the relationship between age and strength have studied concentric or isometric muscle actions. Eccentric muscle performance has been studied to a much lesser extent and not until recently have the more significant findings been reported.

Murray and coworkers (32, 33) investigated PT and maximal voluntary contraction (MVC) of concentric isokinetic and isometric muscle actions. The angular velocities selected were 36 and 0°/s. Strength was recorded from knee extensors and flexors in 72 women and 72 men divided into three age groups: 20 to 35, 50 to 65, and 70 to 86 for the females and 20 to 35, 42 to 61, and 70 to 86 for the males. For the males, the average of the PT measures was greatest in the youngest group and lowest in the eldest group for each of the two muscle action types. The middle age group of males displayed isometric MVC efforts at levels of 75 to 80% of the youngest group, and the middle group's concentric isokinetic effort was 65 to 75% that of the youngest group. When the efforts of the eldest male group were compared to the youngest male group, isometric MVC was 55 to 65% that of the youngest group and concentric isokinetic efforts were 45 to 64% those of the youngest group. Murray and coworkers (33) also revealed that average isometric strength of the knee extensors in the male middle group was significantly greater than that of the oldest male group, whereas no significant difference was observed between the oldest and middle groups with regard to isokinetic concentric muscle performance. Murray and coworkers (32) revealed similar results in females. The observed decreases in strength correlated significantly with increasing age. Again, as in the males, the youngest females' performance was greatest for each muscle action type. When comparisons were made among the age groups, the middle female group displayed values 77 to 95% of the youngest group while the eldest female group performed at 56 to 78% of the level of the young. Additionally, the oldest females showed only 69 to 88% of the performance level measured in the middle group. Murray and coworkers (32) compared the gender performances across all age groups and asserted that knee strength of the females was generally 74% that of the males.

In a somewhat similar comparison to those completed by Murray and associates (32, 33), Young, Stokes, and Crowe (52, 53) assessed isometric strength of the quadriceps in males and females of varying ages. They studied 25 females, 71 to 81 years of age, and 25 females, 20 to 29 years of age, for MVC of the knee extensors (52). Peak MVC of the older female subjects was 35% less than for the comparative group of younger females. Likewise, in the male test groups, 12 younger subjects (21–28 years of age) were compared to 12 older subjects (70–79 years of age) for MVC of the quadriceps (53). Data revealed that the average MVC in the older group was 39% less than the young male group. The percentage decrease in MVC from younger to older was similar for both males and females; however, the older male subjects performed at a level 43% better than the older female group for the same activity (53).

Johnson (22) studied concentric isokinetic and isometric quadriceps efforts in 30 female subjects in two age groups, 20 to 29 and 50 to 80 years of age. When intergroup performances were compared, isokinetic concentric efforts were 41% lower in the older group, and similarly, the isometric values generated by the older subjects were lower by 40% than for the younger subjects. Johnson's (22) findings were in agreement with those of Young, Stokes, and Crowe (52). In another comparison, Clarkson, Kroll, and Melchionda (12) studied quadriceps strength in two age groups with mean ages of 64.5 and 23.2 years. They found a significant correlation between increasing age and MVC, as a 47% decrease in strength was recorded in the older group.

Whipple, Wolfson, and Amerman (51) investigated intraage class PT during concentric quadriceps efforts in two groups of subjects with mean ages of 82.2 and 84.6 years. In the study, they compared "fallers" (a faller was defined as a person having one or more falls per year) with controls who did not fall. Angular velocities of 60 and 120°/s were selected, and the strength of the fallers was uniformly observed to be less than that of the controls. At 60°/s, the fallers performed at 57% of the level of controls, and at 120°/s the PT of fallers was 61% that of the controls.

Harries and Bassey (16) provided further data when they assessed quadriceps strength of women in their third and seventh decades. An average 35% decrease over all velocities was noted in the older women. A study by Stanley and Taylor (44) assessed concentric knee extensor strength in women in their third, fourth, sixth, and seventh decades with angular velocities ranging from 60 to 400°/s. Their findings supported Harries and Bassey (16), indicating a definitive decline in isokinetic strength with increasing age. Stalberg and co-workers (43) also recorded concentric and isometric knee extensor strength using male and female subjects, 20 to 70 years of age. Their findings revealed a decrease in isometric strength of 35% for older males and 29% for older females. Concentric strength was observed to decline by 30% and 39% for older males and females, respectively.

Additional information regarding age-related changes in muscle was provided from a study which assessed 111 men and women, 20 to 100 years of age, for the effects of aging on isometric strength of muscles of the ankle (50). Decreases in MVC were initially observed to decline in the sixth decade for both genders. Specifically, strength of the dorsi- and plantarflexors in the male 80- to 100-year-old group decreased 44% and 45%, respectively, compared to the 20- to 32-year-old group, and the strength in the female 80- to 100-year-old group decreased 37% and 52%, respectively. The authors concluded that a decrease in muscle mass specific to the older subjects was entirely responsible for the decreased strength in the older subjects.

# Isokinetic Muscle Performance With Age: "Eccentric"

Eccentric muscle performance in advanced age has been relatively unstudied. This paucity of material is obvious when compared to the amount of literature available on concentric and isometric muscle effort. Vandervoort, Kramer, and Wharram (49) reported some of the original data on eccentric performance in aged populations. Twenty-six females aged 20 to 29 were compared to 26 females 66 to 89 years of age during concentric and eccentric efforts at 45 and 90°/s. At 45°/s, the older subjects' eccentric peak torque values were 71% those of the younger group. Likewise, the older subjects' eccentric peak torque at 90°/s was recorded at only 75% of the value recorded from the younger subjects. Concentric strength of the older group at 45°/s revealed a 46% decline compared to the younger group and at 90°/s a 44% decrease was observed in concentric strength of the aged. The researchers contend that eccentric muscle performance is less affected by increasing age than is concentric muscle performance, when comparisons of isokinetic torque production are used as the basis of comparison (49).

In a study comparing concentric and eccentric quadriceps strength in males and females 15 to 34 years of age, Highgenboten, Jackson, and Meske (17) revealed that concentric muscle performance has a more significant relationship with age than does eccentric muscle performance. This was discovered when a group of young subjects, ages 15 to 24, performed significantly better during concentric activity than did the older subjects, 25 to 34 years of age. However, no significance was observed between the strength of younger subjects and older subjects during eccentric activity. Between gender differences were also observed. In general, female performances during eccentric quadriceps activity were 18% less than male performances, and concentric efforts in the females were 23% less than in the males. Older females were 12% weaker than the older males during eccentric quadriceps efforts. Likewise, the younger females displayed a decrease of 23% during eccentric performances as compared to the younger male group.

More recent investigations of the relationship between eccentric muscle performance and aging have yielded interesting data. In a study by Poulin and coworkers (40), eccentric strength appeared to be less affected by age than concentric strength. Males 23 to 32 years of age were compared to males 60 to 75 years of age. The data revealed a 31% decline in elbow and 32% decline in knee concentric strength in the older males. For eccentric elbow strength, the older males were 21% weaker than the younger males. In contrast, knee eccentric strength did not differ from the values recorded in the younger males.

Hortobagyi and coworkers (20) assessed males and females ranging from 18 to 80 years for eccentric, concentric, and isometric strength of the knee extensors. Their results revealed a significant 30 N/decade decline in concentric and isometric strength, yet only a 9 N/decade decline in eccentric strength. Two investigations by Porter and associates (38, 39) support the findings of Hortobagyi and coworkers (20). An earlier study of younger and older males and females demonstrated a general decrease in all quadriceps strength parameters, but a less significant effect was noted with eccentric strength. Their later study revealed that the eccentric strength of the ankle plantar- and dorsiflexors is also maintained as older females demonstrated eccentric strength values 97% and 100% of the younger females, whereas concentric measures of the older females were 74% and 89% those of the younger females. The findings of these authors suggest there is a relative maintenance or preservation of eccentric strength during aging that is not present for concentric and isometric strength.

## Isokinetic Assessment of the Older Person

The ability of isokinetic testing to specifically assess individual muscle action types supports its use among older subjects. Comparisons between individual action types may provide useful information in the examination of the functional status of the aging muscular system. Isokinetic assessment techniques possess the specificity required to ascertain muscular performance characteristics under concentric, isometric, and eccentric conditions that may be more latent when individual action types are not assessed.

Numerous investigations have suggested that the relationship between aging and skeletal muscle performance is linear, that is, skeletal muscle performance declines as age increases. These same studies also suggest that age is associated with a muscle action specificity such that the linear decline in strength is not equivalent for each action type, but rather, eccentric muscle performance is less affected by aging than are concentric and isometric muscle performances. However, data regarding eccentric strength in the aging is clearly lacking in the literature, and only recently have investigators begun to ascertain the relationship between aging and eccentric muscle function under any conditions whether functional or isokinetic. The ability to test individual muscle action types makes isokinetics useful in the older population.

Use of isokinetics in the older population has revealed certain assessment characteristics. From the limited amount of eccentric isokinetic data available from investigators such as Hortobagyi and coworkers (20), Poulin and coworkers (40), and Vandervoort, Kramer, and Wharram (49), the data do reveal that the underlying physiological response of aging muscle does conform to the torque-velocity relationship (9). This relationship implies that the force (torque) developed in a shortening (concentric) action is less than the maximal isometric force and that the force developed during a lengthening (eccentric) activation is greater than the maximal isometric force by 50 to 100% (9). Therefore, it appears that the effects of aging do not compromise the basic physiological performance characteristics of aging muscle specific to the torque-velocity relationship when assessed by isokinetics.

Investigations into aging and eccentric muscle performance have suggested that not only does older muscle maintain normal physiological performance regarding the torque-velocity curve but that eccentric performance is sustained despite declining concentric and isometric strength (20, 40, 49). These investigations have suggested that eccentric strength is preserved or less affected by advancing age. The functional implications of this eccentric preservation warrant further assessment of age-related muscle action-specific changes in muscle performance in the older individual. This, therefore, should be one role of isokinetic investigation.

The necessity for muscle action-specific testing in older individuals is further supported by evidence of preferential fiber type selectivity that is likewise action dependent. Nardone, Romano, and Schieppati (35) and Albert (1) have asserted that eccentric activation of skeletal muscle imposes a preferential recruitment of type II fibers. Nardone, Romano, and Schieppati provided data that revealed that fast twitch, type II skeletal muscle fibers are selectively recruited during voluntary tasks in which controlled lengthening of the active muscle is completed. Furthermore, they suggested that these fibers might be relatively inactive during shortening actions as well as sustained activity and are activated only under lengthening conditions. These results were presented without plausible explanation for the possible neural pathways responsible for their observed phenomenon.

The aforementioned necessity for muscle action–specific testing in older individuals centers on the assertions of Nardone, Romano, and Schieppati (35) and Albert (1) that type II fibers are preferentially recruited with eccentric actions. As noted, morphological studies of aging muscle have detailed declines in type II fiber number, size, and area. Therefore, a collective evaluation of the literature presents a conundrum. If aging is associated with an attenuation of type II fibers, and type II fibers are selectively recruited with eccentric actions, then older individuals would appear at risk for declining eccentric performance secondary to loss of type II fibers. However, more recent investigations of eccentric performance of skeletal muscle in older individuals have shown maintenance of eccentric strength in older subjects. These conflicting observations require some unifying answer to explain the apparent contradictions, which should not be left to mere conjecture. Rather, additional evidence needs to be provided from scientific investigation.

# Functional Indications for Use of Isokinetics in Older Individuals

The significance of ascertaining the degree of change in muscle action specificity of older individuals is evidenced by the functional use of eccentric actions, the current data on falls among older individuals, and the implications that preserved eccentric performance may have on older individuals. Eccentric muscle performance is often considered to serve a shock-absorbing function, that is, forces are dissipated rather than generated, as in concentric muscle effort (45). An example of eccentric muscle performance is a "step-down" maneuver, when an individual descends a step and transfers load to the lower extremity on the step below. The quadriceps muscle group must absorb the forces and decelerate the increasing load as the weight-bearing limb stabilizes under the load. Insufficient absorption, or dissipation, of this load may expose to tremendous forces the noncontractile elements within the musculoskeletal system, in particular the weight-bearing bones. Overloading the bones' capacity to accept force may lead to fracture.

From this example, one might postulate that a potentiating cause for fracture is an insufficient dissipation of forces by eccentric muscle effort. Fractures in the older population are only one of many concerns, since skeletal trauma, primarily of the hip, pelvis, and spine, is one of the most common causes of bed rest in this group (7). The prevalence of femur fractures in the elderly is high and often correlated with falling (46). Safety during ambulation is a matter of great concern in the elderly population, and reports by the National Safety Council state that falls are one of the leading causes of accidental death among individuals aged 65 and over (18). Researchers have reported that the decreases observed in skeletal muscle in advanced age lead to a fourfold increase for the chances of falling (36). Some authors contend that one-third to one-half of the population age 65 years and over will suffer a fall at some point during the year (10, 46). Considering that eccentric muscle activation is largely used during gait for stability and force dissipation, further functional importance of eccentric muscle activation is noted. Preliminary data support a differential response of genders in eccentric function at higher velocities, possibly placing females at greater risk as they age (3).

Loss of fast twitch fibers in older subjects has been correlated to femur fractures in this population. Aniansson and coworkers (2) biopsied the quadriceps of 52 subjects who had suffered recent femur fractures. The test group was compared to an age-matched control group. Following analysis, the test subjects demonstrated significantly greater evidence of FT fiber atrophy than did the age-matched group. A correlation may be evident between the observation of Aniansson and coworkers and the prevalence of femur fractures in the elderly. This correlation may provide insight into the importance of eccentric muscle performance in the elderly and thus the necessity for isokinetic testing in the older population. These factors indicate that training programs for lower extremity conditions of elderly individuals should include activities to enhance speed of activation and eccentric function. Fortuitously, the existing data do support higher velocities and maximal efforts in the application of isokinetic exercise. Ideally, the training sequence can be designed to fit the needs of the individual cognizant of his or her special needs.

Therefore, the ability of isokinetics to assess individual muscle action types supports its use in the older population. The necessity for ascertaining the functional performance capacity of these individual muscle action types, and specifically eccentric muscle actions, is evidenced by the preponderance of data detailing the relationship between age-related type II fiber loss, preferential recruitment of type II fibers with eccentric activation, and maintenance of eccentric strength with aging.

## Summary

Although the available literature regarding the age-related changes of skeletal muscle is plentiful, it does contain some potentially conflicting and presently unexplained data. Much of the conflicting information is centered in three distinct, yet inherently related areas: (1) type II fibers are lost with advancing age at a rate disproportionate to type I fibers, (2) type II fibers are selectively recruited during eccentric activation, and (3) eccentric strength is maintained or is less affected by age than concentric or isometric strength in older individuals. More recent investigative findings in these three areas are largely responsible for the conflicting information. This may suggest that the investigative interest in this area of age-related changes in skeletal muscle is progressive, providing important yet not fully understood information. Much more investigative work is necessary if accurate conclusions are to be available. The impetus is obvious when considering the growing population of older individuals. Only direct investigative efforts will yield the required knowledge.

## References

1. Albert M. 1991. Eccentrics: Clinical program design and DOMS. In *Eccentric muscle training in sports and orthopaedics*, 39. New York: Churchhill Livingstone.

2. Aniansson A, Zetterberg L, Hedberg M et al. 1984. Impaired muscle function with aging: A background factor in the incidence of fractures of the proximal end of the femur. *Clin Orthop* 191: 192–210.

3. Bellew JW, Malone TR, Nitz AJ, Hart AL. 1998. Gender specificity in the age-related decline of strength: Concentric versus eccentric. *Isokin Exerc Sci* 7: 1–9.

4. Bemben MG. 1998. Age-related alterations in muscular endurance. *Sports Med* 25(4): 259–69.

5. Bemben MG, Boileau RA, Misner JE, Bemben DA, Massey BH. 1996. Isometric intermittent endurance of four muscle groups in men aged 20–74 years. *Med Sci Sports Exerc* 28(1): 145–54.

6. Birren JE, Woods AM, Williams MV. 1979. Speed of behavior as an indicator of age changes and the integrity of the nervous system. In *Brain function in old age*, ed. Hoffmeister F, Miller C. New York: Springer-Verlag.

7. Booth FW, Weeden SH. 1993. Structural aspects of aging human skeletal muscle. In *Musculoskeletal soft-tissue aging: Impact on mobility*, ed. Buckwalter JA, Goldberg VM, Woo S L-Y. Rosemont, IL: American Academy of Orthopedic Surgeons.

8. Bosco C, Komi PV. 1980. Influence of aging on the mechanical behavior of the leg extensor muscles. *Eur J Appl Physiol* 45: 209–19.

9. Brooks GA, Fahey TD, White TP. 1996. Skeletal muscle structure and contractile properties. In *Exercise physiology*. 2d ed. Mountain View, CA: Mayfield.

10. Brooks SV, Faulkner JA. 1994. Skeletal muscle weakness in old age: Underlying mechanisms. *Med Sci Sports Exerc* 26: 432–39.

11. Brown WF. 1972. A method for estimating the number of motor units in thenar muscles and the changes in motor unit count with aging. *J Neurol, Neurosurg, and Psychiatry* 35: 845–52.

12. Clarkson PM, Kroll W, Melchionda AM. 1981. Age, isometric strength, rate of tension development, and fiber composition. *J Geront* 36: 648–53.

13. Edström L, Larsson L. 1987. Effects of age on contractile and enzyme histochemical properties of fast and slow twitch single motor units in the rat. *J Physiol (Lond)* 392: 129–45.

14. Graves JE, Pollock ML, Carroll JF. 1994. Exercise, age, and skeletal muscle function. *Southern Med J* 87(Suppl): 18–22.

15. Grimby G, Danneskiold-Samsoe B, Hvid K, Saltin B. 1982. Morphology and enzymatic capacity in arm and leg muscles in 78–81 year old men and women. *Acta Physiol Scand* 115: 125–34.

16. Harries UJ, Bassey EJ. 1990. Torque-velocity relationships for the knee extensors in women in their 3rd and 7th decades. *Eur J Appl Physiol* 60: 187–190.

17. Highgenboten CL, Jackson AW, Meske NB. 1988. Concentric and eccentric torque comparisons for knee extension and flexion in young adult males and females using the Kinetic Communicator. *Am J Sport Med*: 16: 234–37.

18. Hindmarsh JJ, Estes EH. 1989. Falls in older persons: Causes and intervention. *Arch Intern Med* 149: 2217.

19. Hopp JF. 1993. Effects of age and resistance training on skeletal muscle. *Phys Ther* 73: 361–73.

20. Hortobagyi T, Donghai Z, Weidner M, Lambert NJ, Westbrook S, Houmard JA. 1995. The influence of aging on muscle strength and muscle fiber characteristics with special reference to eccentric strength. *J Geront: Med Sci* 50A(6): B399–406.

21. Israel S. 1992. Age-related changes in strength and special groups. In *Strength and power in sport*, ed. Komi PV, 319–28. Oxford, UK: Blackwell Scientific.

22. Johnson T. 1982. Age-related differences in isometric and dynamic strength and endurance. *Phys Ther* 62: 985–89.

23. Larsson L. 1983. Histochemical characteristics of human skeletal muscle during aging. *Acta Physiol Scand* 117: 469–71.

24. Larsson L, Grimby G, Karlsson J. 1979. Muscle strength and speed and movement in relation to age and muscle morphology. *J Applied Physiol* 46: 451–56.

25. Larsson L, Karlsson J. 1978. Isometric and dynamic endurance as a function of age and skeletal muscle characteristics. *Acta Physiol Scand* 104: 129–36.

26. Larsson L. 1978. Morphological and functional characteristics of the aging skeletal muscle in man. *Acta Physiol Scand* 457(Suppl): 1–36.

27. Larsson L, Sjödin B, Karlsson J. 1978. Histochemical and biochemical changes in human skeletal muscle with age in sedentary males age 22 to 65 years. *Acta Physiol Scand* 103: 31–39.

28. Lennmarken C, Bergman T, Larsson J, Larsson LE. 1985. Skeletal muscle function in man: Force, relaxation rate, endurance, and contraction time dependence on sex and age. *Clin Physiol* 5: 243–55.

29. Lexell J, Taylor CC, Sjöström M. 1988. Total number, size, and proportion of different fiber types studied in whole vastus lateralis muscle from 15- to 83-year-old men. *J Neurol Sci* 84: 275–94.

30. Lexell J, Downham D, Sjöström M. 1986. Distribution of different fiber types in human skeletal muscles. *J Neurol Sci* 72: 211–22.

31. Lindstrom B, Downham D, Gerdle B, Lexell J. 1997. Skeletal muscle fatigue and endurance in young and old men and women. *J Geront: Med Sci* 52(1): B59–66.

32. Murray PM, Duthie EH, Gambert SR, Sepic SB, Mollinger LA. 1985. Age-related differences in knee muscle strength in normal women. *J Geront* 40: 275–80.

33. Murray PM, Gardner GM, Mollinger LA, Sepic SB. 1980. Strength of isometric and isokinetic contractions: Knee muscles of men aged 20 to 86. *Phys Ther* 60: 412–19.

34. Nakao M, Inoue Y, Murakami H. 1989. Aging process of leg muscle endurance in males and females. *Eur J Appl Physiol* 59: 209–14.

35. Nardone A, Romano C, Schieppati M. 1989. Selective recruitment of high-threshold human motor units during voluntary isotonic lengthening of active muscles. *J Physiol* 409: 451–71.

36. Pendergast DR, Fisher NM, Calkins E. 1993. Cardiovascular, neuromuscular, and metabolic alterations with age leading to frailty. *J Geront* 48: 61–67.

37. Petrofsky JS, Lind AR. 1975. Aging, isometric strength and endurance, and cardiovascular responses to static effort. *J Appl Physiol* 38: 91–95.

38. Porter MM, Myint A, Kramer JF, Vandervoort AA. 1995. Concentric and eccentric knee extension strength in older and younger men and women. *Can J Appl Physiol* 20(4): 429–39.

39. Porter MM, Vandervoort AA, Kramer JF. 1997. Eccentric peak torque of the plantar and dorsiflexors is maintained in older women. *J Geront: Med Sci* 52 (2): B125–31.

40. Poulin MJ, Vandervoort AA, Paterson DH, Kramer JF, Cunningham DA. 1992. Eccentric and concentric torques of knee and elbow extension in young and older men. *Can J Sport Sci* 17(1): 3–7.

41. Serratrice G, Raux H, Aquaron R. 1968. Proximal muscular weakness in elderly subjects. *J Neurol Sci* 7: 275–99.

42. Social Security Administration. 1988. *Social Security area population projections* (actuarial study No. 102, SSA Publ. No. 11-11549). Baltimore: Social Security Administration.

43. Stalberg E, Borges O, Ericsson M, Essen-Gustavsson B, Fawcett PRW, Nordesjo LO, Nordgren B, Uhlin R. 1989. Quadriceps femoris muscle in 20- to 70-year-old subjects: Relationship between knee extension torque, electrophysiological parameters, and muscle fiber characteristics. *Muscle & Nerve* 12: 382–89.

44. Stanley SN, Taylor NAS.1993. Isokinematic muscle mechanics in four groups of women of increasing age. *Eur J Appl Physiol* 66: 178–84.

45. Stauber WT. 1989. Eccentric action of muscles: Physiology, injury, and adaptation. *Exerc Sport Sci Rev* 17: 157–85.

46. Tineti ME. 1986. Performance-oriented assessment of mobility problems in elderly patients. *J Am Geriatr Soc* 34: 119–26.

47. Tomonaga M. 1977. Histochemical and ultrastructural changes in human skeletal muscle. *J Am Geriatr Soc* 25: 125–31.

48. U. S. Bureau of the Census. 1987. Estimates of the population of the United States by age, sex, and race 1980 to 1986. Current populations report (series P-25, No. 1000). Washington, DC: U.S. Bureau of the Census.

49. Vandervoort AA, Kramer JF, Wharram ER. 1990. Eccentric knee strength of elderly females. *J Geront* 45: 125–28.

50. Vandervoort AA, McComas AJ. 1986. Contractile changes in opposing muscles of the human ankle joint with aging. *J Appl Physiol* 61: 361–67.

51. Whipple RH, Wolfson LI, Amerman PM. 1987. The relationship of knee and ankle weakness to falls in nursing home residents: An isokinetic study. *J Am Geriatr Soc* 35: 13–20.

52. Young A, Stokes M, Crowe M. 1984. The size and strength of the quadriceps muscle of old and young women. *Eur J Clin Invest* 14: 282–87.

53. Young A, Stokes M, Crowe M. 1985. The size of the quadriceps muscles of old and young men. *Clin Physiol* 5: 145–54.

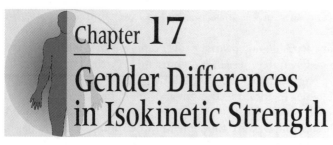

## Chapter 17
# Gender Differences in Isokinetic Strength

Joan M. Eckerson

Gender-related differences in muscle strength have been reported to vary from 40 to 80% depending upon the measurement protocol used, subjects studied, and body segment tested (25). Although force production has been shown to be highly related to muscle cross-sectional area (CSA) in both sexes, several studies (25, 26, 41) have indicated that females continue to exhibit lower force than males even when expressed per unit CSA. The greater force output demonstrated by males has been attributed to several factors including differences in the musculoskeletal system, morphology and fiber distribution, electromechanical responses and neural activation, hormone concentrations, and physical activity patterns.

## Differences in Muscle Morphology, Fiber Distribution, and Quality of Strength

Komi and Karlsson (29) compared skeletal muscle characteristics, metabolic profiles, and physical performance using young (15–24 yr) male and female twins as subjects. Comparative data were obtained for muscle strength, mechanical power, maximal oxygen consumption, electrical activation, fiber composition of the vastus lateralis (VL), and skeletal muscle enzyme concentrations. Females exhibited a 100% longer rise time in isometric force, and in functional tests their performance was 61.1 to 84.6% that of males. Histological findings indicated that slow twitch (ST) fiber distribution was significantly higher in males (55.9 ± 11.9%) than in females (49.1 ± 7.7%), and males also demonstrated significantly higher concentrations of calcium-stimulated ATPase, creatine phosphokinase, phosphorylase, and lactate dehydrogenase. The differences in the enzyme concentrations explain, in part, differences observed in the force-time characteristics between males and females and may be due to hormonal influences or adaptations to different physical activity patterns. The authors suggested that the lower neuromotoric efficiency (represented by force-time relationships in combination with the qualitative and quantitative differences in muscle mass resulted in lower muscular power in females.

In a related study, Ryushi and coworkers (41) reported that maximal force per CSA is influenced by differences in training status as well as by gender. In their study, male strength athletes were significantly different from physically active males and females in absolute strength and size of muscle fibers and in maximal force per CSA of the quadriceps muscle. Force production per CSA was greatest in athletes, and was two times greater when compared to females, indicating that differences in force are due to factors other than muscle mass. There were no significant differences in the ST fiber distribution among the three groups, which is in contrast to the results of Komi and Karlsson (29) for untrained females. However, when examining fiber size, the male strength athletes demonstrated larger fast twitch b (FTb) fiber areas vs. ST fiber areas compared with physically active males and females, and females showed larger ST fiber areas vs. FT fiber areas when compared to both male groups. Differences in force-time curves indicated that the rate of maximal force development in females was lower than in both male groups, which suggests that females are not able to recruit their available motor unit (MU) pool. Because the rate of force production largely depends upon the rate of neural activation (29), it is likely that the slower rate of force production leads to lower force output during dynamic muscle actions in females. The authors suggested that neural activation is important in increasing strength per CSA and that the differences in fiber size and neural activation between genders may be due to lower levels of testosterone in females or differences in daily activity patterns.

Kanehisa, Ikegawa, and Fukunaga (26) also reported that untrained males exhibited significantly greater force per CSA for isokinetic knee extension (KE) and knee flexion (KF) measured at 1.05 rad/s compared to females. However, no significant differences existed between the sexes when strength was expressed per CSA for the elbow flexors and extensors at the same speed. This finding is interesting, given the fact that the difference in muscle CSA between the sexes is smaller in the thigh when compared to the upper arm. The authors suggested that the greater quadriceps (Q) angle in females might be responsible, in part, for the lower force production per CSA in the lower extremity. This may be particularly true for KE since a greater Q angle presents a biomechanical disadvantage when transferring force to the lower leg via the patella during KE. Based upon the findings of others (29, 41), Kanehisa, Ikegawa, and Fukunaga (26) also hypothesized that untrained females may lack the ability to recruit their entire MU pool in large muscle groups such as the quadriceps and hamstrings during maximal dynamic muscle actions for which contraction time is restricted, as in the isokinetic condition.

In contrast to Kanehisa, Ikegawa, and Fukunaga (26) and Ryushi and coworkers (41), Castro and associates (7) reported that muscle quality (peak torque (PT) per CSA) is equal between genders and that increases in strength per unit area, which occur with resistance training, are not gender dependent. In their study maximum isometric torque (TQ) per unit muscle and bone (M+B) cross-sectional area was measured in the upper arm and thigh of 26 trained (n = 13 males + 13 females) and 26 untrained (n = 13 males + 13 females) young adults (18–30 yr). Maximal isometric TQ of the elbow flexors and extensors (60° and 80°, respectively) and knee flexors and extensors (20° and 60°, respectively) was recorded by a Lido isokinetic dynamometer. The results revealed no significant differences in mean upper arm or thigh TQ per unit M+B CSA between trained or untrained males and females. However, mean TQ per CSA was significantly greater for trained subjects of both genders compared with untrained subjects for the arm and the thigh. Percentage comparisons of mean strength and CSA values showed that women had 75.5% of the thigh strength of men and 76.4% of the men's thigh CSA. Correspondingly, women had 57.1% of the men's arm strength and 60.2% of their arm CSA. Miller and coworkers (35) also reported that the CSA of the arm and thigh of females was 57.5% and 72.5%, respectively, that of the males. These results indicate that gender differences in absolute strength are primarily explained by differences in lean body mass (LBM) distribution. Castro and associates (7) suggested that the greater peak isometric TQ per M+B CSA of the trained subjects of both genders was most likely due to neuromuscular adaptations or a genetic predisposition.

## Differences in Electromechanical Activity

As indicated in the studies previously described, at least part of the gender differences in maximal strength may be attributed to differences in electromechanical activity. To gain a better understanding of the potential differences in electromechanical responses and rate of force development between the sexes, Bell and Jacobs (2) compared total reaction time, premotor time, electromechanical delay (EMD), and rate of force development during isometric maximal voluntary contractions (MVC) of the elbow flexors in 40 women and 46 men (19–46 yr). Subjects were divided into four groups based upon their MVC and were categorized as either weak or strong. Neither total reaction time nor premotor time was significantly different across groups; no significant differences were observed between groups in the times required to reach various percentages of their MVC force. However, the EMD for both male groups was significantly shorter than for the female groups. The researchers found weak, but significant, negative relationships between EMD and MVC and the rate of force development, which suggests that part of the differences in strength between men and women may be associated with differences in EMD response times. Komi and Karlsson (29) have suggested that the lower rate of force development in females compared to males may be a result of "structural differences between males and females in muscle elastic tissue". Therefore, Bell and Jacobs (2) speculated that series elastic components in the male muscle are more resistant to stretching compared to in the female muscle, which results in shorter EMD. The greater stiffness in male musculature may be attributed to higher levels of physical activity or daily activities that elicit a strength-training effect.

In a similar study, Ives, Kroll, and Bultman (24) examined gender-related differences in rapid movement kinematics and triphasic EMG patterns during elbow flexion (EF) in 10 males and 10 females (18–26 yr). Subjects were asked to move their forearms as fast as possible through 90° EF and stop as sharply as possible at a terminal end point. An electromagnet was set to 0, 40%, and 70% of each subject's maximal isometric TQ to provide resistance and initiate quick release movements. The results indicated that males were 30 to 40% faster in all movement times and accelerations when compared to females. Marked differences in qualitative and temporal EMG of the biceps and triceps indicated that the performance differences were due, in part, to neuromuscular coordination mechanics. Males showed a more rapid increase in neural activation, shorter EMG burst duration, and faster reciprocal activation of agonist and antagonist muscles. The faster kinematics in males suggests that they are better able to provide braking by the antagonist, whereas females are more neurally constrained with regard to rapid EMG activation of the triceps and thus have limited braking capabilities.

Gender differences in force production and fatigability during repeated maximal isokinetic muscle actions have also been investigated. Kanehisa and coworkers (25) assessed the force generation capacity during 50 maximal KE actions at 3.14 rad/s in untrained males (n = 27) and females (n = 36) (18–25 yr) and measured the CSA of the quadriceps. Measurements included the mean force (F) of all 50 and every 5 consecutive contractions and the percent decline (% D) in F. Females exhibited lower F than males even when F was expressed per unit CSA. The % D of F was also greater in females when the force output per unit muscle CSA during the first to fifth contraction were made, indicating that contractions were more fatigable in women. The differences observed between the sexes were attributed to differences in EMG activity, EMD, and rate of force development.

# Differences in Torque-Velocity Relationships

Gender differences in the isokinetic torque-velocity (TQ-V) relationship have been well studied (8, 14, 15, 39, 44). For concentric (CON) muscle actions, the TQ-V curves are similar between genders with both sexes demonstrating decreases in force with increasing velocity (8, 14, 17). However, the relationship between eccentric (ECC) TQ and angular velocity has not been well studied. In addition, there is conflicting data regarding the effects of gender and muscle groups on the relationship between CON and ECC TQ, as well as ECC-CON TQ velocity relationships. Griffin and coworkers (18) have attributed the discrepancies in the literature regarding ECC TQ-V relationships and ECC-CON TQ-V relationships to differences in dynamometers and methodology among studies such as use of gravity correction, separation of maximal ECC and CON efforts, amount of activation force employed and choice of angle velocities, and the criterion measure for TQ. Because average TQ represents the maximal voluntary effort throughout a range of movement (ROM) vs. a single point in the movement (i.e., PT), it has been suggested to be a better index of dynamic muscle performance (30). However, the criterion measure that best reflects muscle performance and functional capacity has not been well established (30).

Griffin and coworkers (18) measured average TQ for CON and ECC KE, KF, and EF at 30° and 120°/s in 50 untrained females and 40 males (21–67 yr) and found that the TQ-V relationships were similar for each muscle group and gender. Females generated greater ECC TQ relative to CON TQ when compared to males in both the upper and lower extremity muscle groups. For both genders, ECC average TQ did not change as a function of velocity, whereas CON TQ decreased as velocity increased. The results for the ECC TQ-V relationship for the females are in contrast to those of Colliander and Tesch (8), who reported that ECC PT increased with increasing speed. The differences in the ECC TQ-V curves between the two studies may have been due to differences in the subjects tested or to differences in the criterion measure used to develop the TQ-V curves. In Griffin's study, which measured average TQ, subjects were untrained and had a large range in age, whereas subjects in Colliander and Tesch's study were measured for PT and were young (mean age = 27 yr) and physically active. Further research is warranted to clarify the effect of preexisting strength levels and training status in ECC and CON TQ-V patterns.

# Bilateral Eccentric and Concentric Torque

Colliander and Tesch (8) assessed maximal bilateral ECC and CON TQ of the quadriceps and hamstring muscles in 13 females and 27 males. Measures included PT of bilateral muscle actions at 0.52, 1.57, and 2.61 rad/s. The results indicated that bilateral ECC PT was greater than CON PT and that the CON KF/KE ratio is higher than the ECC KF/KE ratio for both sexes. Concentric and ECC PT were 60% and 41% greater, respectively, in males than in females. When adjusted for BW, the CON differences were reduced (to 23%) but were still significant, whereas the ECC differences were nearly eliminated (8%). The major findings were that bilateral ECC PT is greater than CON PT in both males and females, and females displayed greater quad ECC PT relative to quad CON PT than males. Griffin and coworkers (18) also reported that women demonstrate greater ECC TQ values compared to CON TQ values for the lower extremity, as well as the upper extremity. The muscle mechanical responses to ECC muscle actions relative to CON muscle actions appear to differ between the sexes. Possible reasons for gender differences include differences in central nervous system (CNS) inhibition of maximal voluntary contractions (i.e., females are unable to recruit their entire MU pool during CON actions) or differences in the structure of muscle tissue, with females demonstrating a greater ability to utilize stored elastic energy (8, 18).

# Gender Differences in the Quadriceps/Hamstring Ratio

The quadriceps/hamstring (Q/H) torque ratio has been reported to range from 43 to 90% depending on the population tested and the velocities used for testing (20). Wyatt and Edwards (46) compared quadriceps and hamstring TQ values during isokinetic exercise in 50 females and 50 males (25–34 yr) on a Cybex II. Both knees were tested at 60, 180, and 300°/s. Peak quadriceps TQ usually occurred during the second and third extension effort, suggesting that it takes several repetitions to reach maximal TQ output. Nondominant and dominant limb TQ values were significantly different for males but not for females, which is in contrast to the findings of Hageman, Gillaspie, and Hill (20), who reported that there was no difference in TQ values between dominant and nondominant knees during CON and ECC exercise at 30 and 180°/s using a Kin-Com in physically active males and females. The Q/H torque ratios in Wyatt and Edwards's study ranged from 72% (60°/s) to 83% (300°/s) for the males and 71% (60°/s) to 85% (300°/s) for the females. These values are higher than those reported in other studies for untrained female subjects but are lower than those reported for trained females. Di Brezzo and coworkers (13) established normative strength data for KE and KF in 241 untrained females (18–28 yr) and reported an approximate Q/H torque ratio of 2:1 (53.6%) at 60°/s without gravity correction. Moffroid and coworkers (36) also reported a similar ratio (50%) in 48 untrained women. In contrast, Hageman, Gillaspie, and Hill (20) reported Q/H torque ratios ranging from 84 to 87% for females at 180°/s.

In the study by Wyatt and Edwards (46), dominant to nondominant knee torque ratios were 97 to 98% in males and 97 to 104% in females, and there were no significant differences between limbs. Hageman, Gillaspie, and Hill (20) reported similar results for trained females but found that the Q/H torque ratios in trained males were significantly greater in the nondominant limb during both ECC and CON muscle actions at 30 and 180°/s. Inconsistencies between studies may be attributed to differences in the dynamometers used to measure TQ as well as differences in testing protocols. Possible reasons for differences between and within genders in the Q/H relationship may be due to training status, muscle actions tested, or perhaps the structural and physiological differences between men and women.

It is well known that the Q/H torque ratio decreases with increasing speeds, and Wyatt and Edwards (46) have suggested that at test speeds greater than 300°/s, hamstring TQ may exceed quadriceps TQ. Klopfer and Greij (28) examined Q/H performance at high velocity isokinetic performance (300, 330, 360, 400, and 450°/s) in untrained women (n = 32) and men (n = 23) (19–37 yr) using the Biodex B-2000. In both males and females, the Q/H torque ratio decreased with increasing velocities (female ratio = 92.4–98.9%, male ratio = 102.9–137.1%). Hamstring TQ output exceeded the quadriceps TQ output in the female subjects, which is in agreement with the suggestion of Wyatt and Edwards (46). There was wide variability among PT values for each gender; however, variability was markedly reduced when TQ was expressed as a percentage of BW. Hageman, Gillaspie, and Hill (20) also reported that there were no significant differences in TQ/BW ratio between the dominant and nondominant knees during ECC and CON exercise at 30 and 180°/s. These results suggest that percent TQ/BW may be more helpful for setting goals for athletes.

# Effect of Velocity and Gender on Load Range

Brown and coworkers (5) examined gender differences in load range (LR), acceleration, and deceleration during KE and KF across a velocity spectrum. Load range decreased with increasing velocity and males exhibited greater load range and less acceleration ROM than females at 240, 360, and 450°/s, while deceleration ROM was not significantly different between genders at any speed. The differences in LR may be neuromuscular, with females demonstrating lower neuromotoric efficiency. Females produced less LR than males during KE and KF at speeds greater than 240°/s; therefore, high speed exercise in females may not be effective. Results suggest that researchers need to consider velocity during KF and KE when LR is a concern. Future research should focus upon angle-specific strength gains in LR over the velocity spectrum and identify an increase in LR as a function of high speed exercise. In addition, there is a need to identify the reason for variation in LR between genders, including the effect of fiber type.

# Effect of Stabilization on Torque

Stabilization during isokinetic testing has been shown to increase TQ, however, few studies have examined the effect of handgrip when testing the knee extensors and flexors. Merriam and coworkers (34) examined the effects of handgrip stabilization on TQ output (60, 180, and 300°/s) and EMG activity of the quadriceps and hamstrings during KE and KF in 15 men (24 ± 3 yr) and 15 women (25 ± 4 yr) using a Cybex 6000. Subjects performed the tests in both a stabilized (handgrips used) and unstabilized (arms folded across the chest) condition. The results indicated a significant interaction for TQ in the males and reflected an 8.4% increase in KE TQ and a 0.2% increase in KF TQ in the stabilized condition. In contrast, stabilization did not significantly effect TQ for the females. This finding is in agreement with Hanten and Ramberg (21), who reported no significant difference between minimal and maximal stabilization for CON and ECC contractions of the quadriceps in 15 women who were similar in age (mean age = 24.7 yr) using the Kin-Com. In the study by Merriam and coworkers (34), the EMG analysis did not show corresponding changes with the TQ data, indicating that TQ differences were not due to differences in activation and, therefore, were most likely due to mechanical factors such as altered length-tension relationships secondary to pelvic positioning. In addition, the researchers suggested that the nonadjustable handgrips and lumbar roll on the Cybex 6000 might not allow persons with shorter stature to generate their maximal isokinetic TQ. These findings indicate that researchers need to be consistent with handgrip stabilization and that gender differences in TQ production can be affected by the use of handgrips.

# Gender Differences in Strength and Fiber Characteristics With Age

Reductions in strength and muscular performance with age, in both men and women, may be attributed to decreases in physical activity as well as to changes in muscle morphology and neural activity (1). Average declines in strength with age for men and women have been reported to be approximately 40% for leg muscles and 30% for arm muscles, with a similar decrease in muscle mass (33%) from age 30 to age 80 (9). Anatomical and physiological changes with age that may account for decreases in strength include a decrease in LBM and an increase in fat content within and between muscle groups (4, 38). Muscle biopsies from 60- to 96-year-olds show more fat and connective tissue than do biopsies from younger subjects and more fiber atrophy, especially in type II fibers (4). A decrease in MU functioning has also been observed in older subjects (4). Although men and women both experience age-associated declines in strength, there appear to be differences between genders with regard to the rate of strength loss depending upon the contraction type and muscle group as well as differences in the atrophy and distribution of type II muscle fibers.

Borges (4) examined isometric and isokinetic KE and KF TQ in males (n = 139) and females (n = 141) aged 20 to 70 yr. Subjects were placed in groups by decade and both legs were measured at 0, 12, 90, and 150°/s. No significant differences in PT were found between the right and left leg. Torque was greater in males across all age groups, while isometric and isokinetic TQ decreased with age in both sexes. Torque significantly decreased between 20 and 30 yr in males and between 40 and 50 yr in females at all velocities tested, whereas maximal isometric TQ significantly decreased between 60 and 70 yr in both sexes. Borges (4) suggested that the decrease in TQ with age occurred as a result of a decrease in fiber area, loss in the number of fibers between 30 and 70 yr, and changes in the neuromuscular system with progressive declines in trophic function of the nerve cell in old age. In females, isokinetic KE TQ varied between 59% (150°/s) and 69% (12°/s) of that in males. In KF, females varied between 44% (150°/s) and 71% (12°/s) of that in males. Muscle biopsies in 31 females and 34 males showed that the area of type II fibers decreases with age. Females, in particular, experienced marked decreases in both type IIa and IIb fibers, whereas males only showed decreases in type IIa fibers. When the influence of the type II area on TQ was statistically eliminated, there was still an inverse correlation between fiber area and TQ, suggesting that other factors such as increased fat and connective tissue and a loss in muscle fibers and MUs also contribute to strength declines.

Freedson and coworkers (14) also examined TQ produced by age group and gender to provide descriptive PT values for the back, shoulders, and knees of male and female industrial workers. Subjects (1,196 females and 3,345 males; 17–62 yr) were divided into the following age groups: < 21, 21–30, 31–40, 41–50, 50+ yr. Males were consistently stronger in all measures across all ages, and females exhibited faster strength loss across age. For females, the highest PT values were observed for KF and KE under age 31 yr, whereas the shoulder and back measures were highest between 31 and 40 yr. For the males, the highest PT values were all observed under age 31 yr. The females showed their highest rates of decline in strength for the shoulders, knees, and back between the later decades (i.e., between 41–50 and 50+). The results were similar for the men for the shoulder and back; however, knee TQ measures remained more stable with age. Women also showed significantly greater KF/KE torque ratios at the higher speeds compared to the men. Freedson and coworkers (14) suggested that the data might be useful for comparative purposes in strength evaluations but warned that further research is necessary before determining appropriate standards for use as strength guidelines.

Although several studies have examined gender-related differences in isometric and CON strength, few have examined changes in ECC strength with age. The relationship between ECC strength and age has important functional implications since ECC muscle actions have a significant role in ambulation by providing stabilization and deceleration forces (33). Lindle and coworkers (33) assessed age and gender differences in muscle strength, isometric, CON, and ECC PT of the knee extensors at 30°/s and 180°/s in 654 males (n = 346) and females (n = 308) (20–93 yr) using a Kin-Com. In addition, the stretch-shortening cycle (SSC) was measured in a subsample of 47 subjects. The results demonstrated significant ($p < .001$) age-related reductions in CON and ECC PT for men and women at both speeds; however, no differences were observed between the gender groups or velocities. Age-associated CON losses started in the fourth decade for both genders at a rate of approximately 8 to 10% per decade. The decline in ECC strength was also similar for men and women; however, ECC strength loss appeared at least a decade later (in the 50s) in women. Age was better for explaining losses in CON strength when compared to ECC strength, accounting for 30% (CON) vs. 19% (ECC) of the variance in males and 28% (CON) vs.11% (ECC) in females. When CON and ECC PT were related to muscle quality (strength per kg of regional fat free mass), both genders showed losses in CON strength. However, for ECC strength, only the males showed a significant age-related decline. Differences in the mechanical and elastic properties of the muscle may explain, in part, the greater preservation of ECC strength with age in women. The results of this study also showed that the SSC in older women (70 yr) was significantly enhanced when compared to men of similar age as well as to younger men and women, indicating that older women have a greater capacity to store and utilize elastic energy.

Hortobagyi and associates (23) also reported a gender difference in the relationship of ECC strength and age but found no age-related alterations in muscle quality in men or women when using ECC strength values. In their study, older men (70 ± 1.5 yr) produced 20% less ECC KE strength than younger men (29.5 ± 1.5 yr), whereas older women (69 ± 1.8 yr) exceeded young women (29.3 ± 1.8 yr) by approximately 10%. This is in contrast to the results of Lindle and coworkers (33), who found an age-related decline in ECC KE strength of approximately 31% and 22% in men and women, respectively. The conflicting results between the two studies may be attributed to differences in sample size or methodology. Hortobagyi and associates (23) reported angle-specific peak force, whereas Lindle and coworkers (33) corrected peak force for the length of the lever arm and reported strength as PT.

Recently, Bellows and coworkers (3) examined gender-specific differences in the decline of quadriceps strength in 60 males (n = 30) and females (n = 30). Subjects were gender matched to three age groups (20–29, 40–49, and 60–69 yr), with 10 subjects in each gender-age group, and performed CON and ECC knee extensions at 60 and 120°/s on a Cybex 6000. Females demonstrated a greater rate of decline in ECC strength vs. CON strength at 120°/s compared to males, which suggests that ECC muscle strength is affected by aging at a different rate than CON strength at faster speeds. These results are in contrast to those of Lindle and coworkers (33), who reported that women showed a greater decline in CON (35%) vs. ECC (22%) strength with age; however, the difference was not significant. Bellows and associates (3) also reported that males appear to lose CON strength at a greater rate than females at 120°/s (42.6% vs. 38.1%, respectively); however, this difference was not statistically significant ($p = .09$). Murray and coworkers (38) also found that the percentage decline of knee muscle strength was lower in women compared to men and suggested that this may be due to a smaller decline in LBM with age for women. Bellows and coworkers (3) theorized that the decline in ECC strength in females was possibly due to both structural and functional changes with age such as osteoporotic changes in the skeletal system or a decreased ability to dissipate force during ECC contraction.

# Age-related Differences in Morphology and Enzyme Activity

Aniansson and associates (1) examined gender differences in isometric and isokinetic strength (30, 60, 120, and 180°/s), muscle morphology, and enzyme activity of the quadriceps in 52 males (66–76 yr) and 13 females (61–71 yr).

Peak TQ was significantly lower in women vs. men at all velocities. Body cell mass (via K⁺ counting) was significantly greater in males and was highly correlated to strength in both sexes. Although type I fiber distribution was approximately the same between males (48%) and females (54%), there was a significant difference in type IIb distribution (18% vs. 4% for the males and females, respectively). No sex differences were observed for $Mg^{++}ATPase$, myokinase, LDH, and phosphate (ATP and PC) content, and there was no correlation between these variables and strength, suggesting that differences in strength are due to differences in cell mass. The histological findings are in contrast to those of Komi and Karlsson (29) for younger men and women. Although the distribution of ST fibers for both sexes appears to be similar between the two studies, Komi and Karlsson (29) reported that the ST distribution in men (55.9%) was significantly higher than that in women (49.1%). In addition, men had significantly higher concentrations of ATPase and LDH. The finding by Aniansson and coworkers (1) of no significant differences with age in enzyme and phosphate concentrations may be due to changes in hormone concentrations, such as a decrease in testosterone in men, or to similar levels of physical activity in older males and females.

More recently, Frontera and coworkers (16) also suggested that age- and gender-related differences in strength are primarily due to differences in muscle mass (MM). In their study, isokinetic strength of the elbow and knee extensors and flexors was assessed in 200 healthy 45- to 78-year-old men and women to determine the relationship between muscle strength, age, and body composition. Peak TQ was measured at 60 and 240°/s at the knee, and at 60 and 180°/s at the elbow on a Cybex II. The absolute strength of the women ranged from 42.2 to 62.8% of that in males. When expressed per kg of muscle mass, the gender differences for KE, KF, and EE PT were eliminated; however, EF PT remained significantly lower, indicating that factors other than MM may account for decreases in upper body strength. Danneskiold-Samsoe and others (9) also reported that the KE strength of elderly females (78–81 yr) was 43 to 64% of that in males, while the largest differences were observed for EF/EE. The differences in absolute strength were similar to those reported by Murray and associates (38), who reported that the KE strength in women aged 20 to 86 yr was 74% that of males, and Borges (4), who found that women in different age groups have approximately 65.7% and 53% the isokinetic PT of males in KE and KF, respectively. In agreement with Aniansson and coworkers (1), the findings of Frontera and associates (16) suggest that age- and gender-related differences in strength are primarily due to differences in muscle mass and not muscle function.

# Age-Related Differences in Range of Motion

Fugl-Meyer, Gustafsson, and Burstedt (17) assessed isometric and isokinetic maximal plantarflexion (PF) TQ in 69 females and 66 males (20–65 yr). Fifteen subjects of each sex represented each decade < 60 yr. Each leg was tested at 30,

60, 90, 120, and 180°/s with the knees flexed at 0° and 90°. For females up to age 49 yr, ROM at the ankle was significantly greater when compared to the corresponding male groups. Range of motion decreased with age for both sexes; however, there was no age dependence for ROM when the knees were in 90° of flexion. The authors suggested that the greater ROM for the women in both knee positions might be reflected by anatomical differences such as smaller crural circumference and foot length.

Many of the gender-related differences in strength observed in young males and females appear to persist with age. Although it has been suggested that age- and gender-related differences in isometric and isokinetic strength are primarily due to differences in LBM, other factors such as FT fiber distribution (particularly IIb), amount of intramuscular fat and connective tissue, level of physical activity, and anatomical differences may also contribute. In addition, there is conflicting data with regard to age-related declines in PT between genders, especially for ECC muscle actions, indicating a need for further study.

## Eccentric and Concentric Isokinetic Training

The effect of ECC and CON training on functional performance has not been well studied. However, studies that have examined the effects of ECC and CON training for improving muscular strength indicate that the greatest training effects are demonstrated when tests are of the same type as the training program (37). Higbie and coworkers (22) examined the effects of CON and ECC training on muscle strength, CSA, and neural activation in 54 females (18–35 yr). Maximal CON and ECC KE strength was determined pretraining at 60°/s on the Kin-Com. Subjects trained either concentrically or eccentrically three times per week for 10 weeks, and performed three sets of 10 repetitions for a total of 30 sessions. During the first week of training, the subjects were required to meet or exceed a force marker on the Kin-Com screen, which was set at the pretest peak force measured during the ECC or CON muscle actions. The force marker placement was subsequently adjusted each week based upon strength tests. The results posttraining showed that ECC training was more effective than CON training for developing ECC strength, and CON training was more effective than ECC training for developing CON strength, suggesting that gains in strength following CON and ECC training are highly dependent upon the muscle action used for testing and training. The CSA (via MRI) of the quadriceps increased more with ECC training (+ 6.6%) vs. CON training (+ 5.0%), and the increases by ECC training with ECC testing (+ 36.2%) were greater than the increases by CON training with CON testing (+ 18.4%). Morrissey and associates (37) have suggested that the greater improvement in ECC strength with ECC training may be due to an increased learning effect, since subjects are less familiar with ECC exercise. Both the CON and ECC training groups experienced increases in EMG activity when compared to a control group; however, there were no significant differences in

EMG responses between the two training groups. The researchers concluded that muscle hypertrophy and neural adaptations contribute to strength increases following both CON and ECC training.

Ryan, Magidow, and Duncan (40) determined the velocity-specific and mode-specific effects of ECC isokinetic training of the hamstrings in 34 females (21–40 yr). Subjects trained eccentrically at 120°/s three times per week for six weeks and were tested pre- and posttraining at 60, 120, and 180°/s using both ECC and CON contractions. The results demonstrated that ECC training of the hamstrings at 120°/s significantly increased ECC strength at all velocities tested and significantly increased CON strength at 120 and 180°/s, indicating that ECC isokinetic training is neither mode nor velocity specific.

## Velocity Training

Although there are inconsistencies in the literature regarding specificity of velocity training, it is likely that training at both fast and slow speeds is necessary for optimal gains in functional performance. Because increases in muscle growth and contractile strength are related to the amount of tension developed within the muscle, slow velocity training by athletes who perform high velocity movements appears necessary to stimulate maximum adaptations within the muscle (42). Therefore, when training for speed and power, velocity spectrum training is recommended since fast movements train the nervous system and slow movements train the muscles (42). Emphasis should also be placed on the contraction type (ECC, CON, isometric) to provide the appropriate stimulus for neural adaptation (42). Range of motion specificity is also important since strength increases are the greatest at the joint angles or angular ROM exercised (37).

## Functional Performance

Although many studies have examined the effects of isokinetic training protocols on muscular performance using laboratory strength tests, there are virtually no studies that have determined the effects of isokinetic training on functional performance in men or women. In a study by Van Oteghen (43) the effectiveness of isokinetic training at two speeds for improving vertical jump (VJ) was examined in 48 collegiate volleyball players. Subjects were randomly assigned to a fast speed training (n = 16), slow speed training (n = 16), or a control group (n = 16). Subjects performed 3 sets of 10 repetitions on a Compensator leg press machine (Robar Mini-Gym, Inc.), 3 days per week for 8 weeks. Both the slow and fast speed groups had significantly greater VJ performance vs. the controls following training, and there was no significant difference in VJ between the two training groups. The results indicated that neither fast nor slow training was superior to the other for improving VJ performance.

Given the physiological differences between genders discussed earlier in this chapter, it is recommended that, in future studies, data not be pooled and that findings are reported specific to gender.

# Unilateral Training and Cross-Transfer

Krotkiewski and coworkers (31) determined the effect of unilateral isokinetic strength on local adipose and muscle tissue morphology, thickness, and enzymes in 10 females (24–29 yr). Subjects completed one-legged KE exercise for 5 weeks and performed 3 sets of 10 repetitions daily at 60°/s. Strength was assessed on both legs pre- and posttraining at 30, 60, 120, and 180°/s. Endurance was also measured using 30 reps at 180°/s and was expressed as the percentage decline in PT from the first 3 contractions to the last 3 contractions. Training resulted in an increase in quadriceps force of 14 to 26% in the trained leg and 4 to 13% in the untrained leg indicating that a crossover effect occurred. The training also resulted in a significant increase in muscle thickness, type II fiber area, and enzyme changes that were consistent with changes related to increased contractility and glycolytic capacity in the trained leg. There was a decrease in subcutaneous fat in the trained leg; however, it occurred as a consequence of the change in leg geometry (i.e., the same amount of fat surrounds an increased muscle volume). Therefore, five weeks of training did not result in regional fat mobilization.

Kannus and coworkers (27) examined the effect of one-legged exercise on strength, power, and endurance of the contralateral leg using isometric and concentric isokinetic training in 20 untrained males and females. Following seven weeks of training, isometric and isokinetic strength significantly increased in both the trained and untrained legs. The mean strength benefit in the untrained limb was 36% (hamstrings) and 58% (quadriceps) of that achieved in the trained limb. The untrained hamstring muscles showed greater benefits in the endurance parameters than in the strength power measures, whereas the opposite was true for the quadriceps. It was concluded that neuromuscular facilitation improved strength and power in the untrained limb by a certain amount; however, further improvement in the trained limb will not result in increases in the untrained limb since hypertrophy cannot play a role.

In contrast to Krotkiewski and coworkers (31) and Kannus and coworkers (27), Weir and coworkers (45) found no crossover effect when they determined the effects of unilateral isometric strength training on joint angle specificity and cross-training in 17 females. Subjects trained by performing 2 sets of 10 repetitions of isometric leg extension at 80% of their maximal isometric TQ at a joint angle of 0.79 rad below the horizontal plane for 6 weeks. Training resulted in a significant increase in TQ output at 0.79 and 1.31 rad in the trained limb; however, there was no increase in strength in the untrained limb. In addition, there was no significant increase in EMG of the VL or vastus medialis in association with the joint angle-specific strength increases. The authors hypothesized that the joint angle specificity was due to a decrease in antagonistic cocontraction or hypertrophy of the quadriceps at specific levels.

In summary, it is important to consider the concept of specificity of training when designing an isokinetic strength-training program. Ideally, the training exercises should mimic the sport movement as closely as possible with regard to movement pattern, velocity of movement, contraction type, and contraction force (42). It is also important to consider that, in the case of sport movements performed at high velocities, training at low velocities is necessary to induce maximal adaptations within the muscle (42).

# Effects of Menstrual Cycle on Muscular Performance

Research examining the effect of the menstrual cycle on muscular performance indicates that active women with a normal cycle experience no significant change in strength, work performance, or rating of perceived exertion as a result of cycle changes. In addition, although BW has been reported to vary between 0.5 and 1.0 kg during the menstrual cycle, these changes do not appear to affect strength performance (6, 12).

Di Brezzo, Fort, and Brown (11) examined the relationships among strength, endurance, BW, and body fat (% fat) during three phases of the menstrual cycle (luteal, ovulation, menses) in 21 females (18–36 yr). In general, they reported that different phases of the cycle had little or no effect upon the correlations among BW, percentage fat, and KE and KF at 60, 180, and 240°/s. High correlations among most strength measures at the three speeds were found for each phase during the cycle ($r$ range = .80–.95) and between the cycle phases ($r$ = .64–.89).

Di Brezzo and coworkers (10) also examined dynamic strength of the knee flexors and extensors at 180 and 240°/s and the rate of perceived exertion (RPE) in active (n = 9) and sedentary (n = 9) women during menses, ovulation, and the luteal phase. Although the PT values were significantly higher in the active women, there were no significant differences in percent fat, PT, endurance ratios, and RPE throughout the cycle phases. These results suggest that the differences in strength were a function of activity level as opposed to effects of the menstrual cycle.

In a more recent study, Lebrun and associates (32) examined the effects of menstrual cycle phase (follicular and midluteal) on aerobic capacity, anaerobic capacity, isokinetic strength, and high intensity exercise in 16 physically active women (18–40 yr; $\dot{V}O_2$max 50 ml/kg/min). Peak TQ for KF and KE was assessed at 240°/s on a Cybex II. No significant differences were observed in BW, percent fat, sum of skinfolds, or PT between phases. Absolute and relative $\dot{V}O_2$max were slightly lower ($p$ = .04–.06) in the luteal phase, indicating that cyclic increases in steroid hormones may have a slight, deleterious effect on aerobic capacity, with potential implications for individual subjects.

Few studies have examined the effect of the menstrual cycle on ECC isokinetic strength. Gur (19) assessed the reproducibility of CON and ECC tests of KE and KF at 60°/s (4 repetitions) and 240°/s (20 repetitions) and determined the reciprocal moment ratios at different phases of the menstrual cycle (menses, luteal, and follicular) in 16 sedentary women (24–35 yr). The results showed no significant differences among the phases for ECC and CON PT, total work, and their reciprocal ratios for the dominant knee. The ICC values for CON and ECC PT were moderate to excellent, ranging from .49 to .94

during the cycle. These findings were in agreement with others and suggest that menstrual cycle phases do not need to be considered in isokinetic measurement.

In summary, although many women report feelings of bloating and weight gain during ovulation, the fluctuations do not appear great enough to affect strength measures. Therefore, stages of the menstrual cycle do not need to be monitored during strength testing unless gross weight changes are suspected. For training studies, however, it may be advisable to standardize the cycle phase during which testing is performed to eliminate potentially confounding effects as a result of variations in steroid hormone concentrations (32).

# Summary

Differences in electromechanical activity, in combination with qualitative and quantitative variations in muscle mass, may account for several gender-related differences in strength. It appears that women exhibit lower neuromotoric efficiency and neuromuscular coordination mechanics, which may be attributed to hormonal influences, structural differences in muscle (i.e., muscle stiffness), and patterns of physical activity or training. Differences in enzyme activity as well as in the distribution and size of muscle fiber types (particularly type II fibers) may also contribute to differences in strength between the sexes. Because factors other than muscle mass account for gender-related differences in strength, it is recommended that data not be pooled and that findings be reported specific to gender. In addition, there is a need for future research that examines the relationship between ECC TQ and angular velocity, as well as the effect of ECC and CON training on functional performance.

# References

1. Aniansson, A., G. Grimby, M. Hedberg, and M. Krotkiewski. 1981. Muscle morphology, enzyme activity, and muscle strength in elderly men and women. *Clin. Physiol.* 1: 73–86.

2. Bell, D., and I. Jacobs. 1986. Electromechanical response times and rate of force development in males and females. *Med. Sci. Sports Exerc.* 18: 31–36.

3. Bellows, J.W., T.R. Malone, A.J. Nitz, and A.L. Hart. 1998. Gender specificity in the age-related decline of strength: Concentric versus eccentric. *Isok. Exerc. Sci.* 7: 1–9.

4. Borges, O. 1989. Isometric and isokinetic knee extension and flexion torque in men and women aged 20 to 70. *Scand. J. Rehab. Med.* 21: 45–53.

5. Brown, L.E., M. Whitehurst, R. Gilbert, and D. Buchalter. 1995. The effect of velocity and gender on load range during knee extension and flexion exercise on an isokinetic device. *J. Ortho. Sport Phys. Ther.* 21: 107–12.

6. Byrd, P.J., and T.R. Thomas. 1983. Hydrostatic weighing during different stages of the menstrual cycle. *Res. Q. Exerc. Sport.* 54: 296–98.

7. Castro, M.J., D.J. McCann, J.D. Shaffrath, and W.C. Adams. 1995. Peak torque per unit cross-sectional area differs in strength-trained and untrained young adults. *Med. Sci. Sports Exerc.* 27: 397–403.

8. Colliander, E., and P. Tesch. 1989. Bilateral eccentric and concentric torque of quadriceps and hamstring muscles in females and males. *Eur. J. Appl. Physiol.* 59: 227–32.

9. Danneskiold-Samsoe, B., V. Kofod, J. Munter, G. Grimby, P. Schnohr, and G. Jensen. 1984. Muscle strength and functional capacity in 78- to 81-year-old men and women. *Eur. J. Appl. Physiol.* 52: 310–14.

10. Di Brezzo, R., I.L. Fort, M.L. Boorman, and B. Oglesby. 1994. Dynamic strength and perceived exertion in active and sedentary women during the menstrual cycle. *Clin. Kines.* 84–89.

11. Di Brezzo, R., I.L. Fort, and B. Brown. 1991. Relationships among strength, endurance, weight, and body fat during three phases of the menstrual cycle. *J. Sports Med. Phys. Fitness.* 31: 89–94.

12. Di Brezzo, R., I.L. Fort, and B. Brown. 1988. Dynamic strength and work variations during three stages of the menstrual cycle. *J. Ortho. Sports Phys. Ther.* 10: 113–16.

13. Di Brezzo, R., B.E. Gench, M.M. Hinson, and J. King. 1985. Peak torque values of the knee extensor and flexor muscles of females. *J. Ortho. Sports Phys. Ther.* 7: 65–68.

14. Freedson, P., T. Gilliam, T. Mahoney, A. Maliszewski, and K. Kastango. 1933. Industrial torque levels by age group and gender. *Isok. Exerc. Sci.* 3: 34–42.

15. Froese, E.A., and M.E. Houston. 1985. Torque-velocity characteristics and muscle fiber type in human vastus lateralis. *J. Appl. Physiol.* 59: 309–14.

16. Frontera, W.R., V.A. Hughes, K.J. Lutz, and W.J. Evans. 1991. A cross-sectional study of muscle strength and mass in 45- to 78-year-old men and women. *J. Appl. Physiol.* 71: 644–50.

17. Fugl-Meyer, A.R., L. Gustafsson, and Y. Burstedt. 1980. Isokinetic and static plantar flexion characteristics. *Eur. J. Appl. Physiol.* 45: 221–34.

18. Griffin, J., R. Tooms, R. Vander Zwaag, T. Bertorini, and M. O'Toole. 1993. Eccentric muscle performance of elbow and knee muscle groups in untrained men and women. *Med. Sci. Sports Exerc.* 25: 936–44.

19. Gur, H. 1997. Concentric and eccentric isokinetic measurements in knee muscles during the menstrual cycle: A special reference to reciprocal moment ratios. *Arch. Phys. Med. Rehabil.* 78: 501–5.

20. Hageman, P., D.M. Gillaspie, and L.D. Hill. 1988. Effects of speed and limb dominance on eccentric and concentric isokinetic testing of the knee. *J. Ortho. Sports Phys. Ther.* 10: 59–65.

21. Hanten, W.P., and C.L. Ramberg. 1988. Effect of stabilization on maximal isokinetic torque of the quadriceps femoris muscle during concentric and eccentric contractions. *Phys. Ther.* 68: 219–22.

22. Higbie, E., K. Cureton, G. Warren III, and B. Prior. 1996. Effects of concentric and eccentric training on muscle strength, cross-sectional area, and neural activation. *J. Appl. Physiol.* 81: 2173–81.

23. Hortobagyi, T., D. Zheng, M. Weidner, N.L. Lambert, S. Westbrook, and J.A. Houmard. 1995. The influence of aging on muscle strength and muscle fiber characteristics with special reference to eccentric strength. *J. Gerontol. A Biol. Sci. Med.* 50: B399–406.

24. Ives, J., W. Kroll, and L. Bultman. 1993. Rapid movement kinematic and electromyographic control characteristics in males and females. *Res. Q. Exerc. Sport* 64: 274–83.

25. Kanehisa, H., H. Okuyama, S. Ikegawa, and T. Fukunaga. 1996. Sex difference in force generation capacity during repeated maximal knee extensions. *Eur. J. Appl. Physiol.* 73: 557–62.

26. Kanehisa, H., S. Ikegawa, and T. Fukunaga. 1994. Comparison of muscle cross-sectional area and strength between untrained women and men. *Eur. J. Appl. Physiol.* 68: 148–54.

27. Kannus, P., D. Alosa, L. Cook et al. 1992. Effect of one-legged exercise on the strength, power, and endurance of the contralateral leg. *Eur. J. Appl. Physiol.* 64: 117–26.

28. Klopfer, D., and S. Greij. 1988. Examining quadriceps/hamstrings performance at high velocity isokinetics in untrained subjects. *J. Ortho. Sports Phys. Ther.* 10: 18–22.

29. Komi, P.V., and J. Karlsson. 1978. Skeletal muscle fiber types, enzyme activities, and physical performance in young males and females. *Acta Physiol. Scand.* 103: 210–18.

30. Kramer, J.F., and J. MacDermid. 1989. Isokinetic measures during concentric-eccentric cycles of the knee extensors. *Aust. J. Physiother.* 35: 9–14.

31. Krotkiewski, M., A. Aniansson, G. Grimby, P. Bjorntorp, and L. Sjostrom. 1979. The effect of unilateral isokinetic strength training on local adipose and muscle tissue morphology, thickness, and enzymes. *Eur. J. Appl. Physiol.* 42: 271–81.

32. Lebrun, C.M., D.C. McKenzie, J.C. Prior, and J.E. Taunton. 1995. Effects of menstrual cycle phase on athletic performance. *Med. Sci. Sports Exerc.* 27: 437–44.

33. Lindle, R.S., E.J. Metter, N.A. Lynch et al. 1997. Age and gender comparisons of muscle strength in 654 women and men aged 20 to 93 years. *J. Appl. Physiol.* 83: 1581–87.

34. Merriam, S.J., K.R. Nies, A.L. Smith, D.J. Sprugeon, and J.P. Weir. In press. Effect of stabilization on isokinetic knee extension/flexion torque and electromyographic activity. *Phys. Ther.*

35. Miller, A.E.J., J.D. MacDougall, M.A. Tarnopolsky, and D.G. Sale. 1993. Gender differences in strength and muscle fiber characteristics. *Eur. J. Appl. Physiol.* 66: 254–62.

36. Moffroid, M., R. Whipple, J. Hokfosh, E. Lowman, and H. Thistle. 1969. A study of isometric exercise. *Phys. Ther.* 49: 735–46.

37. Morrissey, M., E. Harman, and M. Johnson. 1995. Resistance training modes: Specificity and effectiveness. *Med. Sci. Sports Exerc.* 27: 648–60.

38. Murray, P.M., E. Duthie Jr., S. Gambert, S. Sepic, and L. Mollinger. 1985. Age-related differences in knee muscle strength in normal women. *J. Gerontol.* 40: 275–80.

39. Perrine, J., and V.R. Edgerton. 1978. Muscle force-velocity and power-velocity relationships under isokinetic loading. *Med. Sci. Sports Exerc.* 10: 159–66.

40. Ryan, L., P. Magidow, and P. Duncan. 1991. Velocity-specific and mode-specific effects of eccentric isokinetic training of the hamstrings. *J. Ortho. Sports Phys. Ther.* 13: 33–39.

41. Ryushi, T., K. Hakkinen, H. Kauhanen, and P. Komi. 1988. Muscle fiber characteristics, muscle cross-sectional area, and force production in strength athletes, physically active males and females. *Scand. J. Sports Sci.* 10: 7–15.

42. Sale, D., and J.D. MacDougall. 1981. Specificity in strength training: A review for the coach and athlete. *Can. J. Appl. Sports Sci.* 6: 87–92.

43. Van Oteghen, S. 1973. Two speeds of isokinetic exercise as related to the vertical jump performance of women. *Res. Q.* 46: 78–84.

44. Wagner, L.L., T.J. Housh, J.P. Weir, and G.O. Johnson. 1992. Gender differences in the isokinetic torque-velocity relationship. *Isok. Exerc. Sci.* 2: 110–15.

45. Weir, J., T. Housh, L. Weir, and G. Johnson. 1995. Effects of unilateral isometric strength training on joint angle specificity and cross training. *Eur. J. Appl. Physiol.* 70: 337–43.

46. Wyatt, M., and A. Edwards. 1981. Comparison of quadriceps and hamstring torque values during isokinetic exercise. *J. Ortho. Sports Phys. Ther.* 3: 48–56.

# Chapter 18

# Isokinetic Testing and Training in Tennis

Todd S. Ellenbecker and E. Paul Roetert

The sport of tennis requires repetitive upper and lower extremity muscular activity, which can lead to overuse injury. Muscular activity to stabilize the trunk is also inherent in tennis play and links the upper and lower extremity segments. The specific physiological and mechanical stresses imparted to the body during tennis play produce characteristic anatomical adaptations and injury patterns (14). Knowledge of these characteristic anatomical adaptations as well as the inherent demands and physiological loads placed upon the human body during tennis play will assist in the evaluation and design of optimal conditioning programs for performance enhancement and injury prevention.

Match analyses indicate that over 300 to 500 bursts of energy are required over the course of a tennis match (9). Heart rates during tennis play among accomplished tennis players range between 60 and 90% of maximum during singles play (11). Work-to-rest ratios for tennis players range between 1:2 and 1:3, with the average time spent rallying during points being less than 10 s and the maximum rest period allowed between points being 25 s (48).

Analysis of epidemiological studies in tennis shows a high prevalence of shoulder and elbow overuse injuries (26, 29, 32, 39, 51). Incidence of shoulder injuries among elite junior players ranges from 10 to 30% (14, 29, 32, 39). One interesting statistic taken from epidemiological literature is from Priest and Nagel (37), who studied 84 world-class tennis players: 74% of men and 60% of women had a history of shoulder or elbow injuries, with 21% of men and 23% of women reporting injuries to both the shoulder and elbow of the dominant arm. This injury pattern illustrates the important interrelationship between the shoulder and elbow and provides rationale for total arm strength and conditioning, for both performance enhancement as well as injury prevention.

In addition to the repetitive physiological demands listed previously, tennis requires explosive movement patterns and highly intensive maximal-effort concentric and eccentric muscular work. One prime example is the explosive internal rotation of the shoulder that has been reported to occur during the acceleration phase of the serve at speeds ranging between 1,074 and 2,300°/s (10, 45). Elbow extension and wrist flexion have been reported to occur at 1,700° and 315°, respectively (45). Because of the high velocities inherent in tennis, the use of isokinetic testing and training is indicated to more specifically emulate the type of concentric and eccentric muscular work that occurs during tennis play.

All of these physiological factors play an important role in the application of isokinetic testing and training for the tennis player. This chapter outlines the strength and endurance literature specific to tennis players, and allows sports medicine and sport science professionals to apply objectively based isokinetic data to optimally design testing and training programs and track progress in tennis players.

# Specific Joint Testing for the Tennis Player

The musculoskeletal demands of tennis play affect the entire body, encompassing virtually all regions. The use of isokinetic testing has been applied to many specific regions in the tennis player; it has provided descriptive data and identified unique muscular adaptations and imbalances.

## Glenohumeral Joint Testing

The primary pattern of testing and training for the glenohumeral joint in the tennis player is internal and external rotation (8, 14) (see figure 18.1). Elliot, Marsh, and Blanksby (21) used three-dimensional cinematography to quantify motion at the glenohumeral joint during the tennis serve. They found average abduction angles of 83° during the cocking phase of the serve. The sports medicine professional must use a 90° abduction angle for shoulder rotational testing to closely simulate the specific functional length-tension implications of the musculature (2).

Further testing specifics for the glenohumeral joint include proper stabilization and isolation of test segments, utilization of a standardized range of motion pattern and end stops, and a standardized testing protocol (8, 50). The reader is referred to Wilk, Arrigo, and Andrews (50) and chapter 1 of this book for a full description of the critical components of a standardized isokinetic testing protocol. The range of motion used to generate the data in this chapter for shoulder rotation was 0 to 90° external rotation and 0 to 65° internal rotation. This arc of motion was chosen to utilize a full 155° arc of rotational movement. Researchers have reported alterations in shoulder rotation range of motion with repetitive tennis play, specifically dominant arm internal rotation range of motion loss and total rotation range of motion loss (5, 19, 28, 42); these alterations have implications for injury (25).

The velocity spectrum chosen for three-speed bilateral testing is 90, 210, and 300°/s, and 210 and 300°/s are chosen for two-speed bilateral testing.

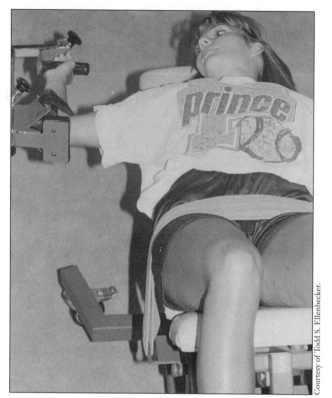

Courtesy of Todd S. Ellenbecker.

**Figure 18.1**    Isokinetic test position for glenohumeral joint internal and external rotation with 90° of glenohumeral joint abduction.

Repetitions for data generation of strength testing are five maximal repetitions, based on the research by Arrigo, Wilk, and Andrews (1). They reported that subjects had their peak performance between testing repetitions two and four. Thus, using five repetitions allows those peak repetitions to be sandwiched within the testing sequence. Rest intervals when testing tennis players have been 30 s, which is similar to the rest interval during tennis play between points in a match. Endurance testing of shoulder internal and external rotation uses similar stabilization procedures but involves the use of 20 maximal concentric repetitions at 300°/s.

Table 18.1 lists the normative data from testing 60 male and 38 female elite junior players between the ages of 12 to 17 years. Testing was completed on a Cybex 6000 isokinetic dynamometer. Normalized data relative to body weight is presented to allow interpretation. These data have been subjected to statistical analysis (12, 13), and results indicate significantly greater dominant arm internal rotation with no significant difference between extremities in external rotation. This finding is consistent with other studies measuring internal and external rotation strength in junior, collegiate, and adult tennis players (4, 14,

**Table 18.1    Shoulder Rotation Isokinetic Peak Torque and Single-Repetition Work/Body Weight Ratios**

| Motion (Mean, °/s) | Dominant arm | | Nondominant arm | |
|---|---|---|---|---|
| | Peak torque (%) | Work (%) | Peak torque (%) | Work (%) |
| External rotation | | | | |
| Males, 210 | 12 | 20 | 11 | 19 |
| Males, 300 | 10 | 18 | 10 | 17 |
| Females, 210 | 8 | 14 | 8 | 15 |
| Females, 300 | 8 | 11 | 7 | 12 |
| Internal rotation | | | | |
| Males, 210 | 17 | 32 | 14 | 27 |
| Males, 300 | 15 | 28 | 13 | 23 |
| Females, 210 | 12 | 23 | 11 | 19 |
| Females, 300 | 11 | 15 | 10 | 13 |
| External rotation:internal rotation ratio | | | | |
| Males, 210 | 51 | 64 | 80 | 78 |
| Males, 300 | 70 | 65 | 81 | 80 |
| Females, 210 | 70 | 66 | 79 | 82 |
| Females, 300 | 67 | 69 | 77 | 80 |

A Cybex 6000 series isokinetic dynamometer and 90° of glenohumeral joint abduction were used. Data expressed in ft-lb per unit of body weight. Subjects were 60 male and 38 female elite junior tennis players aged 12 to 17.

30). These findings explain the differences in the external/internal rotation ratios between the dominant and nondominant extremities. The lower ratios on the dominant arm indicate selective strength development of the internal rotators without concomitant development of strength in the external rotators. The normal external/internal rotation ratio is reported to be 66% (8, 14). Ratios below this 66% ratio indicate a relative deficiency of external rotation strength, which may subject the athlete to injury (49).

In addition to the typical shoulder rotation strength measures that identify characteristic adaptations from repetitive tennis play, fatigue testing of the shoulder internal and external rotators has also been studied. Ellenbecker and Roetert (20) found no significant bilateral differences in the relative fatigue ratios in internal and external rotation in 72 elite junior tennis players. Of significance, however, was the finding of differences between the fatigue responses of the internal and external rotators. Over 20 repetitions, the internal rotators fatigued to a level of 83% while the external rotators fatigued to 69%. The fatigue ratio is calculated as the work in the first half of the testing repetitions divided by the work in the second half (7, 8). This finding is particularly significant since prior isokinetic studies (4, 12–14, 30, 31) have demonstrated relative weakness of the external rotators, and this study (20) demonstrates a greater fatigue response of the external rotators when compared to the opposing internal rotation musculature. Isokinetic research studies such as these provide rationale for the use of conditioning programs for the external rotator musculature to improve not only strength but also muscular endurance and ultimately muscle balance. The use of isolated joint testing, which is inherent in isokinetic testing, has allowed researchers to identify this muscular imbalance in the glenohumeral joint of elite tennis players.

## Isokinetic Training of the Glenohumeral Joint

Isokinetic dynamometers have also been used for training the glenohumeral joint internal and external rotation musculature. A six-week bout of isokinetic training using a velocity spectrum format produced significant improvements in both concentric and eccentric internal and external rotation strength in collegiate (15) and adult tennis players (34). One modification these authors have found helpful for isokinetic training of the internal and external rotators is the use of the seated, scapular plane training position (see figure 18.2).

The scapular plane training position utilizes a stable chair placed next to the elevated dynamometer, which allows the athlete to train with approximately 80 to 90° of glenohumeral joint abduction. The chair is tilted (front inward) at a 30° angle to place the glenohumeral joint in the scapular plane (44). The scapula is free to move and rotate, and the seated position forces the external rotators to work against gravity as the shoulder is exercised through a range of 90° of external rotation and 35° of internal rotation. Research comparing the seated, scapular plane training position did not show significant differences to coronal plane testing with respect to force generation (16). However, other studies have compared planes of testing for internal and external rotation and found differences between abduction angles, and coronal, scapular, and frontal plane data generation (46).

Ng and Kramer (35) tested and compared the dominant arm internal and external rotation strength in healthy female control subjects to a group of female collegiate tennis players using a seated, scapular plane testing position. They found no significant difference between dominant arm internal and external rotation strength in the healthy control subjects. In the collegiate tennis players internal rotation strength exceeded external strength, and eccentric strength exceeded concentric strength measured at 60°/s on a Kin-Com dynamometer system.

Additional comparative research was published by Mikesky and coworkers (33), who tested baseball pitchers and tennis players using a Kin-Com with 90° of glenohumeral joint abduction. Baseball pitchers showed greater strength in the internal and external rotators but had lower external/internal rotation ratios compared to the tennis population. As with all isokinetic testing and training, care should be taken to carefully position the subject using repeatable and objective methods and positions that allow reliable interface to the dynamometer, to optimize testing and training with isokinetics.

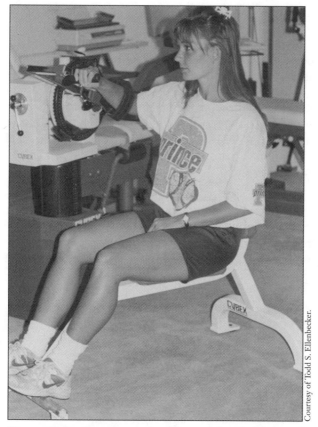

Courtesy of Todd S. Ellenbecker.

**Figure 18.2** Seated, scapular plane training position used only for isokinetic training of the shoulder internal and external rotators.

# Isokinetic Training and Testing Velocity

An additional factor important in the application of isokinetic exercise and testing is velocity. Since isokinetics have an inherent accommodating resistance level and constant velocity that is manipulated by the practitioner or scientist, selection of an appropriate exercise and testing velocity is of paramount importance. Brown and coworkers (3, see chapter 5 for full discussion) tested 12 elite junior tennis players using a Biodex isokinetic dynamometer to determine the effects of testing velocity on the subjects' ability to sustain the preset angular velocity through the range of motion. The portion of the range of motion where subjects were able to sustain the preselected velocity was termed load range. They tested subjects for internal and external shoulder rotation at speeds ranging between 60 and 450°/s and found an inverse relationship between isokinetic angular velocity and isokinetic load range. Acceleration and deceleration portions of the isokinetic torque curve statistically increased as angular velocity of performance increased (3). These results indicate that care must be taken to choose isokinetic training or testing velocities that allow the individual to benefit from the stimulus provided by the sustained velocity load range while utilizing more functional velocities. We recommend use of the velocity spectrum training and testing protocols proposed by Davies (8) to provide an optimal training stimulus.

Additional testing of the glenohumeral joint has been published on elite tennis players using the pattern of shoulder extension and flexion (12). A range of motion of 0 to 120° was used to prevent impingement and yet allow a large excursion of motion. The velocity spectrum of 90, 210, and 300°/s was again used. Results of the testing are listed in table 18.2, *a* and *b*.

### Table 18.2a    Shoulder Flexion/Extension Isokinetic Strength in Highly Skilled Adult Male Tennis Players

|  | Motion/speed (%) | Dominant | Nondominant |
|---|---|---|---|
| Shoulder flexion |  |  |  |
| Peak torque | 90 | 34 | 32 |
|  | 210 | 31 | 28 |
|  | 300 | 26 | 23 |
| Work | 90 | 27 | 26 |
|  | 210 | 10 | 12 |
|  | 300 | 7 | 7 |
| Shoulder extension |  |  |  |
| Peak torque | 90 | 48 | 41 |
|  | 210 | 41 | 34 |
|  | 300 | 32 | 26 |
| Work | 90 | 36 | 32 |
|  | 210 | 13 | 11 |
|  | 300 | 6 | 5 |

*All numbers expressed in % of ft-lb relative to body weight in lb.

### Table 18.2b    Unilateral Strength Ratios: Shoulder Flexion/Extension in Highly Skilled Adult Male Tennis Players

|  | Ratio/speed (%) | Dominant | Nondominant |
|---|---|---|---|
| Peak torque | 90 | 71 | 78 |
|  | 210 | 78 | 83 |
|  | 300 | 82 | 88 |
| Work | 90 | 76 | 81 |
|  | 210 | 83 | 107 |
|  | 300 | 113 | 163 |

Significantly greater dominant arm flexion and extension strength were measured isokinetically, with even greater differences noted for dominant and nondominant shoulder extension. The powerful concentric internal rotation and extension movement pattern exhibited on the serve and overhead in tennis most likely created this unilateral strength development in adult highly skilled male players (12, 40).

# Elbow Joint Testing

Isokinetic normative data for the elbow joint is sparse in the current literature. The authors of this chapter are currently studying the important relationship between the elbow extensors and flexors in elite junior tennis players (see table 18.3, *a* and *b*).

A specific parameter important in testing the elbow joint for these athletes is the use of an extension stop 10° from full extension, due to the presence of

**Table 18.3a Elbow Extension/Flexion Peak Torque and Single-Repetition Work/Body Weight Ratios in Elite Junior Tennis Players Generated on a Cybex 6000 Isokinetic Dynamometer—Males**

| | Motion/speed (%) | Dominant arm | Nondominant arm |
|---|---|---|---|
| Flexion | | | |
| Peak torque | 90 | 20 | 20 |
| | 210 | 18 | 17 |
| | 300 | 18 | 18 |
| Work | 90 | 28 | 28 |
| | 210 | 18 | 18 |
| | 300 | 14 | 14 |
| Extension | | | |
| Peak torque | 90 | 21 | 18 |
| | 210 | 20 | 17 |
| | 300 | 20 | 17 |
| Work | 90 | 30 | 26 |
| | 210 | 20 | 17 |
| | 300 | 16 | 14 |
| Flexion/extension ratios | | | |
| Peak torque | 90 | 97 | 108 |
| | 210 | 92 | 102 |
| | 300 | 93 | 101 |
| Work | 90 | 95 | 106 |
| | 210 | 90 | 107 |
| | 300 | 84 | 97 |

**Table 18.3b   Isokinetic Elbow Extension/Flexion Peak Torque and
Single-Repetition Work/Body Weight Ratios in Elite Junior Tennis
Players Generated on a Cybex 6000 Isokinetic Dynamometer—Females**

|  | Motion/speed (%) | Dominant arm | Nondominant arm |
|---|---|---|---|
| Flexion |  |  |  |
| Peak torque | 90 | 15 | 16 |
|  | 210 | 15 | 15 |
|  | 300 | 15 | 15 |
| Work | 90 | 22 | 21 |
|  | 210 | 13 | 19 |
|  | 300 | 9 | 8 |
| Extension |  |  |  |
| Peak torque | 90 | 19 | 17 |
|  | 210 | 18 | 15 |
|  | 300 | 18 | 15 |
| Work | 90 | 25 | 22 |
|  | 210 | 15 | 13 |
|  | 300 | 11 | 9 |
| Flexion/extension ratios |  |  |  |
| Peak torque | 90 | 93 | 97 |
|  | 210 | 85 | 105 |
|  | 300 | 90 | 101 |
| Work | 90 | 89 | 99 |
|  | 210 | 90 | 113 |
|  | 300 | 87 | 102 |

an elbow flexion contracture of at least 5 to 10° degrees on the dominant, tennis-playing arm in many players (6, 17). Care is taken to be sure the athlete is not forcefully extending into end range of motion due to the possible impingement by posterior osteophytes (17).

A range of motion of –10° to 125° is normally targeted unless the athlete cannot achieve this range of motion comfortably in a pretesting evaluation with a universal goniometer. Speeds of 90, 210, and 300°/s are used for three-speed bilateral testing, with speeds of 210 and 300°/s used for two-speed bilateral testing. Similar testing on professional baseball players did not show a significant difference between the throwing and nonthrowing extremity in either elbow flexion or extension strength. A ratio of approximately 1:1 was found between the elbow extensor and flexor musculature (17). Further research is clearly needed in this area to better define the elbow extension/flexion strength and unilateral strength ratio in this population. Research using professional baseball players by Wilk, Arrigo, and Andrews (50) has reported a

10 to 20% dominance factor for the elbow flexors and a 5 to 15% dominance factor for the elbow extensors using a Biodex isokinetic dynamometer.

# Forearm and Wrist Testing

Ellenbecker (12) performed research involving isokinetic testing of the wrist flexors and extensors and forearm pronators and supinators. He tested the wrists and forearms of 22 highly skilled adult tennis players at 90, 210, and 300°/s. He measured significantly greater wrist flexion, extension, and forearm pronation for the dominant arm using bilateral velocity spectrum testing on a Cybex II dynamometer (see tables 18.4 and 18.5). Testing specifics included

### Table 18.4a  Isokinetic Wrist Extension/Flexion Normative Data From Highly Skilled Adult Male Tennis Players

|  | Motion/speed (%) | Dominant | Nondominant |
|---|---|---|---|
| Wrist extension |  |  |  |
| Peak torque | 90 | 6 | 5 |
|  | 210 | 5 | 4 |
|  | 300 | 4 | 3 |
| Work | 90 | 5 | 4 |
|  | 210 | 2 | 1 |
|  | 300 | 1 | 1 |
| Wrist flexion |  |  |  |
| Peak torque | 90 | 8 | 8 |
|  | 210 | 8 | 7 |
|  | 300 | 7 | 6 |
| Work | 90 | 8 | 7 |
|  | 210 | 3 | 2 |
|  | 300 | 1 | 1 |

All numbers expressed in % of ft-lb relative to body weight in lb.

### Table 18.4b  Unilateral Wrist Extension/Flexion Ratios From Highly Skilled Adult Tennis Players

|  | Ratio/speed (%) | Dominant | Nondominant |
|---|---|---|---|
| Peak torque | 90 | 71 | 68 |
|  | 210 | 64 | 61 |
|  | 300 | 63 | 58 |
| Work | 90 | 64 | 61 |
|  | 210 | 61 | 57 |
|  | 300 | 62 | 55 |

### Table 18.5a Forearm Pronation/Supination Normative Data From Highly Skilled Adult Tennis Players

|  | Motion/speed (%) | Dominant | Nondominant |
|---|---|---|---|
| Forearm pronation |  |  |  |
| Peak torque | 90 | 6 | 5 |
|  | 210 | 5 | 4 |
|  | 300 | 4 | 3 |
| Work | 90 | 6 | 5 |
|  | 210 | 2 | 2 |
|  | 300 | 1 | 1 |
| Forearm supination |  |  |  |
| Peak torque | 90 | 5 | 5 |
|  | 210 | 4 | 4 |
|  | 300 | 3 | 3 |
| Work | 90 | 5 | 5 |
|  | 210 | 2 | 4 |
|  | 300 | 1 | 3 |

All numbers expressed in % of ft-lb relative to body weight in lb.

### Table 18.5b Unilateral Forearm Supination/Pronation Ratios From Highly Skilled Adult Tennis Players

|  | Ratio/speed (%) | Dominant | Nondominant |
|---|---|---|---|
| Peak torque | 90 | 93 | 98 |
|  | 210 | 88 | 104 |
|  | 300 | 83 | 101 |
| Work | 90 | 86 | 97 |
|  | 210 | 80 | 103 |
|  | 300 | 75 | 103 |

isolating the distal upper extremity by using a forearm strap and upper body-testing table provided by Cybex. A range of motion of 35° of wrist extension and 55° of wrist flexion were targeted using range of motion stops (12). Forearm pronation and supination testing took place, using 50° of forearm pronation and 50° of forearm supination range of motion secured with stops.

These results show that repetitive tennis play stimulates the development of muscular strength as measured on an isokinetic dynamometer. Nirschl and Sobel (36) initially reported a dominance factor in the distal upper extremity of 5% in recreational and 10 to 15% in competitive, elite level tennis players. The data from the 22 adult highly skilled players are in agreement with Nirschl and Sobel's findings, with a dominance factor of up to 30% measured at some speeds. Tables 18.4, *a* and *b*, and 18.5, *a* and *b*, also list the unilateral strength ratio that is calculated by the dynamometer's data reduction system by dividing the weaker muscle group into the stronger muscle in agonist/antagonist pairings. The extension/flexion ratios range between 60 and 70% for the dominant extremity, with supination/pronation ratios ranging between 75 and 80%. The increased activation of the forearm flexors and pronators during the acceleration phase of the serve and forehand provide a stimulus for the development of this characteristic flexor/pronator strength adaptation (6, 12, 17, 36, 40). This unilateral development of the distal upper extremity has been referred to as "King Kong" arm and is objectively quantified with distal isokinetic testing in this elite level population (17). Comparison of the dominant unilateral extension/flexion ratios between baseball players (50–59%) and tennis players (60–70%) shows much greater wrist extension strength development relative to the wrist flexors in the tennis players tested (12, 17). This increased activation of the wrist extensor musculature is prevalent in the backhand, forehand, and serve with biomechanical testing of elite players with EMG (40). The increased load on the wrist extensors in tennis players is thought to be one etiological factor in lateral humeral epicondylitis (36).

## Knee Joint Testing

Testing of the lower extremity has been done in tennis players. Ellenbecker and Roetert (18) tested 87 elite junior tennis players (62 male and 25 female) on a Cybex 6000 series dynamometer system. Testing took place at 180 and 300°/s with 5 repetitions used for data generation. Gravity correction and stabilization were used according to manufacturer's recommendations (7). A random determination of starting limb was followed to minimize the effects of learning.

Table 18.6, *a* and *b*, displays the knee extension/flexion data and hamstring/quadriceps unilateral strength ratios from the testing (18). Analysis of knee extension/flexion testing shows no significant bilateral difference, which is in contrast to most of the upper extremity isokinetic normative data reported previously in this chapter. Hamstring/quadriceps ratios range between 60 and 70% for peak torque and between 50 and 60% for single repetition work values. Read and Bellamy (38) tested 11 elite adult tennis players and compared them to age-matched track athletes. They found less power and lower work/body weight ratios in the tennis players, as well as no bilateral differences among tennis players using a Lido isokinetic dynamometer. No other lower extremity isokinetic studies on tennis players are currently available in the literature for discussion. In general, these data indicate that bilateral symmetry with respect to the hamstrings and quadriceps should be expected in tennis players.

## Trunk Testing

Earlier discussion in this chapter provided detailed descriptions and normative data on upper and lower extremity testing in the tennis player. The trunk

**Table 18.6a    Isokinetic Knee Extension/Flexion Peak Torque, Single-Repetition Work/Body Weight Ratios, and Unilateral Strength Ratios From Elite Junior Tennis Players Generated on a Cybex 6000 Isokinetic Dynamometer—Males**

| Parameter/speed | Left | | Right | | | |
|---|---|---|---|---|---|---|
| | Mean | SD | Mean | SD | t-value | Sig |
| Knee extension | | | | | | |
| Torque/BW 180 | 60.2 | 21.7 | 60.5 | 22.5 | 0.30 | 0.766 |
| Torque/BW 300 | 53.8 | 6.8 | 54.0 | 8.8 | 0.22 | 0.827 |
| Work/BW 180 | 61.4 | 23.5 | 62.1 | 24.5 | 0.47 | 0.644 |
| Work/BW 300 | 54.1 | 12.7 | 52.8 | 12.6 | 1.72 | 0.090 |
| Knee flexion | | | | | | |
| Torque/BW 180 | 36.6 | 13.5 | 36.0 | 13.5 | 1.04 | 0.305 |
| Torque/BW 300 | 33.7 | 5.9 | 32.6 | 5.9 | 1.41 | 0.168 |
| Work/BW 180 | 35.2 | 13.6 | 35.2 | 14.3 | 0.03 | 0.973 |
| Work/BW 300 | 29.5 | 8.1 | 29.5 | 7.7 | 0.06 | 0.954 |

All values expressed in ft-lb relative to body weight in lb.

**Table 18.6b    Isokinetic Knee Extension/Flexion Peak Torque, Single-Repetition Work/Body Weight Ratios, and Unilateral Strength Ratios From Elite Junior Tennis Players Generated on a Cybex 6000 Isokinetic Dynamometer—Females**

| Parameter/speed | Left | | Right | | | |
|---|---|---|---|---|---|---|
| | Mean | SD | Mean | SD | t-value | Sig |
| Knee extension | | | | | | |
| Torque/BW 300 | 44.4 | 5.5 | 47.4 | 6.7 | 2.31 | 0.049 |
| Work/BW 300 | 43.3 | 7.6 | 42.6 | 7.2 | 0.60 | 0.554 |
| Knee flexion | | | | | | |
| Torque/BW 300 | 30.7 | 6.1 | 31.3 | 4.9 | 0.57 | 0.584 |
| Work/BW 300 | 27.2 | 7.0 | 26.5 | 5.9 | 0.96 | 0.348 |

All values expressed in ft-lb relative to body weight in lb.

plays an integral role in the kinetic chain by linking the lower body to the upper body (23, 41). The trunk must transfer force, arriving through the legs and hips from the ground, to the upper body to allow effective stroke production (23, 41, 48). Fabrocini (22) found that without this transfer of force via trunk rotation, the tennis strokes lacked both power and control.

To date, only one study has been undertaken to isokinetically document trunk extension and flexion strength in elite junior tennis players. Roetert and coworkers (43) tested 60 nationally ranked junior tennis players between the ages of 13 and 17 using a Cybex TEF modular component system. Testing speeds of 60 and 120°/s were chosen due to their predominance in the isokinetic spinal testing literature (47). Following a standardized warm-up, subjects performed 5 repetitions at 60°/s and 15 repetitions at 120°/s. A 30 s rest period was again used between testing speeds for specificity reasons (48).

Results of the testing are listed in table 18.7, *a* and *b*. Of particular significance was the finding that the trunk flexors were consistently stronger than the trunk extensors. Unilateral trunk flexion/extension ratios ranged from 102 to 122%. This is in contrast to the findings of Timm (47), who consistently reported greater trunk extensor strength in 28,176 normal subjects compared to trunk flexor strength. The forceful trunk flexion movement pattern that occurs during the acceleration phase of the tennis serve is immediately preceded by an eccentric stretch to the abdominals, which may explain this strength adaptation by the trunk flexor musculature in these elite tennis players.

These findings are a prime example of how isokinetic strength data has influenced the design and execution of conditioning programs for tennis players.

### Table 18.7a Trunk Flexion/Extension Data, and Trunk Flexion/Extension Ratios for Males and Females

| | Data | | | | Ratios |
|---|---|---|---|---|---|
| | Peak torque/body weight | | Work/body weight | | Peak torque/ body weight |
| | Flexion | Extension | Flexion | Extension | |
| Males | | | | | |
| 60°/s | 126.4% | 123.6% | 82.7% | 88.6% | 102% |
| 120°/s | 118.6% | 105.2% | 69.5% | 75.8% | 112% |
| Females | | | | | |
| 60°/s | 99.8% | 90.3% | 70.6% | 66.6% | 110% |
| 120°/s | 97.4% | 79.8% | 61.0% | 53.9% | 122% |

### Table 18.7b Unilateral Trunk Flexion/Extension Ratios From Elite Junior Tennis Players

| Ratios (%) | Peak torque | Work |
|---|---|---|
| Males 60°/s | 102 | 93 |
| Males 120°/s | 112 | 92 |
| Females 60°/s | 110 | 106 |
| Females 120°/s | 122 | 113 |

Due to the high incidence of lower back injuries in recreational and professional tennis players (24), sports medicine and sport science professionals are now recommending trunk extension strengthening exercises along with the standard abdominal routines used for years (48). It is generally agreed that the use of trunk extension exercises will promote a greater degree of balance between the muscles that flex and extend the trunk and provide greater stabilization of the spine during the rotational and flexion/extension movement patterns that are inherent in tennis strokes (24, 48).

Further research is clearly indicated in many areas developed in this chapter. A greater understanding of trunk rotation strength is of prime importance due to the rotational forces imparted to the trunk with tennis play (24).

# Isokinetic Testing and Functional Performance in Tennis

In all areas of isokinetic exercise and testing applications, the role and relationship between isolated joint testing and functional performance is of prime importance and interest. Several studies involving tennis players and isokinetics have examined the relationship between isolated joint testing and functional performance. Ellenbecker, Davies, and Rowinski (15) tested and trained 22 collegiate tennis players over a six-week period using either concentric-only or eccentric-only internal and external rotation. Following the six-week training paradigm, significant strength improvements were measured in both the concentric and eccentric training groups, but only the group that trained concentrically for the six-week study period had a significant increase (mean = 8.42 mph) in postimpact ball velocity measured with cinematography. The eccentric training group showed no significant improvement in postimpact ball velocity with over half of the subjects actually showing a decrease in the speed of their serve. The direct cause of this increase in ball velocity could not be attributed solely to increased strength in the shoulder internal and external rotators, since the tennis serve consists of a complex series of timed rotations and of whole body segment contributions.

Further research was performed by Ellenbecker (12), who tested shoulder internal/external rotation, shoulder flexion/extension, and wrist flexion/extension and forearm pronation to attempt to find a correlation between isokinetically measured strength and ball velocity measured with a radar gun. No significant correlation was found between any movement pattern tested isokinetically in 22 adult tennis players and average or peak serving velocity. Mont and coworkers (34) performed a similar concentric and eccentric training study. With the addition of a control group, Mont and coworkers (34) tested and trained 30 elite adult tennis players using a concentric-only or eccentric-only training program for isokinetic shoulder internal and external rotation. They found increases of greater than 11% in both the concentric and eccentric training groups, as well as increased strength. An improvement in muscular endurance was also measured among the trained subjects, who were able to maintain their serve velocity in a functional fatigue serving protocol greater than the control group. The results of these studies show that a six-week period of isokinetic training does increase concentric and eccentric shoulder internal and external rotation strength (15, 34) but that a direct mechanism for this increased serving velocity has not been proven from the isolated training literature.

One final investigation studied the relationship between isokinetic testing and a functional "on court" test. Roetert and coworkers (43) tested 60 tennis players for trunk extension and flexion strength and compared the strength results with the subjects' ability to throw a six-pound medicine ball using forehand, backhand, and overhead and reverse overhead tosses. The study revealed significant correlations ($r$ = .42–.82) for the medicine ball tosses and the isolated isokinetic trunk test.

# Eccentric Testing Implications for the Tennis Player

Eccentric isokinetic training and testing has been performed on tennis players (15, 27, 34) but to a much lesser extent than concentric isokinetic testing and training. Eccentric training over a six-week period produced significant concentric strength improvements in both the internal and external rotators in one study using collegiate tennis players (15), while eccentric training produced 11% improvements in both concentric and eccentric internal and external rotation strength in adult players (34).

Kennedy, Altchek, and Glick (27) tested both concentric and eccentric external rotation strength at 150°/s using a Lido isokinetic dynamometer. Results of their testing showed a significant difference, 1.46 vs. 1.19, in the eccentric/concentric ratio between the dominant and nondominant extremity, respectively. Ellenbecker (15) also found eccentric/concentric external rotation ratios to average 1.68 through the velocity spectrum on the dominant arm. Only the dominant arm was tested in that study so bilateral comparisons could not be made.

These findings suggest a mode-specific strength improvement on the dominant arm with respect to eccentric external rotation. Since the rotator cuff is highly active during the follow-through phase following impact of the ball, indicating eccentric decelerative work, a dominance effect is only present in the external rotators with eccentric testing. Application of this research again has ramifications for conditioning programs of tennis players. Any training regimen should include both concentric and eccentric muscular actions, in particular for muscle groups like the external rotators, which specifically function in an eccentric decelerative pattern (40, 48). Further research must be done to better understand the eccentric muscular capabilities in the tennis player and to delineate better parameters for the application of eccentric isokinetic training for tennis players and other athletes.

# Summary

Review of the available literature on isokinetic muscular performance of tennis players demonstrates selective strength development and muscular adaptations due to the inherent stresses in the game of tennis. Repetitive tennis play produces muscular imbalances that may subject the tennis player to injury and negatively affect performance. Significantly greater strength has consistently been measured in the dominant arm of tennis players in the shoulder internal rotators, flexors, and extensors, wrist flexors and extensors, as well as forearm pronators. No bilateral differences have been measured in shoulder external rotation strength. Symmetrical strength has been measured in the quadriceps and hamstrings musculature in the lower extremity. Muscular imbalances have been identified in the shoulder and trunk, with characteristic muscular adaptations secondary to the inherent movement patterns required for successful tennis play. Baseline isokinetic testing can also assist in designing training programs to help prevent injuries and increase performance. Further research is needed on all populations of tennis players, from the elite junior to the competitive senior player, as well as a greater understanding of eccentric isokinetic muscular responses and ultimately their relationship to both functional performance and injury prevention.

# References

1. Arrigo CA, Wilk KE, Andrews JR. 1994. Peak torque and maximum work repetition during isokinetic testing of the shoulder internal and external rotators. *Isok Exerc Sci* 4(4): 171–75.

2. Bassett RW, Browne AO, Morrey BF, An KN. 1990. Glenohumeral muscle force and moment mechanics in a position of shoulder instability. *J Biomechanics* 23: 405.

3. Brown LE, Whitehurst M, Findley BW, Gilbert R, Buchalter DN. 1995. Isokinetic load range during shoulder rotation exercise in elite male junior tennis players. *J Strength Cond Res* 9(3): 160–64.

4. Chandler TJ, Kibler WB, Stracener EC, Ziegler AK, Pace B. 1992. Shoulder strength, power, and endurance in college tennis players. *Am J Sports Med* 20: 455–58.

5. Chandler TJ, Kibler WB, Uhl TL et al. 1990. Flexibility comparisons of junior elite tennis players to other athletes. *Am J Sports Med* 18: 134–36.

6. Chinn CJ, Priest JD, Kent BE. 1974. Upper extremity range of motion, grip strength, and girth in highly skilled tennis players. *Phys Ther* 54: 474–82.

7. Cybex Inc., a division of Henley Healthcare. 1992. *Cybex applications manual.* Austin, TX: Cybex.

8. Davies GJ. 1992. *A compendium of isokinetics in clinical usage.* 4th ed. La Crosse, WI: S & S.

9. Deutsch E, Deutsch SL, Douglas PS. 1988. Exercise training for competitive tennis. *Clin Sports Med* 7: 417–27.

10. Dillman CJ. 1991. The upper extremity in tennis and throwing athletes. Paper presented at the United States Tennis Association annual meeting at Tucson, Arizona.

11. Docherty D. 1982. A comparison of heart rate responses in racquet games. *Br J Sports Med* 1(6): 96–100.

12. Ellenbecker TS. 1991. A total arm strength isokinetic profile of highly skilled tennis players. *Isok Exerc Sci* 1(1): 9–21.

13. Ellenbecker TS. 1992. Shoulder internal and external rotation strength and range of motion of highly skilled junior tennis players. *Isok Exerc Sci* 2: 1–8.

14. Ellenbecker TS. 1995. Rehabilitation of shoulder and elbow injuries in tennis players. *Clin Sports Med* 14(1): 87–110.

15. Ellenbecker TS, Davies GJ, Rowinski MJ. 1988. Concentric versus eccentric isokinetic strengthening of the rotator cuff: Objective data versus functional test. *Am J Sports Med* 16: 64–69.

16. Ellenbecker TS, Feiring DC, DeHart RL, Rich M. 1992. Isokinetic shoulder strength: Coronal versus scapular plane testing in unilaterally dominant upper extremity athletes. *Phys Ther* 72(Suppl): 580.

17. Ellenbecker TS, Mattalino AJ. 1996. *The elbow in sport*. Champaign, IL: Human Kinetics.

18. Ellenbecker TS, Roetert EP. 1995. Concentric isokinetic quadriceps and hamstring strength in elite junior tennis players. *Isok Exerc Sci* 5: 3–6.

19. Ellenbecker TS, Roetert EP, Piorkowski PA, Schulz DA. 1996. Glenohumeral joint internal and external rotation range of motion in elite junior tennis players. *J Orthop Sports Phys Ther* 24(6): 336–41.

20. Ellenbecker TS, Roetert EP. 1999. Isokinetic muscular fatigue testing of shoulder internal and external rotation in elite junior tennis players. *J Orthop Sports Phys Ther* 29: 275-281.

21. Elliot B, Marsh T, Blanksby B. 1986. A three-dimensional cinematographic analysis of the tennis serve. *Int J Sport Biomechanics* 2: 260–71.

22. Fabrocini B. 1995. The planning of a powerful trunk for tennis. *Strength and Conditioning* 17: 25–29.

23. Groppel JL. 1992. *High tech tennis*. Champaign, IL: Human Kinetics.

24. Hainline B. 1995. Low back injury. *Clin Sports Med* 14(1): 241–65.

25. Harryman DT, Sidles JA, Clark JM et al. 1990. Translation of the humeral head on the glenoid with passive glenohumeral motion. *J Bone Joint Surg (Am)* 72: 1334–43.

26. Kamien M. 1989. The incidence of tennis elbow and other injuries in tennis players at the Royal Kings Park Tennis Club of Western Australia from October 1983 to September 1984. *Aust J Sci Med Sport* 21: 18–22.

27. Kennedy K, Altchek DW, Glick IV. 1993. Concentric and eccentric isokinetic rotator cuff ratios in skilled tennis players. *Isok Exerc Sci* 3(3): 155–59.

28. Kibler WB, Chandler TJ, Livingston BP, Roetert EP. 1996. Shoulder range of motion in elite tennis players. *Am J Sports Med* 24(3): 279–85.

29. Kibler WB, McQueen C, Uhl T. 1988. Fitness evaluation and fitness findings in competitive junior tennis players. *Clin Sports Med* 7: 403–16.

30. Koziris LP, Kraemer WJ, Triplett NT, Fry J, Bauer JG, Pedro A, Clemson A, Connors J. 1991. Strength imbalances in women tennis players [abstract]. *Med Sci Sports Exerc* 23(Suppl): 253.

31. Kraemer WJ, Triplett NT, Fry AC, Koziris LP, Bauer JE, Lynch JM, McConnell T, Newton RU, Gordon SE, Nelson RC, Knuttgen HG. 1995. An in-depth sports medicine profile of women college tennis players. *J Sports Rehab* 4(2): 79–98.

32. Lehman RC. 1988. Shoulder pain in the competitive tennis player. *Clin Sports Med* 7: 309–27.

33. Mikesky AE, Wigglesworth JK, Edwards JE, Roetert EP. 1993. Comparison of rotational shoulder strength between baseball pitchers and tennis players. *Med Sci Sports Exerc* 25(5) (S171): 963.

34. Mont MA, Cohen DB, Campbell KR, Gravare K, Mathur SK. 1994. Isokinetic concentric versus eccentric training of shoulder rotators with functional evaluation of performance enhancement in elite tennis players. *Am J Sports Med* 22(4): 513–17.

35. Ng LR, Kramer JS. 1991. Shoulder rotator torques in female tennis and nontennis players. *J Orthop Sports Phys Ther* 13(1): 40–46.

36. Nirschl RP, Sobel J. 1981. Conservative treatment of tennis elbow. *Phys Sports Med* 9: 43–54.

37. Priest JD, Nagel DA. 1976. Tennis shoulder. *Am J Sports Med* 4: 28–42.

38. Read MTF, Bellamy MJ. 1990. Comparison of hamstring/quadriceps isokinetic strength ratios and power in tennis, squash, and track athletes. *Br J Sports Med* 24: 178–82.

39. Reece LA, Fricker PA, Maguire KF. 1986. Injuries to elite young tennis players at the Australian Institute of Sport. *Aust J Sci Med Sports*.

40. Rhu KN, McCormick J, Jobe FW et al. 1988. An electromyographic analysis of shoulder function in tennis players. *Am J Sports Med* 16: 481–85.

41. Roetert EP, Ellenbecker TS, Chu DA, Bugg BS. 1997. Tennis-specific shoulder and trunk strength training. *Strength and Condition* 19(3): 31–39.

42. Roetert EP, Ellenbecker TS, Brown SW. In press. Shoulder internal and external rotation range of motion in elite junior tennis players: A longitudinal analysis. *J Strength Cond Res*.

43. Roetert EP, McCormick TJ, Brown SW, Ellenbecker TS. 1996. Relationship between isokinetic and functional trunk strength in elite junior tennis players. *Isok Exerc Sci* 6: 15–20.

44. Saha AK. 1983. Reprint. Mechanism of shoulder movements and a plea for the recognition of "zero position" of glenohumeral joint. *Clin Orthop Rel Res* 73: 3–10.

45. Shapiro R, Stine RL. 1992. Shoulder rotation velocities. Technical report submitted to the Lexington Clinic, Lexington, KY.

46. Soderberg GJ, Blaschak MJ. 1987. Shoulder internal and external rotation peak torque production through a velocity spectrum in differing positions. *J Orthop Sports Phys Ther* 8(11): 518–24.

47. Timm KE. 1995. Clinical Applications of a normative database for the Cybex TEF and torso spinal isokinetic dynamometers. *Isok Exerc Sci* 5: 43–49.

48. United States Tennis Association, Roetert EP, Ellenbecker TE. 1998. *Complete conditioning for tennis.* Champaign, IL: Human Kinetics.

49. Warner JJP, Micheli LJ, Arslanian LE et al. 1990. Patterns of flexibility, laxity, and strength in normal shoulders and in shoulders with instability and impingement. *Am J Sports Med* 18: 366–75.

50. Wilk KE, Arrigo CA, Andrews JR. 1991. Standardized isokinetic testing protocol for the throwing shoulder: The throwers series. *Isokinetics Exerc Sci* 1(2): 63–71.

51. Winge S, Jorgensen U, Neilsen AL. 1989. Epidemiology of injuries in Danish championship tennis. *Int J Sports Med* 10: 368–71.

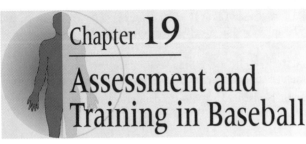

# Chapter 19

## Assessment and Training in Baseball

Joseph F. Signorile and Kiersten Kluckhulm

The particular use of isokinetics as an assessment and training tool for the baseball pitcher is often dictated by the objectives of the researcher or coach. In general, biomechanical studies of the pitching motion have reported extremely high values for both angular velocity and acceleration. These studies have also demonstrated the importance that sequential movements play in producing fastball velocity. However, most isokinetic laboratory evaluations of pitchers have concentrated on evaluations of functional weakness and muscular imbalance. Therefore, they have customarily been performed on isolated joints at low contractile speeds, and researchers typically have not attempted to simulate the high speed, multijoint pattern characteristic of the throwing motion.

This chapter provides a short review of the kinetics, biomechanics, and kinesiology of the pitching motion. It then reviews isokinetic studies performed using specific isolated movements and isokinetic speeds for the purpose of descriptive analyses, diagnostics, injury prevention, and training prescription. Next, studies correlating selected isokinetic variables with ball speed are presented and discussed. In addition, models using isokinetic variables to predict fastball velocity are introduced. Finally, issues such as testing speed and positions, contractile modes, open and closed chain kinetics, isolated versus multijoint movements, and variable selection are addressed in terms of the existing studies and implications for future research.

## Kinematic and Kinetic Analyses as a Template for Isokinetic Testing

To understand the use of isokinetic testing as a functional tool for the analysis of the pitching motion, one must understand the correct form and temporal sequencing pattern associated with the pitch, as well as the forces that cause or limit the related movements. Therefore, this section provides a short review of the kinetics of the pitching motion.

## The Kinetic Chain

Researchers have described pitching as a total body activity that produces velocity through the sequential activation of body parts in a kinetically linked system (23, 36, 54). The additive effects of the segments of the kinetic chain moving in a sequential pattern allow maximal speed to be produced during the pitching motion.

## Movement Phases and Joint Action

Most analyses of the pitching motion describe at least three major phases: cocking, acceleration, and follow-through (see figure 19.1) (36, 58). However, some researchers have described four, five, or six phases (see figure 19.2) (5, 10, 15, 16, 37, 52, 60).

Each phase has specific movement "landmarks," which define it. The stance phase is the preparatory phase preceding the first overt movement in the pitching motion. It is affected by the pitch being thrown (5, 23) and the style of the pitcher (8, 48).

The windup phase begins with the first overt movement and ends when the lead leg is maximally lifted and the throwing hand is removed from the glove (5, 10, 15, 16, 60). In five- and six-phase descriptions, the cocking phase is next. It begins at the end of the windup and ends when the pitching arm reaches maximal external rotation (5, 23). In a three-phase model, the cocking phase incorporates both the stance and windup phases and ends with maximum external shoulder rotation (36). In the six-phase description the cocking phase is further subdivided into a stride phase and an arm-cocking phase. The stride

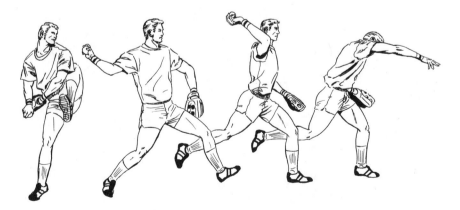

**Figure 19.1** A three-phase model of the pitching motion including, in sequence from left to right, the windup, cocking, and acceleration and follow-through.

From Post 1986.

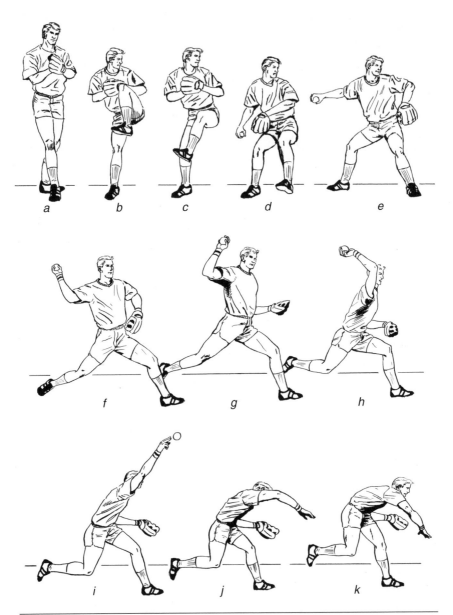

**Figure 19.2** A six-phase model of the pitching motion presenting the wind-up (*a-b*), the stride (*c-e*), arm cocking (*f-h*), arm acceleration (*h-i*), arm deceleration (*i-j*) and follow-through (*j-k*).

From *Journal of Orthopaedic and Sports Physical Therapy* 1993.

phase begins at the end of the windup and ends when the front foot contacts the mound (16). The arm-cocking phase then begins, and it ends with maximal external shoulder rotation (16).

All analyses contain an acceleration phase (10, 15, 16, 60) beginning with the internal rotation of the shoulder following the cocking phase and ending with the release of the ball. In the three-phase and five-phase descriptions the time from ball release until the end of the throwing motion is termed the follow-through (5, 23, 36, 60). In the six-phase description, the final phase is divided into an arm deceleration phase, which ends when the arm reaches maximal internal rotation, and a follow-through phase, which continues from that point to the end of the pitching motion (10, 15, 16, 52, 60).

## Kinetics of the Pitching Phases

The range of motion, torque, speed, and acceleration values during these phases vary considerably and are quite impressive. Reported peak values for angular velocity at the shoulder range from 3,340 to 9,198 °/s (10, 36). Peak elbow angular velocities have been reported between 2,200 and 6,993 °/s (14, 36, 60). Acceleration values of 500,000 °/s$^2$ and -500,000 °/s$^2$ have been reported for the acceleration and deceleration phases, respectively (36). Correlation coefficients of .86 ($p < .01$) and -.97 ($p < .01$) have been reported between ball velocity and the degree of external rotation and the duration of the acceleration phase, respectively (58).

Forces at and about the individual joints have also been examined. High rotary torque (17, 41), varus torque (14, 16, 60), compressive force, and shear force (16) have all been reported at the point of maximal external shoulder rotation. In addition, both shear force and flexion torque have been shown to increase during the acceleration phase (14, 16, 60), and the highest compressive forces on the elbow have been reported during arm deceleration (14, 60). These data are indicative of the impact that sequential activation of body parts within the pitching kinetic link system can have on the stresses produced at the shoulder and elbow.

# Kinesiological Analyses

In addition to understanding the kinetics and kinematics of the pitch, information concerning muscle function during the pitching motion is also helpful in planning a testing protocol. To that end, the following section provides kinesiological and electromyographical analyses of the pitch.

## Muscle Utilization Patterns During Selected Phases

A number of analyses have examined the muscle utilization patterns throughout the pitching motion. While it is beyond the scope of this chapter to provide an exhaustive review of the literature, it may be of interest to provide a short description of these patterns throughout the phases of the pitch.

Electromyographical (EMG) analyses have shown that during the early cocking phase, the activity of the deltoids increases dramatically, and toward the end of this phase the subscapularis, infraspinatus, and teres minor begin to show increasingly greater activity as the joint capsule is prestretched in external rotation (25). The activity levels of all these muscles are then minimized during the acceleration phase as the shoulder releases its stored energy, and the activity of the pectoralis major, latissimus dorsi, serratus anterior, rotators, and muscles of the upper and lower extremities (59) come into play (26). Finally, the rotator cuff muscles and the biceps show maximal activity during the follow-through, presumably in an attempt to decelerate the arm (26).

It has been shown that more skilled pitchers show better sequential utilization patterns than their less skilled counterparts (18, 59). The EMG data from these studies confirm the importance of the successive utilization of functional muscles in a kinetic chain to maximize throwing (2, 23, 35, 54).

# Isokinetic Strength Evaluations of Pitchers

The majority of the studies that have examined isokinetic strength in pitchers have addressed the topic from the point of view of potential injury mechanisms, injury prevention, and treatment. Given this fact, these studies have targeted the anatomical structure most susceptible to injury, the rotator cuff. This is quite understandable due to the forces at and about the shoulder joint that were reported earlier in this chapter (14, 16, 17, 24, 39, 60).

## Isokinetic Evaluations of the Shoulder

Cook and coworkers (7) examined antagonistic strength ratios for the dominant (D) and nondominant (ND) shoulders of 15 college-aged pitchers and 13 age-matched nonpitchers. Testing was performed on a Cybex II dynamometer (Cybex, a division of Lumex, Inc., Ronkonkoma, NY) using the Cybex upper body testing and exercise table (UBXT). The motions tested included shoulder extension and flexion and shoulder internal and external rotation. Shoulder extension/flexion was blocked at 180° of flexion and 0° of extension. Shoulder internal and external rotations were both blocked at 60°. Evaluations were performed at 180°/s and 300°/s. Shoulder range of motion was also evaluated using a standard 360° goniometer. Strength ratios reported were flexion/extension (Flex/Ext) and external rotation/internal rotation (ER/IR).

These researchers reported significant differences for the pitchers' throwing (D) shoulders versus their nonthrowing (ND) shoulders in ER/IR ratios at 180°/s (D = .70, ND = .81) and 300°/s (D = .70, ND = .81). However, the pitchers demonstrated no significant differences in Flex/Ext ratio for either shoulder. For the nonpitchers, no significant differences were seen in ER/IR between the dominant (D) and nondominant (ND) shoulder, but a significant difference in the shoulder Flex/Ext strength ratio was reported at 300°/s (D = .99, ND = .76). The researchers attributed the differences in D versus ND ratios in the pitchers to weaker external rotation strength in the throwing arm versus the nonthrowing arm in the majority of the pitchers. In addition, at 180°/s, five of the pitchers also exhibited increased internal rotational strength that would serve to further decrease the ER/IR ratio. When shoulder strength ratios were compared for the ND shoulder between the pitchers and nonpitchers, no significant differences were reported for any motion or speed. However, for the D shoulder, all strength ratios proved significant between the groups.

In explaining the differences in shoulder rotational strength ratios between the D and ND shoulders of the pitchers, Cook and coworkers (7) cited the theory, presented separately by Jobe and Ling (27) and Pappas, Zawacki, and Sullivan (36), that atrophy of the infraspinatus due to subscapular nerve entrapment may result from repetitive overhead throwing. They also stated that the impact of sport-specific stresses, whether they were the result of training, competing, or both, was punctuated by the fact that the ND shoulders of both the pitchers and nonpitchers exhibited no significant differences in the Flex/Ext or ER/IR ratios, while the pitchers' D shoulder strength ratios were significantly lower than the nonpitchers' for all speeds and directions tested.

The pattern for shoulder range of motion reported by Cook and her coworkers (7) was similar to that presented earlier by King, Brelsford, and Tullos (30). These researchers reported an increase in external shoulder rotation and a decrease in internal shoulder rotation for the dominant shoulder compared to the nondominant shoulder (30). This pattern was not seen in the nonpitchers. Citing the findings of DePalma, Cooke, and Prabhaker (9) and Mottice (34), Cook and her coworkers hypothesized that both the IR/ER ratio imbalances and the Flex/Ext imbalances could be partially explained by simple differences in the muscle volumes between the related muscle groups.

Alderink and Kuck (1) studied 26 high school and collegiate pitchers, ages 14 to 21. They employed a Cybex II and UBXT. Measurements of peak torque during shoulder abduction/adduction, flexion/extension, horizontal abduction/adduction, and external/internal rotation were made for the shoulders of the dominant (D) and nondominant (ND) arms at 90, 120, 210, and 300°/s. Results showed significant differences between the D and ND shoulders for adduction at 90°/s and 120°/s, flexion at 210°/s, extension at all speeds, and external rotation at 210°/s and 300°/s. No significant differences were seen between the D and ND shoulders for horizontal adduction or abduction at any speed tested.

Brown and associates (6) compared isokinetic strength of the internal and external shoulder rotators between pitchers and other major league players. A Cybex II dynamometer was used with the subject in a neutral standing position. Test speeds were 180, 240, and 300°/s. The results showed that, for both motions, the pitchers were capable of producing greater mean peak and mean average torque for both the dominant and nondominant shoulders at all testing speeds. They also reported greater torque production for the D versus ND shoulder for all testing conditions. No differences were found between the rotation ratios for either shoulder in either group at any of the speeds tested.

Wilk and coworkers (61) examined the strength characteristics of the internal and external shoulder rotators. Subjects were 150 professional pitchers (mean age = 23.4 yr, mean weight = 199 lb), and testing was performed on a Biodex multijoint dynamometer (Biodex Corp., Shirley, NY). Testing was performed at 90° of shoulder abduction and 90° of elbow flexion. In addition, the subject was seated in the Biodex accessory chair and was restrained at the waist, shoulders, and upper arm using Velcro strapping. Gravity compensation was employed. Testing was performed at 180°/s and 300°/s. The researchers reported a significant difference in external rotator torque between the throwing shoulder (T) and nonthrowing shoulder (NT) at 180°/s (T = 34.5 ± 6.2 ft-lb, NT = 36.5 ± 6.8 ft-lb) but not at 300°/sec. They also reported a significant difference in the mean torque by body weight ratio of the external rotators at 180°/s (T = 17.5 ± 2.9 ft-lb, NT = 18.7 ± 3.3 ft-lb) (61). No other significant differences were detected between the T and NT shoulders.

The results reported by Wilk and coworkers (61), showing no significant differences in internal rotator torque between the T and NT shoulders, are similar to those that were reported by Alderink and Kuck (1) and Ivey and coworkers (22) but are in opposition to those reported by Brown and associates (6) in professional pitchers and Hinton (21) in high school pitchers. In contrast, the results that showed significant differences in external rotator torque between the T and NT shoulder (61) are in agreement with those of Hinton (21) and Brown and associates (6) but opposed to the results reported by Alderink and Kuck (1). It should also be noted that Wilk, Andrews, and Arrigo (62) and Brown and associates (6) reported no significant differences in rotation ratios between the dominant and nondominant shoulders, while Cook and coworkers (7) did.

A recent study of 125 professional pitchers examined internal and external rotator peak torque and work on a Cybex 300 series dynamometer at 210°/s and 300°/s (11). No significant differences were found in internal rotation peak torque or single repetition work for either speed. However, external rotation peak torque and work were significantly higher in the dominant versus the nondominant arm at both speeds.

In a study examining shoulder abductor and adductor strength in 85 professional baseball pitchers, Wilk, Andrews, and Arrigo (62) reported no significant differences in mean peak torque between the throwing (T) and nonthrowing (NT) side for the shoulder abductors. However, there was a significant difference between the throwing and nonthrowing sides for the adductor values at both 180°/s (T = 68.1 ± 12.6, NT = 62.1 ± 10.5) and 300°/s (T = 61.0 ± 12.5, NT = 54.6 ± 13.2). In addition, there was a significant difference in abductor/adductor ratios at 180°/s (T = 82.5%, NT = 66.0%) and 300°/s (T = 93.8%, NT = 70.3%) (62). They noted that the data reported, showing no significant difference between the T and NT shoulder abductors, were similar to that reported by Alderink and Kuck (1), who also found no significant difference between the abductors of the T and NT shoulders in high school- and college-aged pitchers.

In their evaluation of internal and external rotator strength in professional baseball players reported earlier in this section, Wilk and coworkers (61) noted that testing of the external rotators would be more appropriately done in an isokinetic eccentric mode, and that such a study would be "a significant contribution to the current literature". They cite as the bases for their statement the work of both Jobe and coworkers (25, 26) and Dillman, Fleisig, and Andrews (10) showing that the primary responsibility of the external rotators is the deceleration of the arm during the follow-through. Two studies have provided such eccentric data.

A study by Mikesky and associates (33) examined isokinetic internal and external shoulder rotator strengths and elbow flexion and extension strengths, both eccentrically and concentrically. Twenty-five collegiate baseball pitchers were evaluated at 1.6, 3.7, and 5.3 rad/s (90, 210, and 300°/s). The internal rotators were found to be stronger than the external rotators both eccentrically and concentrically, producing external to internal ratios of between 62% and 81%. The eccentric strength of the rotators averaged 114% of the concentric strength. The concentric and eccentric extension-to-flexion ratios ranged from 71% to 110% and the eccentric values averaged 33% higher than the concentric values.

A later study by Sirota and coworkers (50) evaluated 25 professional pitchers using a Kin-Com isokinetic dynamometer. Testing was performed eccentrically and concentrically at 60 and 120°/s. They reported that eccentric values were significantly higher than concentric values for both internal and external rotation. In addition, they found no significant differences in mean torque for either motion between the throwing and nonthrowing arms.

## Isokinetic Evaluations of the Legs

The legs comprise the initial segments in the kinetic chain that transfers force and velocity to the shoulder girdle through the core muscles of the body. Given this fact, it is surprising that little attention has been dedicated to the evaluation of leg strength in pitchers.

A study by Tippett (52) did examine isokinetic strength and active range of motion in the stance and kicking legs of 16 college baseball pitchers. Subjects were tested on a Cybex II dynamometer. The following motions were evaluated: long-sitting ankle plantar/dorsiflexion at 30°/s and 180°/s, sitting knee extension at 60°/s and 240°/s, supine hip flexion/extension at 60°/s and 240°/s, sidelying hip abduction/adduction at 30°/s and 180°/s, and long-sitting hip internal/external rotation at 30°/s and 180°/s. In the kick leg versus the stance leg, they reported greater strength of the dorsiflexors at 30°/s, the hip flexors at 60°/s and the hamstring at 240°/s. However, the strength of the external rotators on the stance leg was greater than the external rotators of the kick leg at 180°/s. Tippett (52) explained these differences as products of the pitching motion itself as the kick leg is lifted and subsequently planted, and the stance leg rotates to transfer torque and velocity from the lower to the upper extremities.

# Studies Relating Isokinetic Variables to Ball Velocity

Using a Cybex II dynamometer and UBXT to stabilize the trunk and isolate the individual segments of the upper extremity, Pedegana and associates (38) examined the relationship of upper extremity strength to throwing speed. The testing speeds used were 60°/s and 180°/s for the shoulder and elbow and 30°/s and 120°/s for the wrist and forearm. For their analyses it appears that the researchers used the speed that produced the highest torque value for a particular movement. The results of their simple linear regression analysis are reproduced in table 19.1. As can be seen from the table, the movements that showed a significant relationship to ball speed were elbow extension, shoulder external rotation, shoulder extension, shoulder flexion, and wrist extension, with wrist extension explaining nearly twice the variance of any other variable.

Pedegana and associates (38) also developed a predictive equation for ball velocity:

$$V = 94.90 - 0.14 \text{ (ELXT)} - 1.18 \text{ (WEXT)},$$
where: ELXT = elbow extension and WEXT = wrist extension.

This equation accounted for 65% of the variance in ball velocity.

**Table 19.1   Summary of Simple Linear Regression Relating Throwing Speed to Given Variables**

| Movement | t-statistic | $R^2$ |
|---|---|---|
| Elbow flexion | −0.08 | .00 |
| Elbow extension | −2.83[a] | .27 |
| Pronation | 1.17 | .06 |
| Shoulder abduction | −1.02 | .05 |
| Shoulder adduction | 1.22 | .06 |
| Shoulder external rotation | −2.94[a] | .28 |
| Shoulder extension | −2.47[b] | .22 |
| Shoulder flexion | −2.91[a] | .28 |
| Shoulder horizontal extension | −0.88 | .03 |
| Shoulder horizontal flexion | −0.26 | .00 |
| Shoulder internal rotation | 1.21 | .06 |
| Supination | −1.45 | .09 |
| Wrist extension | −4.65[a] | .50 |
| Wrist flexion | −0.44 | .01 |

[a]Significance at 1% level (t > 2.83). [b]Significance at 5% level (t > 2.08). Adapted from *American Journal of Sports Medicine* 1982.

Bartlett, Storey, and Simons (3) evaluated the relationship between upper extremity torque and throwing speed. Using a Cybex II and UBXT at 90°/s, these researchers tested the correlation between throwing speed and upper extremity torque in 11 professional baseball players. The results of their testing are presented in table 19.2. As can be seen from the table, only one variable, shoulder adduction, demonstrated a significant correlation to throwing speed.

A training study comparing isokinetic (IKN) and individualized dynamic variable resistance (IDVR) training in a group of 27 junior and senior high school baseball players indicated a relationship between upper body torque and power and throwing velocity (66). Players were randomly assigned to the IKN, IDVR, or a control (C) group for 5 weeks (15 sessions). Before and after the training subjects were evaluated isokinetically on a Musculoskeletal Evaluation Rehabilitation and Conditioning dynamometer (MERAC, Universal Equipment Co., Cedar Rapids, IA) at 500°/s. Pitching speed was evaluated using a radar gun. The results showed that only the IDVR group made significant increases in isokinetic torque, measured during dominant shoulder internal rotation and external rotation, and power, measured during external rotation. In addition, the IDVR group was the only group to demonstrate increases in throwing velocity. Although no correlation analyses were performed, the similar

### Table 19.2    Summary of Pearson Correlation Coefficients Relating Throwing Speed to Each Motion

| Movement | $r^2$ | P value |
| --- | --- | --- |
| Elbow extension | 0.000 | 0.499 |
| Elbow flexion | −0.307 | 0.179 |
| Pronation | −0.111 | 0.373 |
| Shoulder abduction | −0.283 | 0.200 |
| Shoulder adduction | 0.545 | 0.041 |
| Shoulder external rotation | 0.359 | 0.139 |
| Shoulder extension | 0.459 | 0.078 |
| Shoulder flexion | −0.337 | 0.155 |
| Shoulder horizontal abduction | 0.030 | 0.465 |
| Shoulder horizontal adduction | 0.260 | 0.220 |
| Shoulder internal rotation | 0.098 | 0.387 |
| Supination | −0.208 | 0.270 |
| Wrist extension | −0.109 | 0.375 |
| Wrist flexion | −0.162 | 0.317 |

Reprinted from *American Journal of Sports Medicine* 1989.

patterns of change between fastball velocity and these isokinetic measures offer evidence of a causal relationship.

Two studies from our laboratory, examining the relationship between isokinetic variables and fastball velocity are somewhat unique in the speeds tested, the testing positions employed, and the variables measured. Each study used the same sample of seven collegiate baseball pitchers, ages 18 to 21. The subject characteristics for the sample are presented in table 19.3.

Isokinetic testing was performed on a Biodex System 2 dynamometer (Biodex Corporation, Shirley, N.Y.). Both studies employed a diagonal throwing pattern ($D_2$) as one of the variables (see figure 19.3). This pattern was chosen to allow the sequential use of all body parts in a kinetic chain that simulated the actual pitching motion. In accordance with the set-up and positioning instructions in the Biodex System 2 applications and operations manual, the power head of the dynamometer was oriented at 90° and the sensitivity was set at A. The tilt of the power head was varied between a 20°- and 30°-angle depending on the height of the player. A lightweight shoulder attachment with a spring-loaded handle was used, and the length of the lever arm was adjusted to a range of motion that provided the greatest comfort and performance during the pitcher's simulated pitching motion. Foot position was also chosen to maximize comfort and force production.

Prior to testing, the pitchers were allowed as many trials as necessary to establish the foot position and lever arm length that they felt would optimize their performance. Once established, the power head angle, power head height, and lever arm length were recorded and held constant for all subsequent trials of that individual. In addition, each pitcher's foot position was marked on a grid (see figure 19.3) in front of the Biodex, and this position was held constant for all trials.

To reduce the potential impact that damping and overshoot might have on the data (42, 46, 49) the shoulder attachment used had no mechanical stops,

### Table 19.3　Subject Characteristics

| Subject | Age | Height (in) | Weight (lb) |
|---------|-----|-------------|-------------|
| 1 | 19 | 71.5 | 202.0 |
| 2 | 20 | 74.0 | 191.0 |
| 3 | 19 | 73.0 | 228.0 |
| 4 | 18 | 72.5 | 210.0 |
| 5 | 19 | 69.5 | 187.0 |
| 6 | 21 | 71.0 | 165.5 |
| 7 | 20 | 73.0 | 206.0 |
| Mean | 19.6 | 72.0 | 199.9 |

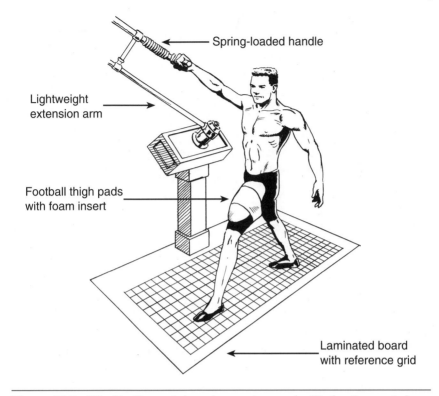

Spring-loaded handle

Lightweight
extension arm

Football thigh pads
with foam insert

Laminated board
with reference grid

**Figure 19.3** The $D_2$ diagonal throwing motion on the Biodex System 2 dynamometer.

and no electromagnetic braking was used to decelerate the limb. In this way the pitcher was allowed a complete follow-through. The necessity to stop the solid lever arm of the machine was addressed by placing a one-inch thick closed-cell foam pad between two football thigh pads and attaching this appliance to the pitcher's lead thigh (see figure 19.3). When the arm followed through across the body, the lever arm of the shoulder attachment struck the pad, terminating the motion. This braking method was tried at all testing speeds prior to being employed in the study, and it was found that contact with the pad produced no discernable discomfort that would cause an anticipatory deceleration of the arm prior to completion of the motion.

### Study I: The $D_2$ Throwing Motion as a Predictor of Fastball Velocity

Our first study had two objectives. The first was to examine the correlation between measures of torque, power, and acceleration recorded at high isokinetic speeds and fastball velocity measured under game conditions. The second objective was to develop a predictive model for fastball velocity (FBV) using these isokinetic evaluations. The $D_2$ diagonal-throwing pattern described earlier was used for this analysis. Tests were administered at speeds of 90, 180,

300, 400, and 450°/s. Five repetitions were collected at each testing speed. The order of the speeds was randomized to reduce the potential impact of order on the results. A minimum rest of 10 min was allowed between trials. The variables analyzed included instantaneous torque (TOR), instantaneous power (POW), work (WK), peak acceleration (ACC), and joint angle at peak acceleration (JA). Ball speed was measured using a radar gun under game conditions.

Correlation and regression analyses were performed using the data from the repetition yielding the highest acceleration for each speed and the highest fastball velocity recorded during the game situation. The strongest correlations seen among the isokinetic variables and FBV were ACC at 400°/s ($r^2 = .75$, $p = .05$), TOR at 300°/s ($r^2 = .77$, $p = .04$), and POW at 400°/s ($r^2 = .87$, $p = .01$).

Mallows' $Cp$ was used to determine the best regression model using all the variables measured. This model contained three variables, acceleration at 180°/s (ACC180), acceleration at 450°/s (ACC450), and instantaneous power at 400°/s (POW400). The predictive model was

FBV = 80.078 − .0010 (ACC180) − .0026 (ACC450) + 0.1204 (POW400).

The model accounted for 98% of the variance in fastball velocity ($r^2 = .9889$, $p = .0007$) (29). A graph showing the measured fastball velocity plotted against the predicted fastball velocities computed using the data from which they were derived is presented in figure 19.4.

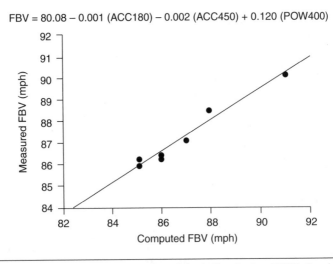

**Figure 19.4**   Measured versus computed fastball velocity (FBV) for the predictive model using the D$_2$ throwing motion. Isokinetic variables are acceleration at 180°/s (ACC180), acceleration at 450°/s (ACC450), and instantaneous power at 400°/s (POW400) ($r^2 = .9889$, $p = .0007$).

## Study II: Additional Factors Used With $D_2$ Data to Predict Fastball Velocity

The purpose of our second study was to include the $D_2$ throwing pattern, hip, knee, wrist, and elbow flexion and extension, shoulder internal and external rotation, and plantar- and dorsiflexion as potential isokinetic variables in a predictive model. The variables we considered for each movement tested were average power (AP) and peak torque (PT). All movements were tested at 90, 180, 300, 400, and 450°/s. In addition to the isokinetic variables, anthropometric measures were also included as potential predictors. The measured segmental lengths used are presented in table 19.4. The FBV values used were those reported in the previous study.

Mallows' $Cp$ yielded three predictive models. The first model included $D_2$ average power at 450°/s ($D_2$450AP), $D_2$ peak torque at 450°/s ($D_2$450PT), and average power for hip extension at 180°/s (HE180AP). The model and a graph of the measured versus predicted FBV values using the data from the study are presented in figure 19.5. This model accounted for approximately 97% of the measured variance in FBV ($r^2 = .9837$, $p = .0012$) (29).

The second model, which used $D_2$ average power at 450°/s ($D_2$450AP) and $D_2$ peak torque at 450°/s ($D_2$450PT), accounted for 90% of the variance ($r^2 = .9517$, $p = .001$) (29). The equation and graph for this model are presented in figure 19.6.

The third model, which explained nearly 99% of the variance ($r^2 = .9949$, $p = .0001$), used two variables, the cervical 7 to acromioclavicular segmental

### Table 19.4 Measured Segmental Lengths

| Abbreviation | Description of segment |
| --- | --- |
| C7Ac | From the spinous process at cervical vertebra 7 to the acromioclavicular articulation |
| AcOl | From the acromion process to the olecranon process of the ulna |
| O1DsR | From the olecranon process to distal styloid process of the radius |
| SrDutP | Distal styloid of the radius to the ungual tuberosity of the distal phalanx of the third finger |
| OlutP | From the olecranon process to the ungual tuberosity of the distal phalanx of the third finger |
| C1Sa | From the spinous process at cervical vertebra 1 to the sacrum |
| ILPa | From the greater trochanter of the femur to the base of the patella |
| MTMM | From the proximal end of the medial border of the tibia to the distal tip of the medial malleolus |
| PCtutP | From the posterior portion of the calcaneal tuberosity to the ungual tuberosity of the distal end of the terminal phalanx of toe one or two |

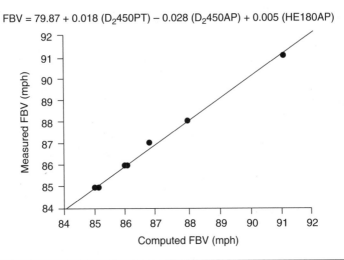

**Figure 19.5** Measured versus computed fastball velocity (FBV) for the predictive model using the $D_2$ throwing motion variables peak torque at 450°/s ($D_2$450PT), average power at 450°/s ($D_2$450AP), and hip extension average power at 180°/s (HE180AP) ($r^2 = .9837$, $p = .0012$).

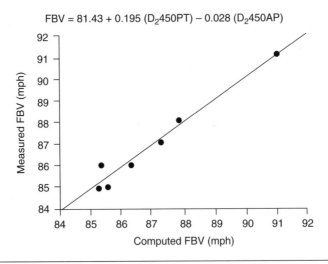

**Figure 19.6** Measured versus computed fastball velocity (FBV) for the predictive model using the $D_2$ throwing motion variables peak torque at 450°/s ($D_2$450PT) and average power at 450°/s ($D_2$450AP) ($r^2 = .9517$, $p = .0010$).

length (C7Ac, see figure 19.7) and $D_2$ average power at 180°/s ($D_2$180AP). The mathematical model and graph for this analysis are presented in figure 19.8.

## Conclusions

The studies cited in this section have provided both correlation data between selected isokinetic testing conditions and fastball velocity and regression models for the prediction of fastball velocity using isokinetic and other supplementary data. These studies differ in terms of speeds tested, joint selection, positioning, and open/closed chain kinetics. The methods employed in each study were chosen to answer specific research questions. Therefore, the methods employed by the researchers differed considerably. For example, the study by Pedegana and coworkers (38) incorporated isolated movements of the wrist, forearm, elbow, and shoulder at speeds between 30 and 180°/s depending on the movement. Bartlett, Storey, and Simons (3) employed isolated movements of the shoulder in their study. They tested at only one speed, 90°/s. Both research groups used a Cybex II and UBXT for their testing. The studies from our laboratory used a standing diagonal throwing motion ($D_2$) with no restraints on the movement other

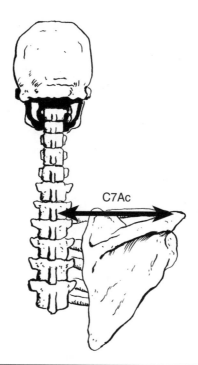

**Figure 19.7** Illustration of the segmental measurement from the spinous process of cervical vertebra 7 to the acromioclavicular joint (C7Ac).

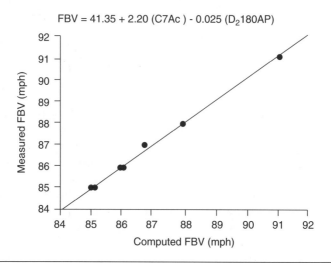

$$FBV = 41.35 + 2.20 (C7Ac) - 0.025 (D_2 180AP)$$

**Figure 19.8**   Measured versus computed fastball velocity (FBV) for the predictive model using the segmental length for C7Ac and the $D_2$ throwing motion variable, average power at $180°/s$ $(D_2 180AP)$ $(r^2 = .9949, p = .0001)$.

than those dictated by the mechanical limits of lever arm and power head. In addition, our testing was performed through a spectrum of higher speeds (90, 180, 300, 400, and 450°/s). In addition to the $D_2$ movement pattern, our second study also incorporated both isolated movements using an accessory chair, support pads, and restraining straps, as well as anthropometric measures of segmental lever arms. Both studies used a Biodex System 2 dynamometer.

While our studies produced both higher correlation values and more descriptive regression models for fastball velocity, the use of the diagonal standing motion without restraint does bring into question test-retest reliability, even when foot position is held constant for individuals. In addition, while analyses using the $D_2$ motion provided a nearly perfect predictive model for fastball velocity, they did not allow the evaluation of the contributions of specific joints, which was possible when isolated movements were employed (3, 38). However, the use of a closed kinetic chain, with limited restraint on the degrees of freedom of the individual segments during a whole body movement, does more closely simulate the functional pitching motion.

As can be seen from this short analysis of isokinetic studies, the methodology used is dependent on the nature of the research question being addressed. In addition, as the biomechanical and kinesiological factors that define the pitching motion are incorporated into testing patterns, further changes in methodology and differences in specific applications can be expected. The final section of this chapter attempts to address some of these methodological considerations.

# Methodological Considerations in Isokinetic Evaluation of Pitching

A number of methodological considerations should be considered in designing an isokinetic-testing program for pitchers. Among the important factors are testing speeds, body positioning, range of motion, contractile mode, variable selection, and the question of isolated versus multijoint testing. Each of these is addressed in the sections that follow.

## Appropriate Speeds for Testing

A decision concerning the correct isokinetic speeds to be used when testing the specific joints and movements related to pitching is complex. It is a simple matter to state that these evaluations should be done at the speeds specific to the pitching motion, but this not only reflects one-dimensional reasoning, it is also impossible given the available isokinetic technology. The average angular velocity reported by Pappas, Zawacki, and Sullivan (36) for the shoulder (6,180°/s) or elbow (4,595°/s) during the pitch is far greater than that available on any isokinetic testing dynamometer.

Cook and associates (7) stated that the top angular velocity of the Cybex II dynamometer used in their study was 300°/s, far below the angular velocity of over 6,000°/s reported for the shoulder during the pitch. However, these researchers did note that for isolated shoulder extension/flexion and internal/external rotation movements on the Cybex UBXT, a speed of 300°/s may have been too fast for either their pitchers or nonpitchers. It must be remembered that these isolated movements do reduce peak velocity by limiting the additive effects of the kinetic chain that would be active during the performance of the actual pitch. These authors (7) also cited the findings of Wallace and coworkers (56) indicating that the best speed of testing for normal shoulder flexion/extension was at approximately 120°/s.

In addition, Cook and associates (7) stated that changes in direction of movement were difficult at 300°/s and that subjects often appeared to show a subconscious attempt to decelerate the arm near the anticipated end of the range of motion of the test. This was presumably an attempt to prevent the abrupt feeling of braking that would be more perceptible at higher speeds. In the studies from our laboratory, we were also concerned with anticipatory deceleration of the throwing motion due to mechanical braking and therefore employed the use of protective padding rather than machine-generated braking to decelerate the movement. This technique might be compared to the use of rubber matting or air bags to help the runners in the 55 m decelerate at the end of the run in New York's Melrose games.

In explaining their use of the testing speed of 90°/s for their study, Bartlett, Storey, and Simons (3) presented both sides of the high speed/low speed argument. First they cited the work of Elsner, Pedegana, and Lang (12), which indicated that speeds of 60°/s or less could result in inaccurate data due to lack of stabilization and fear of injury since substantial braking was necessary to maintain these slow movement speeds.

Bartlett, Storey, and Simons (3) also referred to Sapega and coworkers (46) and Winter, Wells, and Orr (65) in their critique of isokinetic testing performed above 180°/s, citing the erroneously high readings caused by overshoot as the dynamometer reaches its endpoint and is subjected to mechanical braking forces. Bartlett, Storey, and Simons (3) also stated that damping can reduce the impact of overshoot, but it can also suppress significant quantities of true muscular torque. This is in agreement with the statement by Rothstein, Lamb, and Mayhew (42) that the application of a damping force can reduce the overshoot artifact, but it will also distort the shape of the isokinetic curve earlier in the range of motion. In fact, Sinacore and associates (49) have encouraged the use of zero damping when accurate determination of angle-specific torque is desired.

In our analysis of three-dimensional maps reported earlier in this text, we also addressed the problem of deceleration artifact. We noted in creating these three-dimensional surfaces that the artifact grew progressively larger as the speed of testing increased. In our opinion, if high speed full-body movements employing the entire kinetic chain are to be tested, this can best be accomplished if a braking system other than the dynamometer is utilized to stop the motion. In addition, the use of a lightweight testing arm is recommended to reduce the momentum of the test apparatus.

It should be noted that Bartlett, Storey, and Simons (3) also mentioned the use of only a single speed of testing as a possible limiting factor in detecting a correlation between torque and throwing speed. We agree with this statement and encourage the use of multiple speeds in constructing a predictive model or analyzing specific muscle functions.

As can be seen from this abbreviated review addressing speed selection, the testing speeds we choose can be affected by the purpose of the study (for assessments versus predictive models), specific joints and movements (shoulder versus knee, shoulder internal versus external rotation), body position (supine, seated, or standing), number of body segments involved (single versus multijoint evaluations), relative versus absolute values (need for absolute versus comparative data), the braking system employed (hard versus soft stops, or external deceleration), and a number of other factors that may not have been addressed in this section. In the next section we continue to examine testing speed, but with specific emphasis on testing position.

## Testing Position and Speed Interactions

A number of authors have addressed the topic of body position and its impact on isokinetic evaluations. There is little doubt from these studies that the positioning of the body during testing is of extreme importance when considering the questions being addressed and the biomechanical efficiency in specific planes of motion. Obviously, testing performed in a supine position affords greater stabilization and isolation than testing performed in a standing position. However, it also reduces the number of levers that can additively produce movement. Therefore, as was the case with testing speed, no perfect model can be provided for optimal positioning of the body during isokinetic testing for the pitch. The best that we can hope to do in this section is to provide information that will help the reader in his or her decision-making process.

Since the majority of the studies that have examined positioning have also looked at it over a spectrum of test speeds, we present our review using this precedent.

A study by Sodenberg and Blaschak (51) examined peak torque of the internal and external rotators of the dominant shoulders in 20 normal males. Data were collected at six different seated shoulder positions and three different velocities. Regardless of the testing position, torque always declined as speed increased. Tables 19.5 and 19.6 present the data by position. As can be seen by these tables, the positions that should be chosen to maximize results for internal and external rotation are different, but the neutral position does appear to offer a good compromise. The researchers concluded that, since no optimal test position for shoulder external and internal rotation could be determined, different positions could be chosen to attain maximal results for each motion.

Walmsley and Szybbo (57) also presented a study comparing positions and speeds. They used three standing shoulder positions: neutral, 90° of flexion, and 90° of abduction. The speeds employed were 60, 120, and 180°/s. For shoulder internal rotation, there were no significant differences found due to speed. The authors suggest that this may have been due to the small subject number (N = 12) or the range of speeds utilized, which was quite small compared to other studies (13, 51). However, we would also like to present an additional alternative to this explanation. Since the subjects performed in a standing position, it is possible that the use of accessory and synergistic muscles

### Table 19.5 Comparison of Mean Peak Torque Values by Position for Internal Rotation

| Duncan grouping* | Mean peak torque (ft-lb) | N | Position |
|---|---|---|---|
| A | 36.77 | 60 | Neutral |
| B | 34.82 | 60 | Full flexion |
| C  B | 34.03 | 60 | Full abduction |
| C  B | 33.75 | 60 | Midabduction |
| C | 32.73 | 60 | Midposition |
| C | 32.52 | 60 | Midflexion |

*Means with the same letter are not significantly different ($p < .05$) according to Duncan's multiple range test. Reprinted from *Journal of Orthopaedic and Sports Physical Therapy* 1987.

### Table 19.6    Comparison of Mean Peak Torque Values by Position for External Rotation

| Duncan grouping* | Mean peak torque (ft-lb) | N | Position |
|---|---|---|---|
| A | 24.05 | 60 | Full abduction |
| A | 23.58 | 60 | Neutral |
| C  B | 20.75 | 60 | Midposition |
| C  B | 20.10 | 60 | Midabduction |
| C  B | 19.92 | 60 | Full flexion |
| C | 18.68 | 60 | Midflexion |

*Means with the same letter are not significantly different ($p < .05$) according to Duncan's multiple range test. Reprinted from *Journal of Orthopaedic and Sports Physical Therapy* 1987.

could have allowed a greater variance than that which would have occurred in a more isolated and restricted position. Walmsley and Szybbo (57) did report significantly higher torques for the internal rotators in the neutral position than in the other positions tested. For the external rotators, Walmsley and Szybbo (57) reported significantly higher values for 90° of flexion compared to the other two testing positions. For shoulder external rotation there was also a significant effect due to speed of testing, with 60°/s producing significantly higher torques than 180°/s.

An interesting topic addressed by Greenfield and coworkers (19) and later by Tis and Maxwell (53) was the question of testing in the scapular versus the frontal plane (see figure 19.9). Johnson (28) and Poppen and Walker (40) have suggested that the scapular plane is the true functional plane of motion for the shoulder joint. For the purpose of our discussion the comparison of these two planes is important since the scapular plane is the functional plane of motion for the pitch at ball release, given the position of the plant foot.

In promoting the use of the scapular plane for testing, Greenfield and coworkers (19) report the observations of Johnson (28), Poppen and Walker (41), and Saha (45) that the scapular plane is significant since the length-tension relationships of the shoulder abductors and rotators are optimized for elevation in this plane. They also noted that in the plane of the scapula the capsular fibers of the glenohumeral joint are more relaxed. And finally, they cite the work of Poppen and Walker (41) and Saha (43, 44) indicating that this position provides increased joint congruity and stability in the normally functioning rotator cuff.

The data from the Greenfield group's study (19) showed similar Pearson correlation coefficients for repeated tests, with the frontal plane (FP) providing $r$ values of .81 and .92 for external and internal rotation, respectively, and the scapular plane (ScP) providing values of .94 and .92 for the same measures.

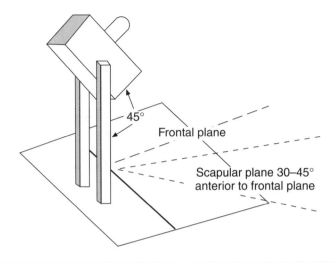

**Figure 19.9** Illustration of the frontal and scapular planes of testing.

As can be seen, the correlation coefficients were somewhat higher for the scapular plane during external rotation.

When torque values were compared in both planes, similar results were produced during internal rotation (ScP = 15.4 ± 5.7 ft-lb, FP = 15.4 ± 5.0 ft-lb). However, the scapular plane produced significantly higher torques than the frontal plane during external rotation (ScP = 14.1 ± 2.9 ft-lb, FP = 12.6 ± 2.8 ft-lb, $p < .001$).

The work of Greenfield and associates (19) was expanded by Tis and Maxwell (53), who examined the difference between the scapular and frontal plane in the dominant and nondominant shoulders of 20 recreationally active females. They evaluated peak torque, average power, and total work at 1.047 (60°/s) and 2.094 rad/s (120°/s). The values produced during testing in the scapular plane were significantly higher than those produced in the frontal plane for all variables under all testing conditions. The researchers suggested that these results indicate that the scapular plane may be a more desirable position for testing.

Each of the studies in this section has implications concerning the positions to be used to optimize results of specific muscle groups. In addition, the concepts of range of motion, stabilization, and isolation, as well as isolated versus multijoint movement, find their conceptual roots in this review of body positioning and isokinetics.

## Range of Motion and Contractile Mode

Range of motion may be one of the most ignored modifying factors in isokinetic testing of the pitching motion and its component parts. Little data has been offered in the literature examining the shapes of the specific torque curves during concentric and eccentric actions of the muscles involved in the pitching motion. For example, internal/external rotational balances have been examined extensively in the literature, but the specific shapes of the related curves have not been comparatively presented. When this factor is combined with the concept of contractile mode (eccentric versus concentric actions) an interesting scenario is presented.

Jobe and coworkers (25, 26) have stated that the external rotators are most active during the follow-through as decelerators of an arm that is releasing the ball at nearly 100 mph. Due to the characteristic triphasic firing patterns exhibited for the agonist/antagonist muscles during high speed ballistic motions (4, 31, 67), it may be that structural adaptations are dictating the imbalances between the external and internal rotators of the shoulder for protective purposes. A number of studies have indicated that the muscle length that produces maximal force can be modified with training and other stresses (20, 32, 63, 64). Given the adaptive changes in the length-tension curve seen with training, some of the imbalances seen in pitchers may be the result of resetting the force-velocity relationship due to the lengthening of the muscles in response to high speed stretching. However, this cannot be confirmed without examining torque throughout the range of motion to determine if modifications in the length-tension relationship have indeed occurred.

A study by Scoville and coworkers (47) has partially addressed the concept of length-specific strength measurements in relation to agonist/antagonist strength ratios for the shoulder. Using a Kin-Com dynamometer these researchers tested individuals through a range of 20° of lateral rotation to 90° of medial rotation at a speed of 90°/s. However, they performed end range of motion analyses for medial rotation at a range from 10° lateral rotation to 20° of medial rotation and for lateral rotation between 60° and 90° of lateral rotation. This study also addressed the concept of eccentric deceleration by examining the strength ratios both concentrically and eccentrically. A third interesting aspect of this study was that torque values were reported as a percentage of the subject's body weight, indicating the researchers' appreciation of relative strength as a meaningful variable when examining performance and injury potential. These researchers reported an end range ratio (60° to 90° of medial rotation) for the medial rotators functioning eccentrically and lateral rotators functioning concentrically of 2.39:1 and 2.15:1 for the dominant and nondominant shoulders, respectively. They also reported an end range ratio (from 10° lateral rotation to 20° of medial rotation) for the lateral rotators functioning eccentrically and medial rotators functioning concentrically of 1.08:1 and 1.05:1 for the dominant and nondominant shoulders, respectively. The authors contended that these measures were more meaningful than previously reported ratios of concentric versus concentric torque measured through the entire range of motion, since they reflect the critical end stage situation using the correct contractile modes for the muscles involved. These data bring into question proposed imbalances reported in earlier studies between the lateral and medial rotators.

Brown and coworkers (6) have intimated that increased range of motion in the external rotators and the resetting of the length-tension curve may be of functional benefit to the pitcher. They stated that during the acceleration phase of throwing "the arm is whipped from a position of extreme external rotation to one of internal rotation." Tullos and King (55) believe that this increase in external rotation helps improve the efficiency of the internal rotator muscles and thus the ball is delivered with greater velocity.

In addition to these considerations, the reader is also reminded of the concepts of overshoot and damping, which are inherent parts of restricting the range of motion during isokinetic testing. The impact that each of these factors can have on isokinetic evaluations has already been discussed.

## Variable Selection

Variable selection is an important aspect of any isokinetic evaluation. The majority of the studies that have evaluated the movements related to pitching have reported torque at varying isokinetic velocities (1, 3, 11, 22, 33, 38, 50, 62). Torque adjusted for body weight has also been reported (47). In some cases, including the work from our laboratory, total work and average power were also included in the data (53). In the predictive studies from our laboratory, acceleration and time to peak torque were also computed. Along with these isokinetic measures, range of motion, segmental length, segment mass, and electromyographical analyses may also be used to further investigate the throwing motion and its component parts. The choice of variables is, once again, dictated by the nature of the assessment and its purpose.

## Isolated Versus Sequential Movement

The necessity for coordinated sequential movements in optimizing ball speed has been sustained by both EMG and biomechanical studies (2, 18, 23, 25, 26, 54, 59). However, the majority of studies using isokinetic devices for evaluation have concentrated on isolated open chain movements rather than the closed chain multijoint movements that simulate the action of the pitch. In addition, little information currently exists on the practical importance of segmental lever length to the production of fastball velocity.

Pedegana and coworkers (38) attributed their lack of perfect statistical correlation between measured isokinetic strengths of the arm and throwing speed to the isolation process itself. They cited the study by Toyoshima and associates (54), who indicated that only 53.1% of throwing speed is the result of the contribution of the arm and that throwing is a complex act involving all body parts. One of the major limitations cited by Cook and associates (7) in their study of isokinetic shoulder strength ratios of pitchers and nonpitchers was the fact that the sequential movements responsible for producing ball velocity during pitching could not be realistically duplicated using the Cybex. Bartlett, Storey, and Simons (3) also indicated that throwing is a complex motion involving all body parts. These researchers cited the work of both Toyoshima and associates (54) and Atwater (2) to substantiate this statement. The relationship between these statements and the kinetic link model should be considered.

A study by Hinton (21) addressed not only the topic of speed and isolation with regard to isokinetic evaluation of the shoulder; it also addressed body position. This researcher presented convincing evidence, using data collected from 26 high school baseball pitchers, that significant differences can occur in the torque values recorded for isolated movements of the shoulder due to body position. He found that external rotation peak torque and total work and external/internal rotation peak torque and total work ratios were higher when measured in a supine, 90° abducted position compared to a standing neutral condition. The standing neutral position, however, produced higher values for internal rotation peak torque and total work.

Each of these studies contributes to the body of information indicating there is a trade-off that exists between measurements made on isolated joints and those produced using multiple body segments. The decision as to which method is more desirable, as with the other modifying factors mentioned, is dependent on the nature of the inquiry.

# Summary

This chapter is presented as a partial review and working consolidation of the literature on pitching and isokinetic testing. It is not intended as an exhaustive review of any of the topics covered, nor does it profess to offer absolute guidelines or testing protocols. We believe that protocols, guidelines, and methods are specific to the information sought by the researcher, practitioner, or coach and should be structured to reflect that information.

# References

1. Alderink, G.J., and Kuck, D.J. 1986. Isokinetic shoulder strength in high school and college-aged pitchers. *J. Orthop. Sports Phys. Ther.* 7(4): 163–72.

2. Atwater, A.E. 1971. Movement characteristics of the overarm throw: A kinematic analysis of men and women performers. PhD diss., University of Wisconsin [University Microfilms no. 71-3448]. Abstract in *Dissertation Abstracts International*, 31.5819A.

3. Bartlett, L.R., Storey, M.D., and Simons, B.D. 1989. Measurement of upper extremity torque production and its relationship to throwing speed in the competitive athlete. *Am. J. Sports Med.* 17(1): 89–91.

4. Behm, D.G., and Sale, D.G. 1996. Influence of velocity on agonist and antagonist activation in concentric dorsiflexion muscle actions. *Can. J. Appl. Physiol.* 21(5): 403–16.

5. Braatz, J.H., and Gogia, P.P. 1987. The mechanics of pitching. *J. Orthop. Sports Phys. Ther.* 9(2): 56–69.

6. Brown, L.P., Niehues, S.L., Harrah, A., Yavorsky, P., and Hirshman, H.P. 1988. Upper extremity range of motion and isokinetic strength of the internal and exter-

nal shoulder rotators in major league baseball players. *Am. J. Sports Med.* 16(6): 577–85.

7. Cook, E.E., Gray, V.L., Savinar-Nogue, E., and Medeiros, J. 1987. Shoulder antagonistic strength ratios: A comparison between college-level baseball pitchers and nonpitchers. *J. Orthop. Sports Phys. Ther.* 8(9): 451–61.

8. Coombs, J. 1949. *Baseball coaching.* New York: Prentice Hall.

9. DePalma, A., Cooke, A., and Prabhaker, M. 1967. The role of the subscapularis in recurrent anterior dislocations of the shoulder. *Clin. Orthop.* 54: 35–49.

10. Dillman, C.J., Fleisig, G.S., and Andrews, J.R. 1993. Biomechanics of pitching with emphasis upon shoulder kinematics. *J. Orthop. Sports Phys. Ther.* 18(2): 402–8.

11. Ellenbecker, T.S., and Mattalino, A.J. 1997. Concentric isokinetic shoulder rotation strength in professional baseball pitchers. *J. Orthop. Sports Phys. Ther.* 25(5): 323–28.

12. Elsner, R.C., Pedegana, L.R., and Lang, J. 1983. Protocol for strength testing and rehabilitation of the upper extremity. *J. Orthop. Sports Phys. Ther.* 4: 229–35.

13. Feiring, D.C., Ellenbecker, T.S., and Dersheid, G.L. 1986. Test-retest reliability of the Biodex isokinetic dynamometer. *J. Orthop. Sports Phys. Ther.* 11: 298–300.

14. Feltner, M.E., and Dapena, J. 1986. Dynamics of the shoulder and elbow joints of the throwing arm during a baseball pitch. *Int. J. Sports Biomechan.* 2: 235–59.

15. Fleisig, G.S., Dillman, C.J., and Andrews, J.R. 1994. Biomechanics of the shoulder during throwing. In *The Athlete's Shoulder,* ed. Andrews, J.R, and Wilk, K.E., 355–68. New York: Churchill Livingstone.

16. Fleisig, G.S., Andrews, J.R., Dillman, C.J., and Escamilla, R.F. 1995. Kinetics of baseball pitching with implications about injury mechanisms. *Am. J. Sports Med.* 23(2): 233–39.

17. Gainor, B.J., Pitrowski, G., Puhl, J., Allen, W.C., and Hagen, R. 1980. The throw: Biomechanics and acute injury. *Am. J. Sports Med.* 8: 114–18.

18. Gowan, I.D., Jobe, F.W., Tibone, J.E., Perry, J., and Moynes, D.R. 1987. A comparative electromyographical analysis of the shoulder during pitching. *Am. J. Sports Med.* 15(6): 586–90.

19. Greenfield, B.H., Donatelli, R., Wooden, M.J., and Wilkes, J. 1990. Isokinetic evaluation of shoulder rotational strength between the plane of the scapula and the frontal plane. *Am. J. Sports Med.* 18(2): 124–28.

20. Herzog, W., Guimaraes, A.C., Anton, M.G., and Carter-Erdman, K.A. 1991. Moment-length relations of rectus femoris muscles of speed skaters/cyclists and runners. *Med. Sci. Sports Exerc.* 23(11): 1289–96.

21. Hinton, R.Y. 1988. Isokinetic evaluation of shoulder rotational strength in high school baseball pitchers. *Am. J. Sports Med.* 16: 274–79.

22. Ivey, F.M., Calhoun, J.H., Rusche, K. et al. 1985. Isokinetic testing of shoulder strength: Normal values. *Arch. Phys. Med. Rehabil.* 66: 384–86.

23. Jacobs, P. 1987. The overhand baseball pitch: A kinesiological analysis and related strength-conditioning program. *NSCA J.* 9(1): 5–13.

24. Jobe, F.W., and Moynes, D.R. 1982. Delineation of diagnostic criteria and a rehabilitation program for rotator cuff injuries. *Am. J. Sports Med.* 10: 336–39.

25. Jobe, F.W., Tibone, J.E., Perry, J., and Moynes, D.R. 1983. An EMG analysis of the shoulder in throwing and pitching: A preliminary report. *Am. J. Sports Med.* 11(1): 3–5.

26. Jobe, F.W., Moynes, D.R., Tibone, J.E., and Perry, J. 1984. An EMG analysis of the shoulder in pitching: A second report. *Am. J. Sports Med.* 12(3): 218–20.

27. Jobe, F.W., and Ling, B. 1986. The shoulder in sports. In *The shoulder: Surgical and nonsurgical management*, ed. Post, M. Philadelphia: Lea & Febiger.

28. Johnson, T.B. 1937. Movements of the shoulder joint: A plea for use of "plane of scapula" as plane of reference for movements occurring at humeroscapula joint. *Br. J. Surg.* 25: 252–60.

29. Kerlinger, F.N. 1986. *Foundations of behavioral research*, 535–45. Fort Worth, TX: Holt, Rinehart & Winston.

30. King, J.W., Brelsford, H., and Tullos, H.S. 1969. Analysis of the pitching arm of the professional baseball player. *Clin. Orthop.* 67: 116–23.

31. Latash, M.L. 1998. *Neurophysiological basis of movement.* Champaign, IL: Human Kinetics.

32. Lynn, R., and Morgan, D.L. 1994. Decline running produces more sarcomeres in rat vastus intermedius muscle than does incline running. *J. Appl. Physiol.* 77(3): 1439–44.

33. Mikesky, A.E, Edwards, J.E., Wigglesworth, J.K., and Kunkel, S. 1995. Eccentric and concentric strength of the shoulder and arm musculature in collegiate baseball pitchers. *Am. J. Sports Med.* 23(5): 638–42.

34. Mottice, M.D. 1982. Determination of the normal isokinetic peak torque ratio of the external to internal shoulder rotator muscles in a normal male adult population. Master's thesis, University of Alabama at Birmingham.

35. Pappas, A.M., Zawacki, R.M., and McCarthy, C.F. 1985. Rehabilitation of the pitching shoulder. *Am. J. Sports Med.* 13: 223–35.

36. Pappas, A.M., Zawacki, R.M., and Sullivan, T.J. 1985. Biomechanics of baseball pitching. *Am. J. Sports Med.* 13(4): 216–22.

37. Pappas, A.M., Morgan, W.J., Schultz, L.A., and Diana, R. 1995. Wrist kinematics during pitching. *Am. J. Sports Med.* 23(3): 312–15.

38. Pedegana, L.R., Elsner, R.C., Poberts, D., Lang, J., and Farewell, V. 1982. The relationship of upper extremity strength to throwing speed. *Am. J. Sports Med.* 10(6): 352–54.

39. Perry, J. 1983. Anatomy and biomechanics of the shoulder in throwing, swimming, gymnastics, and tennis. *Clin. Sports Med.* 2: 247–70.

40. Poppen, N.K., and Walker, P.S. 1976. Normal and abnormal motion of the shoulder. *J. Bone Joint Surg.* 58A: 195–201.

41. Poppen, N.K., and Walker, P.S. 1978. Forces at the glenohumeral joint in abduction. *Clin. Orthop.* 135: 165–170.

42. Rothstein, J.M., Lamb, R.L., and Mayhew, T.P. 1987. Clinical use of isokinetic measurements. *Phys. Ther.* 67: 1840–44.

43. Saha, A.K. 1971. Dynamic stability of the glenohumeral joint. *Acta Orthop. Scand.* 42: 491–505.

44. Saha, A.K. 1973. Mechanics of elevation of the glenohumeral joint. *Acta Orthop. Scand.* 44: 668–78.

45. Saha, A.K. 1983. Mechanics of shoulder movements and a plea for the recognition of "zero position" of glenohumeral joint. *Clin. Orthop.* 173: 3–10.

46. Sapega, A.A., Nicholas, J.A., Sokolow, D., and Saraniti, A. 1982. The nature of torque "overshoot" in Cybex isokinetic dynamometry. *Med. Sci. Sports Exerc.* 14(5): 368–75.

47. Scoville, C.R., Arciero, R.A., Taylor, D.C., and Stoneman, P.D. 1997. End range eccentric antagonist/concentric agonist strength ratios: A new perspective in shoulder strength assessment. *J. Orthop. Sports Phys. Ther.* 25(3): 203–7.

48. Seaver, T. 1984. *The art of pitching.* New York: Hearst Books.

49. Sincore, D.R., Rothstein, J.M., Delitto, A., and Rose, S.J. 1983. Effect of damp on isokinetic measurements. *Phys. Ther.* 63: 1248–50.

50. Sirota, S.C., Malanga, G.A., Eischen, J.J., and Laskowski, E.R. 1997. An eccentric and concentric strength profile of shoulder external and internal rotator muscles in professional baseball pitchers. *Am. J. Sports Med.* 25(1): 59–64.

51. Sodenberg, G.J., and Blaschak, M.J. 1987. Shoulder internal and external rotation peak torque production through a velocity spectrum in differing positions. *J. Orthop. Sports Phys. Ther.* 8(11): 518–24.

52. Tippett, S.R. 1986. Lower extremity strength and active range of motion in college baseball pitchers: A comparison between stance leg and kick leg. *J. Orthop. Sports Phys. Ther.* 8(1): 10–14.

53. Tis, L.L., and Maxwell, T. 1996. The effect of positioning on shoulder isokinetic measures in females. *Med. Sci. Sports Exerc.* 28(9): 1188–92.

54. Toyoshima, S., Hoshikawa, T., Miyashita, M. et al. 1974. Contribution of the body parts to throwing performance. In *Biomechanics IV,* ed. Nelson, R.C., and Morehouse, C.A., 169–74. Baltimore: University Park Press.

55. Tullos, H.S., and King, K.W. 1973. Throwing mechanisms in sports. *Orthop. Clin. N. Am.* 4: 709–20.

56. Wallace, W.A., Barton, M.J., Murray, and Wiley, A. 1984. The power available during movement of the shoulder. In *Surgery of the shoulder,* ed. Bateman, J. and Welsh, R., 1–5. Philadelphia: Decker.

57. Walmsley, R.P., and Szybbo, C. 1987. A comparative study of the torque generated by the shoulder internal and external rotator muscles in different positions and at varying speeds. *J. Orthop. Sport Phys. Ther.* 9(6): 217–22.

58. Wang, Y.T., Ford III, H.T., Ford Jr., H.T., and Shin, D.M. 1995. Three-dimensional kinematic analysis of baseball pitching in acceleration phase. *Perceptual and Motor Skills* 80: 43–48.

59. Watkins, R.G., Dennis, S., Dillin, W.H., Schnebel, B., Schneiderman, G., Jobe, F., Farfan, H., Perry, J., and Pink, M. 1989. Dynamic EMG analysis of torque transfer in professional baseball players. *Spine* 14(4): 404–8.

60. Werner, S.L., Flesig, G.S., Dillman, C.J., and Andrews, J.R. 1993. Biomechanics of the elbow during pitching. *J. Orthop. Sports Phys. Ther.* 17(6): 274–78.

61. Wilk, K.E., Andrews, J.R., Arrigo, C.A., Keirns, M.A., and Erber, D.J. 1993. The strength characteristics of internal and external rotator muscles in professional baseball players. *Am. J. Sports Med.* 21(1): 61–66.

62. Wilk, K.E., Andrews, J.R., and Arrigo, C.A. 1995. Abductor and adductor strength characteristics of professional baseball players. *Am. J. Sports Med.* 23(3): 307–11.

63. Williams, P., and Goldspink, G. 1973. The effect of immobilization on the longitudinal growth of striated muscle fibers. *J. Anat.* 116: 45–55.

64. Williams, P., and Goldspink, G. 1978. Changes in sarcomere length and physiological properties in immobilized muscle. *J. Anat.* 127: 459–68.

65. Winter, D.A., Wells, R.P., and Orr, G.W. 1981. Errors in the use of isokinetic dynamometers. *Eur. J. Appl. Physiol.* 46: 397–408.

66. Wooden, M.J., Greenfield, B., Johanson, M., Litzelman, L., Mundrane, M., and Donatelli, R.A. 1992. Effects of strength training on throwing velocity and shoulder muscle performance in teenage baseball players. *J. Orthop. Sports Phys. Ther.* 15(5): 223–28.

67. Zehr, E.P., and Sale, D.G. 1994. Ballistic movement: Muscle activation and neuromuscular adaptation. *Can. J. Appl. Physiol.* 19(4): 363–78.

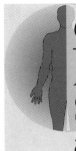

# Chapter 20

# Assessment for Football: Soccer, Australian Rules, and American

Tim V. Wrigley

**A**mong the football codes considered in this chapter—soccer, Australian Rules, and American football—exist many similarities and many differences in physical requirements. In addition, *within* each football code there is a broad range of strength and physiological profiles, and ideal body types for different positional roles, which makes it impossible to consider any football team as a homogeneous group to be judged against the same criteria.

It is in this sense that isokinetic assessment of football athletes presents the major challenge. A similar challenge is encountered in testing many team sports, few of which have a single set of criteria against which athletes can be assessed. Indeed in some cases there may be more similarities among certain physical task requirements across *different* team sports than among the task requirements of different "specialist" positions within the *same* sport. Consequently, there may be as much strength and physiological variability among athletes within football codes as between codes.

However, different positional requirements should not be overemphasized. While they may restrict candidates for certain positions in American football, for example, other positional requirements, and most performance requirements in soccer and Australian Rules, may be somewhat generic or may be met in more than one way. Several body types or physiological profiles may be able to succeed in a given position by employing different playing strategies. Given the fact that not all performance tasks in the football codes are determined solely by player strength, one must bear in mind the many ways in which an athlete may achieve success in football, by strength, speed, speed strength, endurance, skill, and so forth.

Approaches to isokinetic assessment of each football code are not described here separately. Rather, this chapter outlines a general approach to isokinetic assessment of the football codes, as many of the strategies are generic, and can be applied to each football code, rather than being specific to any individual code. Only the results may be different. However, in discussing important issues for isokinetic assessment, a specific football code is typically used as the basis of examples for an issue.

In addition to the performance characteristics of the football codes, they are typically characterized by high rates of injury. At the elite level, it is relatively rare to encounter a player presenting for isokinetic assessment who does not have a significant history of injury, often involving surgery. In such cases, it is impossible to judge players' isokinetic results only in the context of athletic performance. As such, discussion of isokinetic assessment for football would be incomplete without reference to the influence of injury history on isokinetic results and possibly also on future injury likelihood. We will briefly address such issues at the end of this chapter.

## Strength Characteristics of the Football Codes

At the beginning of chapter 3 we discussed the role of strength in various athletic performances. The notion of a strength continuum was introduced (and a strength-power dichotomy avoided), reflecting the extent to which performance in different sports is related to strength. Briefly, at one end of the continuum are sports for which strength is critical—these are the "strength-limited" sports; at the opposite end of the continuum are "strength-independent" sports, for which strength is of minor or no importance. Between these two extremes are the "strength-related" sports, for which strength is of varying importance but not critical to performance success.

However, most sports—including the football codes—are not single-task performances. Rather, they involve a range of tasks and skills. Some of these may depend heavily on strength, while for others, strength may be of little or no importance. Even for a sport with a single success criterion—such as sprint- ing—elite performance may be a result of time-varying strength requirements across different joints and at different velocities (see, e.g., 17). However, it would appear that soccer and Australian Rules football are, in general, strength- related sports. They require both absolute strength (e.g., for kicking and for body contact with opponents) and relative strength (e.g., for running and jump- ing). But while strength is clearly an important asset, players can succeed in these football codes without great levels of strength. However, they usually compensate with other exceptional attributes, such as speed, height, skill, or endurance.

In American football, strength requirements appear to vary by position to a greater extent (15, 27, 35, 76, 89). The linemen, for example, are clearly very different athletes to the running players. Positions on the line are among the most absolute strength limited in any team sport; other positions are also absolute or relative strength limited, but to a lesser extent. As a reflection of these differences in the importance of strength between the football codes, there is clearly a "strength culture" in American football that does not exist to any great extent in Australian Rules and is essentially absent from soccer. Consequently, there is a much greater emphasis on strength training in American football. In soccer, the emphasis is typically on skill; it has been suggested that this has been to the detriment of player fitness, including strength (86).

The football codes include many generic athletic tasks such as sprinting and jumping. In fact, many sports share requirements for performance of these athletic tasks. There is good evidence to suggest that isokinetic strength correlates with these performances (see chapter 3). Most of the football codes share requirements for body contact, in some cases involving tackling. However, the frequency and vigor of the tackling varies greatly among codes.

One of the main distinctions among the football codes is the means by which the ball is conveyed in order to score. In American football, it is generally thrown or carried, but it is occasionally kicked; in soccer it is kicked from the ground; in Australian Rules it is generally kicked at the point of release from the hands. In the codes where the ball is routinely kicked, there is good evidence—mainly for soccer—that kicking success is related to isokinetic strength (see chapter 3). The prevalence of kicking in some codes also raises the possibility of limb dominance for strength. In soccer and Australian Rules, players usually have a preferred kicking leg, although at the elite level they can generally kick with either leg. The next section outlines the apparent lack of evidence for limb strength dominance in soccer.

The work-rest ratios are markedly different among the various codes. In American football, players generally have considerable recovery time between plays and when not on the field (American football is the only code that employs separate offensive and defensive teams). In soccer and Australian Rules play is virtually continuous; however, most players are assigned to particular regions of the field so that they have recovery time whenever the ball is not in their region. However, in both codes, a number of players may be almost continuously involved in the play for extended periods of time with limited opportunities for rest.

## Rationale for Isokinetic Assessment

This section outlines a basis for an isokinetic-testing strategy for football. Indeed, a similar approach should be applied to any sport. Soccer is used as an example, as the scientific literature provides more relevant information for soccer than any other football code. As noted previously, soccer is a strength-related sport, requiring both absolute and relative strength. There are a number of important criteria upon which a strength assessment strategy should be justified:

- Correlation with athletic performance
- Ability to distinguish between players at different levels
- Sensitivity to training adaptations
- Availability of normative data for comparison

- Reliability of test protocols
- Biomechanical analyses of important performance elements

The research evidence to support these criteria for soccer is outlined below.

- *Isokinetic knee and hip strength has been shown to be correlated with kicking velocity and distance* (8, 18, 50, 53, 64) (see chapter 3). This association is evident despite the fact that kicking is a ballistic, multijoint activity, while the isokinetic assessments in these studies were single-joint movements performed at constant angular velocity. One study did not find this correlation (48), although the results were not fully reported, and the small sample size may have explained the lack of a statistically significant correlation. There are many instances in soccer where maximum kick velocity and distance are important (e.g., shots on goal, certain passes). However, it should be noted that in soccer and the other football codes that involve kicking to a significant extent—such as Australian Rules—kicking accuracy is at least as important as kicking distance and velocity.

Many generic athletic tasks within the game of soccer are also common to other sports (e.g., sprinting, jumping). Isokinetic strength has been shown to be related to the performance of these tasks in various athletic groups (see chapter 3), including soccer players (8, 58).

- *Isokinetic strength has been shown to distinguish between elite and subelite performers in soccer* (33, 34, 59, 71, 83) (see figure 20.1). Thus, while soccer might be generally regarded as a strength-related sport, progression to the highest level in soccer may be strength limited to a significant extent.

There is also evidence to suggest that isokinetic assessment is sensitive to some team positional differences in strength among soccer players (16, 57, 83). While there are some discrepancies among the results, it would appear

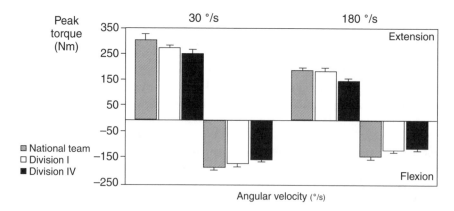

**Figure 20.1**  Concentric knee extension and knee flexion peak torque in Swedish soccer players from different levels.

Modified from *International Journal of Sports Medicine* 1986.

that there is a trend for defenders (including goalkeepers) to have somewhat greater strength than midfielders and forwards. In contrast to the studies mentioned previously, Agre and Baxter (3) were not able to find any such differences.

While results of studies of muscle fiber composition in elite soccer players have been somewhat equivocal (see, e.g., reviews in 66 and 86), it would seem that this may also reflect different physiological requirements of different positions. For example, midfielders resemble endurance athletes to some extent, while the characteristics of forwards may have more in common with sprint-type athletes. Consequently, the quadriceps muscle fiber composition of midfielders may tend more toward slow twitch predominance, while that of forwards may lean more toward fast twitch predominance. As noted in chapter 3, much evidence supports the relationship between muscle fiber composition and isokinetic strength and endurance tests.

- *Isokinetic assessment has been shown to be sensitive to changes in strength over extended training and competition phases in soccer* (74) (see figure 20.2). Sale's (74) data showed that the declines in strength occurred in apparent synchrony with

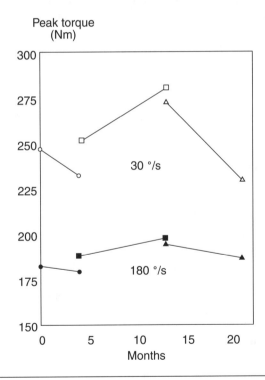

**Figure 20.2**  Variation over time in concentric knee extensor peak torque in soccer players. Not all players were present for each test; same symbols represent same group of players.

Modified from Sale 1991.

increases in maximum oxygen consumption (and vice versa), reflecting the different emphases of training and competition phases.

There are other published and anecdotal reports of a common decline in strength over a competitive season for some sports (30, 62). Whether this is due to more emphasis on strength training in the preseason than during the season, or perhaps reflects a maladaptation (i.e., overtraining), is not clear. However, isokinetic assessment may provide a basis for adjusting the relative training emphases. Decreased concentric knee extensor strength at an intermediate velocity (alone and in comparison to eccentric strength) has recently been found to be an indicator of overtraining in elite athletes (38).

Isokinetic assessment has been shown to be sensitive to changes in strength due to (nonisokinetic) strength training by soccer players in at least one study (18). Furthermore, the strength changes detected isokinetically in this study were associated with changes in sport-specific (kicking) performance, thus indicating sensitivity to function-related strength adaptation. However, such associations may depend on the kicking ability of the players prior to training, that is, the potential for improvement (84). This is only one of a number of considerable problems in establishing a relationship between changes in strength (resulting from any form of strength training) and improvement in any athletic performance (52).

- *Normative data is available on male elite and lower-level soccer players, including juniors* (1–3, 10–12, 16, 19, 22, 33, 34, 36, 39, 43, 44, 46, 49, 57–59, 63, 67, 71, 74, 77, 78, 80, 83, 85, 93). Some female data is also available (13, 20, 47, 56). The majority of this data is for concentric testing of the knee extensors and flexors. Data for eccentric testing is less widely available but can be found, for example, in the work of Aagaard and coworkers (2) and DeProft and associates (18).

- *Isokinetic assessment of the knee extensors and flexors has been shown to be reliable in representative samples of soccer players* (59, 71), albeit with inadequate description of methods. While isokinetic testing has generally been shown to be reliable (25, 54), relatively few reliability studies have been performed with elite athletes.

One should ideally have an understanding of confidence intervals—based on the standard error of measurement (*SEM*)—for isokinetic measurements for different joints, velocities, and muscle actions. An example of the use of the confidence interval is demonstrated with the results of the study by McCleary and Andersen (45). These authors investigated the reliability of concentric knee extension and flexion testing of male collegiate football players at 60°/s on the Biodex dynamometer. They found 95% confidence intervals of around ± 5 to 8% of the group mean peak torque scores. Thus, the "true" score for one of these athletes should lie within this range of their measured score on 95% of occasions.

Such figures—ideally from athletic groups similar to the athlete(s) being tested—may be quoted with each individual score when reporting team data, so that the potential variability in the data is apparent to athletes and coaches.

This is important to prevent too much significance being placed on small differences that are within the bounds of human and test variability. Without some knowledge of the *SEMs* for isokinetic measurement parameters, it is not possible to state whether a change in isokinetic test results over a period of time represents a "true" change or is simply within normal variability (54, 73). Likewise, differences between individual athletes' results may or may not be true differences.

Tests at faster velocities appear to be somewhat less reliable than slower velocity tests (see, e.g., 51). Eccentric test scores also tend to have lower reliability than concentric test scores (32). It is not widely known that the bilateral ratios commonly calculated from absolute isokinetic scores generally have lower reliability than the constituent absolute scores, especially at faster velocities (24, 25, 28, 40, 41, 92). Since bilateral ratios generally form a large part of a test interpretation, it is important that small changes or differences are not overemphasized.

- *Biomechanical analyses of kicking are available that indicate the importance of knee extension and hip flexion*, in particular, to kicking performance (29, 68–70, 87).

# Test Protocols

Soccer, as a strength-related sport, is best suited by a generic protocol. There are relatively few instances where an isokinetic test protocol will be designed specifically for an individual sport. Generally, one will choose the muscle groups that are known to be relevant to a given sport (based on the criteria outlined above) and conduct a standard test protocol for those muscle groups. Most isokinetic dynamometers are capable of testing all major muscle groups in this way. In the rare instances when a special test is deemed to be potentially useful, special adapters have been used where the standard adapters were not adequate. An example of this is the testing of neck strength for American football (72).

A standard concentric protocol involving either continuous, reciprocal movements or discrete, single movements (usually determined by the type of dynamometer available) at two or three angular velocities is generally employed for the football codes. Refer to Wrigley and Strauss (91) for a detailed discussion of procedures that should be followed for testing of all muscle-joint systems.

## Muscle Groups

The extensors and flexors at both the knee and hip have been shown to be important in soccer, especially for kicking (8, 18, 53, 64). While knee extensor/flexor testing is the most commonly performed isokinetic test, hip testing is less common and is associated with a number of special considerations and difficulties related to stabilization and gravitational torque compensation (91). As well as the performance implications of strength in these muscle groups, the knee extensors and flexors, in particular, will often be tested in an injury context. Relevant issues are discussed later in this chapter.

The isokinetic strength of the plantarflexor and dorsiflexor muscle groups has been studied in soccer players (21, 63, 64, 78). Cox (14) reviewed the studies of this muscle group among athletes, including a discussion of the protocols employed.

The need for specialized dynamometer attachments for trunk muscle strength testing has meant that there is relatively little published data on such tests for athletes, including soccer players (4, 88). Furthermore, such testing is fraught with considerable difficulties. These relate to gravitational compensation for the considerable mass of the upper body and the need for increased reliance on absolute and relative torque scores, because bilateral ratios are not available as they are for the limb muscle groups.

## Limb Dominance

Evidence suggests that limb dominance among the lower limb muscle groups of soccer players is not marked, usually amounting to less than a 10% difference between dominant and nondominant limbs (3, 7, 9, 11, 13, 19, 39, 42–44, 48, 53, 78, 80). This essential lack of limb dominance appears to be a consistent finding for most lower limb sports; only unilateral upper limb sports often exhibit strength dominance (91).

## Torque-Velocity and Power-Velocity Relationships

A more comprehensive assessment of strength for the football codes can be derived from testing at a larger range of angular velocities (see, e.g., 1, 2, 33–35) (see figure 20.3). The association between isokinetic strength and muscle fiber type is most apparent at faster velocities, where a higher proportion of fast twitch fibers is associated with greater relative torque production at any given velocity (see chapter 3).

## Anaerobic Muscular Endurance

Many aspects of soccer-specific physiological requirements can be usefully assessed with appropriately designed field tests (5). However, targeted assessment of particular muscle groups and limbs, under standardized conditions, can be addressed by isokinetic testing. Anaerobic muscular endurance testing by isokinetic dynamometry is an example of such targeted testing, which offers options not available via field testing or other forms of anaerobic ergometry. The ability to focus on particular muscle groups in isolated movements may be especially useful where an athlete is recovering from injury.

The intermittent, short-term, high-intensity efforts required in soccer indicate that assessment of short duration anaerobic endurance, and repeat efforts after short recovery periods, is important. Protocols to assess this ability have been described in the literature (26, 75, 81, 82).

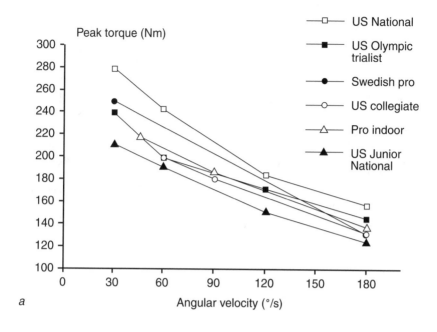

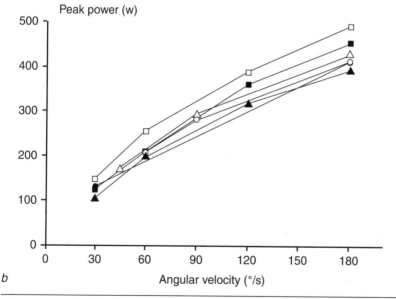

**Figure 20.3** Concentric torque-velocity *(a)* and power-velocity *(b)* relationships for various levels of elite soccer players.

Modified from *The Physician and Sportsmedicine* 1985.

## Other Protocols

The discussion of isokinetic protocols has been limited to those for lower body strength. Isokinetic testing of upper body strength has relatively little relevance to soccer, except in an injury context (e.g., assessing strength after shoulder injury). Upper body strength is more relevant in the other codes, especially American football, but its assessment by isokinetic means will often be similarly limited to clinical situations.

As noted in the discussion of normative data for soccer above, most published data is from concentric testing only, with only a few exceptions (see, e.g., 2, 18). This is largely a reflection of the concentric-only dynamometers that predominated until the late 1980s, rather than a perceived lack of importance of eccentric strength for football. However, more work is required to determine if eccentric isokinetic testing for football yields information that is not provided by the more common concentric test protocols. In some cases, strong athletes can exceed the maximum torque limits of modern isokinetic dynamometers during eccentric muscle actions (e.g., of the knee and hip extensors), thus terminating the test.

More specialized protocols are not routinely performed for the football codes, as they might be for strength-limited sports with a more homogeneous performance requirement such as sprinting, but such protocols do have application in the assessment of particular injuries. For example, hamstring muscle strain injury is particularly common in Australian Rules football (see discussion later), and a hamstring stretch-shortening cycle can be used in the preseason isokinetic assessment and in rehabilitation of such injuries.

# Interpretation of Isokinetic Test Results

The diversity of positional requirements and body types in American football, and the range of physiological types in the other codes, present some challenges for data interpretation. As far as possible, athletes should be compared to their counterparts—this is particularly the case for American football, where players should be compared to those in similar positions. Players in all of the football codes should be assessed on a range of physiological parameters in addition to strength, so that individual physiological strengths and weaknesses can be identified. It is obviously unrealistic to expect all athletes in these codes to score highly on any single physiological test; players will typically score well in some areas but poorly in others.

All of the considerations discussed so far regarding the diversity within each football code suggest that valid comparisons *between* athletes within a team can be somewhat difficult. Therefore, athletes' isokinetic test results should be considered first on an *individual* basis. For example, does an athlete have acceptable left-right balance for the muscle groups tested (i.e., within 15% of opposite limb) (91)? However, an athlete's results must eventually be compared to those of his or her athletic peers, albeit always with recognition of the inherent difficulties for making fair comparisons.

## Torque/Body Mass Ratios

The football codes are similar in requiring both absolute strength (e.g., for kicking and body contact with opponents) and relative strength (e.g., for running and jumping). Relative strength is most commonly expressed as the peak torque/body mass ratio. There are several assumptions underlying the choice of body mass (i.e., to the power of 1.0) as the means of accounting for the effects of body size on strength (see chapter 3). Given the wide range of body masses that are found in American and Australian Rules football, in particular, it is important that this practice is not unfairly biased against particular groups of athletes.

As indicated in chapter 3, the theory underlying the torque/body mass ratio is reasonably well supported (although this issue has not been addressed in great depth in the literature). However, experience suggests that in practice, taller, heavier athletes often seem to score relatively poorly on the torque/body mass ratio. For example, in the data from Rankin and Thompson (65), American football linemen ranked toward the low end among 19 different groups of college athletes (see figure 20.4). While in some cases this may be due to increased relative fat associated with the larger body mass (i.e., less relative muscle mass), this does not always appear to be the explanation. As such, it is suggested that a fairer approach to judging athletes' strength in teams with a large range of body sizes is to separate athletes into body mass groups, so that athletes are compared to their body mass peers (see figure 20.5).

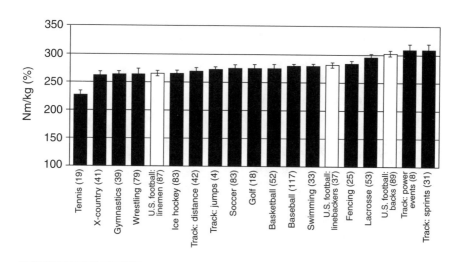

**Figure 20.4**  Peak torque/body mass ratios (Nm/kg, %) for concentric knee extension at 60°/s from male American college athletes. American football player positional groupings are shown as open bars.

Data from *Athletic Training* 1983.

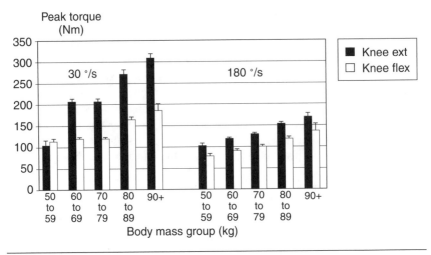

**Figure 20.5** Concentric knee extensor peak torque for high school American football players (15–17 yr) in different body mass categories.

Data from *Archives of Physical Medicine and Rehabilitation* 1979.

## Use of Normative Data

If published normative data is to be employed, the circumstances under which isokinetic data is being collected should match those of the published normative data on the following criteria:

- Type of athletes (e.g., level, positional roles)
- Age, height, weight
- Time during season
- Pretest status (e.g., heavy training, injury excluded?)
- Dynamometer and software used
- Exact test movement performed
- Body position and stabilization
- Test velocity used
- Which limb(s) tested
- Range of motion
- Gravity correction
- Isometric preload and acceleration ramping
- Continuous versus discrete repetitions
- Muscle action type (i.e., concentric or eccentric) and sequence
- Torque measurement parameter used
- Maximum or mean scores used

While there is not sufficient evidence in the research literature to state definitively that results from isokinetic dynamometers made by different companies *cannot* be compared (see review in 91), it is prudent that such comparisons be made with considerable caution. Published normative data is generally only provided as a mean and standard deviation. In that form, the data is of little practical use. Data presented in percentile form is more useful, as one can determine where a given athlete's result falls in relation to a full range of normative team scores. Table 20.1 shows a normative database in percentile form for players from the Australian Football League (the professional Australian Rules football league).

Rather than attempting to use published normative data, it is actually best to construct your own normative data, under your specific measuring conditions. In constructing such a normative database, one should include data only for limbs without a recent injury history or any history of major surgery. In sports with clear differences in positional requirements—such as American football—data should be separated according to position.

It should go without saying that care should be exercised when reporting isokinetic test results, so that coaches and athletes do not draw inappropriate conclusions. Where such caution is not exercised, such tests have been known to affect team selection; this may occur, for example, when isokinetic testing is used to assess recovery from injury. In professional sports, this amounts to

**Table 20.1    Percentile Scores for Absolute and Relative Concentric Knee Extensor Peak Torque at 60°/s Recorded on a Biodex Dynamometer**

|  | Peak torque | |
| Percentile | Nm | Nm/kg |
| --- | --- | --- |
| 0 | 163 | 1.94 |
| 10th | 193 | 2.34 |
| 20th | 209 | 2.46 |
| 30th | 219 | 2.55 |
| 40th | 225 | 2.64 |
| 50th | 233 | 2.74 |
| 60th | 241 | 2.82 |
| 70th | 252 | 2.95 |
| 80th | 268 | 3.04 |
| 90th | 293 | 3.20 |
| 100th | 369 | 3.86 |

Data is based on scores from the stronger leg (injuries excluded) of over 100 Australian Football League players (Isokinetic Dynamometry Laboratory, CRESS, Victoria University).

affecting the athlete's livelihood. In some countries where physical tests—including strength tests—are used for job selection, the conduct and interpretation of these tests are subject to legislation; inappropriate use of such tests is regarded as a human rights violation (55).

# Isokinetic Strength and Football Injuries

Some coaches, athletes, strength and conditioning staff, and medical personnel believe that injury is often the result of weaknesses in particular muscle groups, which can be detected by isokinetic testing. Indeed, detection of such supposed weakness will often be the impetus for isokinetic testing of a football team. Conversely, it is commonly believed that isokinetic testing does not relate closely to athletic performance, per se. As discussed in chapter 3, this second belief would appear to be contradicted by the bulk of the research evidence. Furthermore, as will be discussed, there is little clear evidence to support the utility of isokinetic dynamometry for injury prediction. Therefore, it is likely that isokinetic testing is *more useful* than is widely believed for providing performance-related information but *less useful* for predicting injury.

In assessing isokinetic strength of elite football players, one is regularly confronted with the issue of the possible relationship of the results to past or future injury. Weaknesses *are* often identified by isokinetic testing, but they are almost always associated with a current or previous injury. In fact, the ability to determine whether an athlete still suffers from a residual weakness due to such an injury is one of the more useful aspects of isokinetic dynamometry. It is common to find residual weaknesses from previous injuries when testing athletes (see, e.g., 3, 19, 37).

Bilateral strength differences greater than those that are common among healthy athletes (i.e., up to around 15%) occur so rarely in athletes without an injury history as to challenge the very notion that isokinetic testing might be predictive of injury in previously uninjured athletes; that is, if unexplained weaknesses are present rarely, if ever, then there is no weakness on which to base an injury prediction.

It is possible that more sophisticated test protocols may provide the sensitivity for injury prediction in the future, but existing evidence does not support a role for traditional isokinetic measures in injury prediction. It is beyond the scope of this chapter to review all studies that have examined the relationship between isokinetic strength measures and subsequent injury. However, the evidence in relation to one injury that is common in football will be briefly reviewed.

## Hamstring Muscle Strain Injuries

Hamstring muscle strain injuries are among the most prevalent noncontact injuries in football, particularly Australian Rules. Studies on the association between isokinetic strength and subsequent hamstring injury have been somewhat scarce. The study of professional Australian Rules footballers by Orchard and coworkers (60) reported the association between preseason Cybex 340 concentric peak torque of the knee extensors and flexors (at 60, 180, and 300°/s) and hamstring injury during the subsequent season. Sixteen percent of the 37 players studied suffered a hamstring injury. The bilateral knee flexor ratios at 60°/s were significantly lower in the injured compared to the uninjured players (means of 88% versus 100%, respectively).

While this difference was indeed *statistically* significant, an 88% weaker-to-stronger bilateral knee flexor strength ratio is within the bounds of normal variation among healthy athletes. As such, when testing an individual athlete, his or her individual test result could not reasonably be deemed to be likely to lead to injury, as many athletes would fall into this category. A significant difference in the reciprocal knee flexor/knee extensor ratio (ham-to-quad ratio) was a *secondary* finding in this study, explained by the bilateral knee flexor imbalance mentioned previously and the absence of a bilateral difference in knee extensor strength.

While previous injury history was recorded in this study, the published report did not indicate whether any of the injuries incurred during the season were recurrences. It was noted, however, that previous hamstring injury was not significantly correlated with injury during the season in question. Thus, it remains unclear as to whether the results reflected an association between isokinetic strength and *initial* hamstring injury or inadequate rehabilitation of *previous* hamstring injury, leading to subsequent injury recurrence.

Bennell and coworkers (6) studied preseason concentric and eccentric knee extensor and flexor peak torque in 102 elite Australian Rules footballers, using a Kin-Com dynamometer at 60 and 180°/s. Of the 12 players who suffered a hamstring strain in the subsequent season, 8 were recurrences. Thus only 4 were new injuries, which was insufficient for effective analysis as a separate group. Considering the 12 injuries together, there were no differences in reciprocal or bilateral ratios between the injured and uninjured players.

Therefore, the major difficulty in interpreting the results from such studies—and indeed of other isokinetic and injury studies—is that they have not generally analyzed data separately for new injuries and recurrences of previous injuries. This is unfortunate, as there are two rather different questions here: is isokinetic strength predictive of an initial injury; and having already suffered an injury, is isokinetic strength predictive of a recurrence?

There have been a number of cross-sectional studies comparing isokinetic strength of athletes who have previously suffered a hamstring muscle strain injury to those who have never had such an injury. Some studies have failed to find any significant difference in isokinetic hamstring strength between athletes with and without a history of injury. Worrell and associates (90) found no difference between the concentric or eccentric bilateral ratios for previously injured college athletes and those of uninjured athletes. Paton and coworkers (61) found no difference in concentric flexor/extensor peak torque ratios between a small group of professional soccer players with injury histories and those without. Stephens and Reid (79) found no differences in bilateral or reciprocal ratios between previously injured college football players and those without a previous injury.

Therefore, on the basis of these studies, there did not appear to be any differences in isokinetic strength in previously injured athletes that might be used as a basis for predicting future recurrences. However, in contrast, the study by Jonhagen, Nemeth, and Eriksson (31) on sprinters with a history of very severe hamstring strains did find those athletes to be weaker than uninjured sprinters. Bennell and coworkers (6) also found a difference for Australian Rules footballers with a history of hamstring injury, but those athletes were actually stronger than an uninjured group.

## Summary

Characteristics of three football codes have been discussed: soccer, Australian Rules, and American football. The large volume of isokinetic literature concerning soccer has been used as a basis for an isokinetic testing strategy. While less published information is available for other football codes, a similar approach can be pursued.

Some challenges for data interpretation that are present for sports such as the football codes—with considerable diversity of athletic "types" and performance requirements—have been discussed and approaches to dealing with them have been outlined. Given the high injury rates of the football codes, the use of isokinetic assessment in this clinical context has been briefly outlined. Further work is necessary to clearly elucidate the relationship between isokinetic strength and both new injuries and recurrent injuries.

## References

1. Aagaard, P., E.B. Simonsen, M. Trolle, J. Bangsbo, and K. Klausen. 1994. Moment and power generation during maximal knee extensions performed at low and high speeds. *European Journal of Applied Physiology* 69: 376–81.

2. Aagaard, P., E.B. Simonsen, M. Trolle, J. Bangsbo, and K. Klausen. 1995. Isokinetic hamstring/quadriceps strength ratio: Influence from joint angular velocity, gravity correction, and contraction mode. *Acta Physiologica Scandinavica* 154: 421–27.

3. Agre, J.C., and T.L. Baxter. 1987. Musculoskeletal profile of male collegiate soccer players. *Archives of Physical Medicine and Rehabilitation* 68: 147–50.

4. Andersson, E., L. Sward, A. Thorstensson. 1988. Trunk muscle strength in athletes. *Medicine and Science in Sports and Exercise* 20: 587–93.

5. Balsom, P. 1994. Evaluation of physical performance. In *Football (soccer)*, ed. B. Ekblom, 102–23. Oxford, UK: Blackwell Scientific.

6. Bennell, K., H. Wajswelner, P. Lew, A. Schall-Riaucour, S. Leslie, D. Plant, and J. Cirone. 1998. Isokinetic strength testing does not predict hamstring injury in Australian Rules footballers. *British Journal of Sports Medicine* 32: 309–14.

7. Brady, E.C., M. O'Regan, and B. McCormack. 1993. Isokinetic assessment of un-injured soccer players. In *Science and football II*, ed. T. Reilly, J. Clarys, and A. Stibbe, 351–56. London: Spon.

8. Cabri, J., E. DeProft, W. Dufour, and J.P. Clarys. 1988. The relation between muscular strength and kick performance. In *Science and football*, ed. T. Reilly, A. Lees, K. Davids, and W.J. Murphy, 186–93. London: Spon.

9. Capranica, L., G. Cama, F. Fanton, A. Tessitore, and F. Figura. 1992. Force and power of preferred and nonpreferred leg in young soccer players. *Journal of Sports Medicine and Physical Fitness* 324: 358–63.

10. Chin, M-K., Y.S.A. Lo, C.T. Li, and C.H. So. 1992. Physiological profiles of Hong Kong elite soccer players. *British Journal of Sports Medicine* 264: 262–66.

11. Chin, M-K., R.C.H. So, Y.W.Y. Yuan, R.C.T. Li, and A.S.K. Wong. 1994. Cardio-respiratory fitness and isokinetic muscle strength of elite Asian junior soccer players. *Journal of Sports Medicine and Physical Fitness* 343: 250–57.

12. Chook, K.K., K.C. Teh, and C.K. Giam. 1986. The isokinetic strength of domi-nant quadriceps and hamstring muscles of 47 Singapore national sportsmen. In *Proceedings of 2nd International Sports Science Conference*, ed. C.K. Giam and K.C. Teh, 127–33. Singapore: Singapore Sports Council.

13. Costain, R., and A.K. Williams. 1984. Isokinetic quadriceps and hamstring torque levels of adolescent female soccer players. *Journal of Orthopaedic and Sports Physical Therapy* 54: 196–200.

14. Cox, P.D. 1995. Isokinetic strength testing of the ankle: A review. *Physiotherapy Canada* 472: 97–119.

15. Davies, G.J., D.T. Kirkendall, D.H. Leigh, M.L. Lui, T.R. Reinbold, and P.K. Wilson. 1981. Isokinetic characteristics of professional football players. I. Nor-mative relationships between quadriceps and hamstring muscle groups and rela-tive to body weight [abstract]. *Medicine and Science in Sports and Exercise* 13(2): 76–77.

16. Davis, J.A., J. Brewer, and D. Atkin. 1992. Preseason physiological characteristics of English first and second division soccer players. *Journal of Sports Sciences* 10: 541–47.

17. Delecluse, C., M. Van Leemputte, E. Willems, R. Diels, R. Andries, and H. Van Coppenolle. 1995. Study of performance related strength tests for competition level sprinters. In *Biomechanics in sports XII*, ed. A. Barabas and G. Fabian, 347–50. Budapest: ISBS.

18. DeProft, E., J. Cabri, W. Dufour, and J.P. Clarys. 1988. Strength training and kick performance in soccer players. In *Science and football*, ed. T. Reilly, A. Lees, K. Davids, and W.J. Murphy, 108–13. London: Spon.

19. Ekstrand, J., and J. Gillquist. 1983. The avoidability of soccer injuries. *International Journal of Sports Medicine* 42: 124–28.

20. Fillyaw, M., T. Bevins, and L. Fernandez. 1986. Importance of correcting isokinetic peak torque for the effect of gravity when calculating knee flexor to extensor muscle ratios. *Physical Therapy* 661: 23–31.

21. Fugl-Meyer, A.R. 1981. Maximum isokinetic ankle plantar- and dorsiflexion torques in trained subjects. *European Journal of Applied Physiology* 47: 393–404.

22. Gauffin, H., J. Ekstrand, and H. Tropp. 1988. Improvement of vertical jump performance in soccer players after specific training. *Journal of Human Movement Studies* 15: 185–90.

23. Gilliam, T.B., S.P. Sady, P.S. Freedson, and J. Villanacci. 1979. Isokinetic torque levels for high school football players. *Archives of Physical Medicine and Rehabilitation* 60: 110–14.

24. Gleeson, N., and T. Mercer. 1991. Intrasubject variability in isokinetic knee extension and flexion strength characteristics of adult males: A comparative examination of gravity-corrected and uncorrected data [abstract]. *Journal of Sports Science* 94: 415–16.

25. Gleeson, N.P., and T.H. Mercer. 1996. The utility of isokinetic dynamometry in the assessment of human muscle function. *Sports Medicine* 211: 18–34.

26. Gleeson, N., T. Mercer, and I. Campbell. 1997. Effect of a fatigue task on absolute and relativised indices of isokinetic leg strength in female collegiate soccer players. In *Science and football III*, ed. T. Reilly, J. Bangsbo, and M. Hughes, 162–67. London: Spon.

27. Gleim, G.W. 1984. The profiling of professional football players. *Clinics in Sports Medicine* 3(1): 185–97.

28. Holm, I., P. Ludvigsen, and H. Steen. 1994. Isokinetic hamstrings/quadriceps ratios: Normal values and reproducibility in sport students. *Isokinetics and Exercise Science* 44: 141–45.

29. Huang, T.C., E.M. Roberts, and Y. Youm. 1982. The biomechanics of kicking. In *Human body dynamics*, ed. D.N. Ghista, 409–43. New York: Oxford University Press.

30. Johansson, C., R. Lorentzon, S. Rasmuson, S. Reiz, S. Haggmark, H. Nyman, and A.R. Fugl-Meyer. 1988. Peak torque and OBLA running capacity in male orienteerers. *Acta Physiologica Scandinavica* 132: 525–30.

31. Jonhagen, S., G. Nemeth, and E. Eriksson. 1994. Hamstring injuries in sprinters: The role of concentric and eccentric hamstring muscle strength and flexibility. *American Journal of Sports Medicine* 222: 262–66.

32. Kellis, E., and V. Baltzopoulos. 1995. Isokinetic eccentric exercise. *Sports Medicine* 193: 202–22.

33. Kirkendall, D.T. 1979. Comparison of isokinetic power-velocity profiles in various classes of American athletes. PhD diss., Ohio State University.

34. Kirkendall, D.T. 1985. The applied sport science of soccer. *Physician and Sports Medicine* 134: 53–59.

35. Kirkendall, D.T., G.J. Davies, D.H. Leigh, M.L. Lui, T.R. Reinbold, and P.K. Wilson. 1981. Isokinetic characteristics of professional football players. II. Absolute and relative power-velocity relationships [abstract]. *Medicine and Science in Sports and Exercise* 13(2): 77.

36. Kohno, T., N. O'Hata, M. O'Hara, T. Shirahata, Y. Endo, M. Satoh, Y. Kimura, and Y. Nakajima. 1997. Sports injuries and physical fitness in adolescent soccer players. In *Science and football III*, ed. T. Reilly, J. Bangsbo, and M. Hughes, 185–89. London: Spon.

37. Koutedakis, Y., R. Frischknecht, and N.C.C. Sharp. 1994. Knee flexion to extension peak torque ratios and low back injuries in elite rowers [abstract]. *Journal of Sports Science* 122: 141–42.

38. Koutedakis, Y., R. Frischknecht, G. Vrbova, N.C.C. Sharp, and R. Budgett. 1995. Maximal voluntary quadriceps strength patterns in Olympic overtrained athletes. *Medicine and Science in Sports and Exercise* 274: 566–72.

39. Kramer, J.F., and B. Balsor. 1990. Lower extremity dominance and knee extensor torques in intercollegiate soccer players. *Canadian Journal of Applied Sport Science* 15: 180–84.

40. Kramer, J.F., S. Ingham-Tupper, K. Walters-Stansbury, P. Stratford, and J. MacDermid. 1994. Reliability of absolute and ratio data in assessment of knee extensor and flexor strength. *Isokinetics and Exercise Science* 42: 51–57.

41. Kramer, J.F., D. Nusca, L. Bisbee, J. MacDermid, D. Kemp, and S. Boley. 1994. Forearm pronation and supination: Reliability of absolute torques and nondominant/dominant ratios. *Journal of Hand Therapy* 7: 15–20.

42. Lai, J.S., P.L. Wong, I.N. Lien. 1986. Isokinetic evaluation of soccer players [abstract]. *XXIII FIMS World Congress of Sports Medicine Abstracts*, 138. Canberra: Australian Sports Medicine Federation.

43. Leatt, P., R.J. Shephard, and M.J. Plyley. 1987. Specific muscular development in under-18 soccer players. *Journal of Sports Sciences* 5: 165–75.

44. Mangine, R.E., F.R. Noyes, M.P. Mullen, and S.D. Barber. 1990. A physiological profile of the elite soccer athlete. *Journal of Orthopaedic and Sports Physical Therapy* 124: 147–52.

45. McCleary, R.W., J.C. Andersen. 1992. Test-retest reliability of reciprocal isokinetic knee extension and flexion peak torque measurements. *Journal of Athletic Training* 27(4): 362–65.

46. McHugh, M.P., G.W. Gleim, S.P. Magnusson, and J.A. Nicholas. 1993. A cross-sectional study of age-related musculoskeletal and physiological changes in soccer players. *Medicine, Exercise, Nutrition and Health* 2: 261–68.

47. McKay, L.J., A. Dale, S. Hochstetler, and M.J. Plyley. 1987. Physiological profiles of Canadian varsity women soccer players [abstract]. *Medicine and Science in Sports and Exercise* 192(Suppl.): S48.

48. McLean, B.D., and D.McA. Tumilty. 1993. Left-right asymmetry in two types of soccer kick. *British Journal of Sports Medicine* 274: 260–62.

49. Mercer, T.H., N.P. Gleeson, and J. Mitchell. 1997. Fitness profiles of professional soccer players before and after preseason conditioning. In *Science and football III*, ed. T. Reilly, J. Bangsbo, and M. Hughes, 112–17. London: Spon.

50. Mognoni, P., M.V. Narici, M.D. Sirtori, and F. Lorenzelli. 1994. Isokinetic torques and kicking maximal velocity in young soccer players. *Journal of Sports Medicine and Physical Fitness* 344: 357–61.

51. Montgomery, L.C., L.W. Douglass, and P.A. Deuster. 1989. Reliability of an isokinetic test of muscle strength and endurance. *Journal of Orthopaedic and Sports Physical Therapy* 10: 315–22.

52. Murphy, A.J., and G.J. Wilson. 1997. The ability of tests of muscular function to reflect training-induced changes in performance. *Journal of Sports Sciences* 15:191–200.

53. Narici, M.V., M.D. Sirtori, and P. Mognoni. 1988. Maximal ball velocity and peak torques of hip flexor and knee extensor muscles. In *Science and football*, ed. T. Reilly, A. Lees, K. Davids, and W.J. Murphy, 429–33. London: Spon.

54. Nitschke, J.E. 1992. Reliability of isokinetic torque measurements: A review of the literature. *Australian Journal of Physiotherapy* 382: 125–34.

55. Norman, R.W. 1992. Matching issues in strength measurements. *Canadian Journal of Sports Science* 17: 70–71.

56. Nyland, J.A., D.N.M. Caborn, J.A. Brosky, C.L. Kneller, and G. Freidhoff. 1997. Anthropometric, muscular fitness, and injury history comparisons by gender of youth soccer teams. *Journal of Strength and Conditioning Research* 112: 92–97.

57. Oberg, B., J. Ekstrand, M. Moller, and J. Gillquist. 1984. Muscle strength and flexibility in different positions of soccer players. *International Journal of Sports Medicine* 5: 213–16.

58. Oberg, B., P. Odenrick, and H. Tropp. 1985. Muscle strength and jump performance in soccer players [abstract]. 10th International Congress of Biomechanics, Umea. Abstract book, 311.

59. Oberg, B., M. Moller, J. Gillquist, and J. Ekstrand. 1986. Isokinetic torque levels for knee extensors and knee flexors in soccer players. *International Journal of Sports Medicine* 7: 50–53.

60. Orchard, J., J. Marsden, S. Lord, and D. Garlick. 1997. Preseason hamstring muscle weakness associated with hamstring muscle injury in Australian footballers. *American Journal of Sports Medicine* 251: 81–85.

61. Paton, R.W., P. Grimshaw, J. McGregor, and J. Noble. 1989. Biomechanical assessment of the effects of significant hamstring injury: An isokinetic study. *Journal of Biomedical Engineering* 11: 229–30.

62. Posch, E., Y. Haglund, and E. Eriksson. 1989. Prospective study of concentric and eccentric leg muscle torque, flexibility, physical conditioning, and variation of injury rates during one season of amateur ice hockey. *International Journal of Sports Medicine* 102: 113–17.

63. Poulmedis, P. 1985. Isokinetic maximal torque power of Greek elite soccer players. *Journal of Orthopaedic and Sports Physical Therapy* 6: 293–95.

64. Poulmedis, P., G. Rondoyannis, A. Mitsou, and E. Tsarouchas. 1988. The influence of isokinetic muscle torque exerted in various speeds on soccer ball velocity. *Journal of Orthopaedic and Sports Physical Therapy* 10: 93–96.

65. Rankin, J.M., and C.B. Thompson. 1983. Isokinetic evaluation of quadriceps and hamstrings function: Normative data concerning body weight and sport. *Athletic Training* 18(Summer): 110–14.

66. Reilly, T. 1994. Physiological profile of the player. In *Football (soccer)*, ed. B. Ekblom, 78–94. Oxford, UK: Blackwell Scientific.

67. Rhodes, E.C., R.E. Mosher, D.C. McKenzie, I.M. Franks, and J.E. Potts. 1986. Physiological profiles of the Canadian Olympic soccer team. *Canadian Journal of Sports Science* 11(1): 31–36.

68. Roberts, M.E., and A. Metcalfe. 1968. Mechanical analysis of kicking. In *Biomechanics I*, ed. J. Wartenweiler, E. Jokl, and M. Hebbelinck, 315–19. Basel: Karger.

69. Roberts, M.E., R.F. Zernicke, Y. Youm, and T.C. Huang. 1974. Kinetic parameters of kicking. In *Biomechanics IV*, ed. T. Nelson and C. Morehouse, 157–62. Baltimore: University Park Press.

70. Robertson, D.G.E., and R.E. Mosher. 1983. Work and power of leg muscles in soccer kicking. In *Biomechanics IX-B*, ed. D.A. Winter, R.W. Norman, R.P. Wells, K.C. Hayes, and A.E. Patla, 533–42. Champaign, IL: Human Kinetics.

71. Rochcongar, P., R. Morvan, J. Jan, J. Dassonville, and J. Beillot. 1988. Isokinetic investigation of knee extensors and knee flexors in young French soccer players. *International Journal of Sports Medicine* 9: 448–50.

72. Rogers, B.L. 1984. The development of an interphase connector to isokinetically evaluate rotary cervical spine musculature using the Cybex II dynamometer. *Athletic Training* Spring: 16–18.

73. Rothstein, J.M. 1985. Measurement and clinical practice: Theory and application. In *Measurement in physical therapy*, ed. J.M. Rothstein, 1–46. New York: Churchill Livingstone.

74. Sale, D.G. 1991. Testing strength and power. In *Physiological testing of the high-performance athlete*, 2d ed., ed. J.D. MacDougall, H.A. Wenger, and H.J. Green, 21–106. Champaign, IL: Human Kinetics.

75. Schwendner, K.I., A.E. Mikesky, J.K. Wigglesworth, and D.B. Burr. 1995. Recovery of dynamic muscle function following isokinetic fatigue testing. *International Journal of Sports Medicine* 16: 185–89.

76. Shields, C.L., F.E. Whitney, and V.D. Zomar. 1984. Exercise performance of professional football players. *American Journal of Sports Medicine* 12(6): 455–59.

77. Smith, C., A. Donnelly, J. Brewer, and J. Davis. 1994. An investigation of the specific aspects of fitness in professional and amateur footballers [abstract]. *Journal of Sports Science* 122: 165–66.

78. So, C-H., T.O. Siu, K.M. Chan, M.K. Chin, and C.T. Li. 1994. Isokinetic profile of dorsiflexors and plantarflexors of the ankle: A comparative study of elite versus untrained subjects. *British Journal of Sports Medicine* 281: 25–30.

79. Stephens, D., and J.G. Reid. 1988. Biomechanics of hamstring strains in sprinting events [abstract]. *Canadian Journal of Sports Science* 133: 88P.

80. Svetlize, H.D. 1996. Isokinetic hamstrings and quadriceps evaluation of Argentine elite soccer players [abstract]. *Medicine and Science in Sports and Exercise* 285(Suppl.): S9.

81. Tesch, P.A., and J.E. Wright. 1983. Recovery from short-term intense exercise: Its relation to capillary supply and blood lactate accumulation. *European Journal of Applied Physiology* 52: 98–103.

82. Tesch, P.A., J.E. Wright, J.A. Vogel, W.L. Daniels, D.S. Sharp, and B. Sjodin. 1985. The influence of muscle metabolic characteristics on physical performance. *European Journal of Applied Physiology* 54: 237–43.

83. Togari, H., J. Ohashi, and T. Ohgushi. 1988. Isokinetic muscle strength of soccer players. In: *Science and football*, ed. T. Reilly, A. Lees, K. Davids, and W.J. Murphy, 181–85. London: Spon.

84. Trolle, M., P. Aagaard, E.B. Simonsen, J. Bangsbo, and K. Klausen. 1993. Effects of strength training on kicking performance in soccer. In *Science and football II*, ed. T. Reilly, J. Clarys, and A. Stibbe, 95–97. London: Spon.

85. Tumilty, D.McA., A.G. Hahn, R.D. Telford, and R.A. Smith. 1988. Is "lactic acid tolerance" an important component of fitness for soccer? In *Science and football*, ed. T. Reilly, A. Lees, K. Davids, and W.J. Murphy, 81–86. London: Spon.

86. Tumilty, D.McA. 1993. Physiological characteristics of elite soccer players. *Sports Medicine* 16(2): 80–96.

87. Wahrenberg, H., L. Lindbeck, and J. Ekholm. 1978. Knee muscular moment, tendon tension force, and EMG during a vigorous movement in man. *Scandinavian Journal of Rehabilitation Medicine* 10: 99–106.

88. Williams, C.A., and M. Singh. 1997. Dynamic trunk strength of Canadian football players, soccer players, and middle to long distance runners. *Journal of Orthopaedic and Sports Physical Therapy* 254: 271–76.

89. Wilmore, J.H., R.B. Parr, W.L. Haskell, D.L. Costill, L.J. Milburn, R.K. Kerlan. 1976. Football pros' strengths—and cardiovascular weaknesses—charted. *Physician and Sports Medicine* 4(1): 45–54.

90. Worrell, T.W., D.H. Perrin, B.M. Gansneder, and J.H. Gieck. 1991. Comparison of isokinetic strength and flexibility measures between hamstring injured and noninjured athletes. *Journal of Orthopaedic and Sports Physical Therapy* 133: 118–25.

91. Wrigley, T.V., and G.R. Strauss. 1998. Isokinetic dynamometry: Standardized assessment of strength and power of athletes. In *Test methods manual: Sport specific guidelines for the physiological testing of the elite athlete*, ed. C. Gore. Canberra: Australian Sports Commission.

92. Wrigley, T.V., A. Vasey, L. Watson, and R. Dalziel. 1995. Reliability of clinical isokinetic dynamometry in pathological athletic shoulders. In *Proceedings XIII International Symposium on Biomechanics in Sports*, ed. T. Bauer, 29–33. Budapest: ISBS.

93. Zakas, A., K. Mandroukas, E. Vamvakoudis, K. Christoulas, and N. Aggelopoulou. 1995. Peak torque of quadriceps and hamstring muscles in basketball and soccer players of different divisions. *Journal of Sports Medicine and Physical Fitness* 353: 199–205.

# Chapter 21

# Simulated Space Flight

John F. Caruso and Marcas M. Bamman

As we venture into the 21st century, the National Aeronautics and Space Administration (NASA) and the worldwide space community have goals of inhabiting an international space station and manning missions to Mars. Such projects will expose humans to long periods of weightlessness. Space flight impairs normal human physiology, compromising astronaut safety and performance. Muscle contractile strength is one area of human physiology adversely affected by space flight (10, 30); thus, we must devise countermeasures to strength loss, such as treatments or interventions designed to reduce deconditioning, for man to engage in long-duration space travel. Aerobic exercise, the most widely used countermeasure aboard past space flights, has had little success at maintaining muscle mass or contractile strength (30). Resistance training appears an ideal countermeasure to strength loss based upon its effect in normal gravity (1-g) (6, 8, 9, 13, 20).

## Strength Loss Due to Weightlessness

Data quantifying strength losses resulting from space flight are limited. To date, roughly 65 people have been in outer space for more than one month. Most of those individuals were cosmonauts from the Soviet space program. NASA has some information regarding physiological responses from those space flights, however a lack of data limits their ability to prescribe in-flight resistance training countermeasures. This has led to the development of ground-based research to simulate the effects of weightlessness (3–5, 7, 11, 12, 14–16, 25, 29).

The muscles undergoing the most strength loss from weightlessness are the lower body extensors. Such muscles normally act to maintain posture in 1-g (13, 30) and thus presumably lose strength in the absence of gravity (0-g). The knee (KE) and ankle extensors (AE) are among the lower body extensors most adversely affected by space flight. Unweighting periods of 14 to 16 days, which were designed to examine the impact of a typical space shuttle mission, induced KE strength losses of 12 to 15% (1, 3). The KE strength of astronauts aboard Skylab 2 declined 20% after 28 days of space flight (30), and longer periods of weightlessness have resulted in greater losses (5, 15, 25). The AE undergo similar changes, with longer periods of weightlessness causing greater strength loss (3, 15, 23–25). Both in- and postflight astronaut operational tasks are compromised by such losses. Such deconditioning may also compromise basic locomotor tasks. For instance, while walking, eccentric and concentric AE strength is required during early (heelstrike to midstance) and late (midstance to takeoff) foot support (28). A round-trip manned mission to Mars is projected to last between 15 and 30 months. Such duration of weightlessness is projected to have a profound impact on the muscle mass and strength of astronauts, thereby affecting their in- and postflight performance.

## Countermeasures to Strength Loss

Resistance exercise may be the most appropriate countermeasure to strength losses, based upon its positive effect in 1-g (2, 8). However, little data exists concerning resistance exercise prescription during weightlessness, both in terms of training protocols and space flight equipment. Constant load variable speed training is the most common form of resistance exercise in 1-g. However, conventional equipment depends on gravity for its operation and is therefore useless in outer space. Nonetheless, this form of resistance exercise may serve as an appropriate starting point from which to develop a countermeasure prescription to strength loss. Some researchers suggest that isokinetic dynamometry be employed for space flight (16). Isokinetic dynamometry allows performance of high-tension concentric and eccentric actions without requiring gravity.

Isokinetic dynamometers adapted for use in outer space include the Motomir, a device providing linear concentric and eccentric resistance to the arms and legs. Cosmonauts aboard space station Mir have reportedly used the Motomir; however, little is known regarding its usage in flight.

## Isokinetic Testing of Muscle Performance

Previous space flight–related strength research has examined strength at a single angle (angle-specific torque) (1, 14, 17, 30) or velocity (14, 15, 17, 30) to assess performance. Evaluating contractile strength across an entire range of motion or velocity spectrum from data obtained at a single angle or speed may not adequately represent performance. This may contribute to our lack of knowledge concerning exercise prescription for space flight. Modern-day isokinetic dynamometers quantify muscle performance through an entire range of motion at multiple velocities. Examinations of such performances may be best illustrated using three-dimensional topography, whereby torque is expressed as a function of joint angle and velocity.

An investigation in our lab has examined isokinetic performance before and after a 14-day bed rest. Results are illustrated using three-dimensional topographical (surface) maps to broaden the understanding of strength losses from such a period of simulated weightlessness. Two groups participated in the 14-day bed rest; one refrained from exercise, while the other concurrently engaged in a free weight KE-AE training protocol. Topographical maps were constructed for each group's KE and AE performance before and after the 14-day period. The purposes of the study were to

- quantify torque changes at multiple speeds through an entire range of motion,
- judge the efficacy of the resistance training countermeasure, and
- identify the angles and velocities most susceptible to KE and AE strength loss during a 14-day bed rest.

Twelve male volunteers with physical characteristics similar to the NASA astronaut corps members were recruited. Subjects were obtained through the Test Subject Facility Office in the Medical Sciences Division of NASA's Johnson Space Center. Volunteers were randomly assigned into one of two groups, both undergoing a 14-day bed rest (BR). One group of six subjects concurrently performed a free weight KE-AE training protocol (BR+EX), while six nonexercisers served as controls (BR). To ensure bed rest was examined exclusive of detraining, only individuals who had abstained from strength training for one year prior to the start of the study participated. All subjects passed a comprehensive physical exam. Subject characteristics are presented in table 21.1.

Subjects were housed in the General Clinical Research Center (GCRC) of the University of Texas Medical Branch-Galveston. The GCRC nursing staff continuously monitored subjects to ensure they remained in bed during the 14-day period. The only exception to this rule was for 30 min every other day during supine resistance training (BR+EX) or recumbent out-of-room rest (BR). Subjects were weighed daily and, to ensure no changes in body mass, consumed an isocaloric diet. Protein intake (1.1g/kg/day) remained constant during bed rest. On day 15 subjects were released from the GCRC but did not begin walking until isokinetic posttesting was completed. No subject reported muscle soreness prior to posttesting.

### Table 21.1   Subject Characteristics by Group (Mean ± *SD*)

| Group | Age (yr) | Height (cm) | Preweight (kg) | Postweight (kg) |
|-------|----------|-------------|----------------|-----------------|
| BR | 29.9 ± 6.9 | 177.9 ± 5.8 | 71.5 ± 11.4 | 72.4 ± 10.7 |
| BR+EX | 30.4 ± 6.9 | 178.0 ± 4.0 | 78.2 ± 15.7 | 78.4 ± 15.3 |

Each subject's dominant leg was pre- and posttested on a Lido isokinetic dynamometer (Loredan Biomedical, Inc., Davis, CA). All strength testing occurred at the Johnson Space Center's exercise countermeasures laboratory. The dynamometer was calibrated to ensure accurate measurements. Prior to pretesting, subjects were familiarized with the dynamometer's operation. To limit extraneous body movement, subjects were secured to the Lido with Velcro straps. The KE tests preceded those for the AE. Prior to KE and AE testing, subjects warmed up by performing submaximal repetitions at a constant angular (isokinetic) velocity of 1.04 rad/s. Using only the dominant leg, testing involved three maximal repetitions at each of four (0.52, 1.75, 2.97, 4.19 rad/s) isokinetic velocities. The order in which velocities were examined was randomly assigned for each subject and remained the same at their pre- and posttesting sessions. To minimize error, the final 0.04 radians of flexion and extension were omitted from KE and AE data analysis. With subjects seated upright, KE performance was examined from flexed (1.63 radians) through extended (0.14 radians) angles, relative to a neutral position of 0.78 radians (45° knee angle). Lying supine, AE testing was examined from dorsi- (1.19 radians) through plantarflexion (2.13 radians), relative to a neutral foot position of 1.58 radians. Subjects were encouraged to exert maximal tension throughout concentric and eccentric actions using their extensors exclusively. Following completion of each concentric and eccentric repetition, two-second pauses were given for KE and AE testing. Concentric and eccentric repetitions yielding the highest torque per velocity were analyzed.

# Constant Load Training

In contrast to the BR group, the BR+EX group performed constant load leg and calf presses on a Cybex supine leg press (Cybex Strength Systems, Ronkonkoma, NY). Workouts lasted approximately 30 min every other day. As was the case for testing, KE training always preceded that for the AE. Unlike isokinetic testing, constant load training involved both legs. A single warm-up set, involving high (15+) repetitions performed with a moderate weight, preceded each KE and AE workout. To minimize initial muscle soreness, volume and intensity were progressively increased during the first three workouts until five sets to volitional muscle failure were performed. The KE and AE went through approximately 1.54 (range 3.15–1.62) and 0.95 (range 1.19–2.13) radians of coupled flexion and extension per repetition, respectively. The training load for each set was designed to elicit failure after 8 repetitions (8 RM). If a set did not meet the 8 RM requirement, the weight for the subsequent set was adjusted accordingly. Subjects were instructed to perform the concentric and eccentric phases of each repetition in a slow controlled manner. Rest between sets was limited to 90 s. A certified strength and conditioning specialist (National Strength and Conditioning Association) supervised all training.

# Three-Dimensional Topographic Maps

Three-dimensional topographical (surface) maps provide an in-depth representation of KE and AE performance by treatment group and time. Angle, velocity, and torque are illustrated on the x, y, and z axes, respectively. Figures are composite maps of the six subjects per treatment (BR, BR+EX) group. Pre-bed rest KE and AE topographical maps for the BR and BR+EX groups are shown in figures 21.1 to 21.4. Post-bed rest KE and AE topographical maps for the BR and BR+EX groups are illustrated in figures 21.5 to 21.8. In addition, pre- to post-bed rest KE and AE topographical maps, representing significant torque losses by angle and velocity per group, are shown in figures 21.9 to 21.12. The magnitude of strength loss by treatment condition across each angle and velocity is shown on the z axes of figures 21.9 to 21.12. For instance, figure 21.9 illustrates significant KE torque decrements per angle and velocity between figures 21.1 (pre-BR KE) and 21.5 (post-BR KE). Figure 21.10 (BR+EX KE) represents significant KE torque decrements per angle and velocity between figures 21.2 and 21.6. Figures 21.11 and 21.12, illustrating pre- and post-bed rest AE torque changes per treatment condition, represent similar changes between figures 21.4 and 21.7 (BR) and 21.5 and 21.8 (BR+EX). Map portions of figures 21.9 to 21.12 illustrating no torque (z-axis)

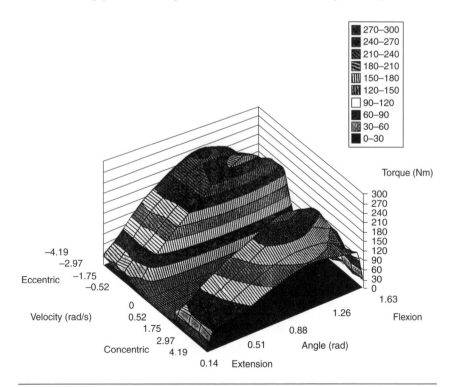

**Figure 21.1**   Pre-bed rest topographical KE map (BR group).

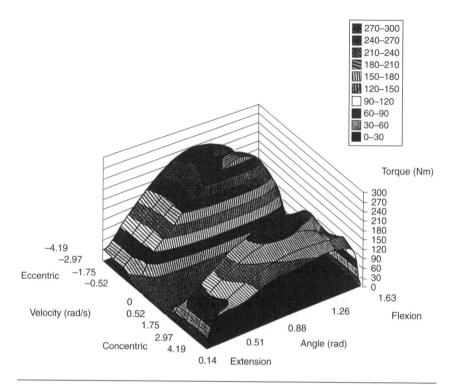

**Figure 21.2**  Pre-bed rest topographical KE map (BR+EX group).

represent nonsignificant strength changes at the corresponding angles and velocities.

Data were analyzed for pre- to post-bed rest differences per treatment assignment. KE and AE data were each treated using a $2 \times 2$ repeated measures ANOVA and Dunnett's a priori contrasts for multiple pairwise comparisons. Significance was established at the .05 level.

The range of motion for KE and AE test repetitions approximated 1.50 and 0.95 radians, respectively. To minimize error, each range of motion was broken down into 10 (KE) and 6 (AE) discrete segments, with average values determined for each velocity and contractile mode. In the presence of an interaction, range of motion segments were compared via a priori contrasts to their corresponding treatment group assignment. Figures 21.9 to 21.12 represent significant pre- to post-bed rest torque decrements by angle and velocity obtained through a priori contrasts.

Pre-bed rest maps for each group (see figures 21.1–21.4) appear similar with respect to the x, y, and z axes. Using the $2 \times 2$ repeated measures ANOVA, group by time interactions occurred for the KE and AE ($p < .05$). At posttesting, significantly fewer range of motion segments noted strength losses in the BR+EX group for both the KE and AE. This points to the efficacy of resistance training as a countermeasure to strength loss during simulated weightless-

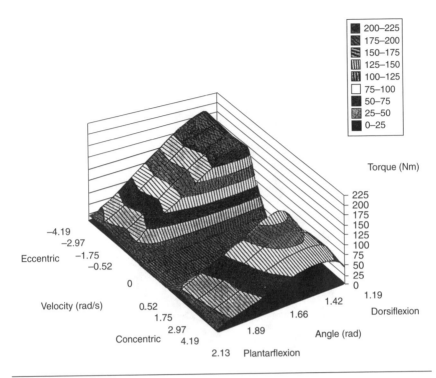

**Figure 21.3** Pre-bed rest topographical AE map (BR group).

ness. Range of motion segments undergoing significant strength losses resulting from simulated weightlessness for each group are illustrated on the z axes of figures 21.9 to 21.12. In addition, this data appears in tabular form in tables 21.2 to 21.5. Significant KE strength losses for the BR and BR+EX groups are shown in tables 21.2 and 21.3, respectively. Significant AE strength losses are shown in table 21.4 (BR group) and table 21.5 (BR+EX).

The KE data for the BR group shows strength maintenance only at the most extended angles at posttesting. In contrast, the BR+EX group shows concentric KE losses only at the slowest (0.52 rad/s) velocity examined. However, eccentric KE losses for the BR+EX group appear to be like those for the BR group. Significant concentric AE torque losses for the BR group occurred during ankle extension at the slowest (0.52 rad/s) velocity examined. Eccentric AE losses for the BR group display significant (at 0.52, 2.97, and 4.19 rad/s) torque losses through a greater range of motion, particularly as the ankle assumed a more flexed posture. The BR+EX group noted significant AE concentric torque losses only during full extension at 2.97 rad/s. No significant eccentric AE losses occurred to the BR+EX group.

Study figures illustrate KE and AE performance, with and without an exercise countermeasure, for specific angles and velocities following a 14-day bed rest. The BR+EX group simulates weightlessness while allowing us to examine

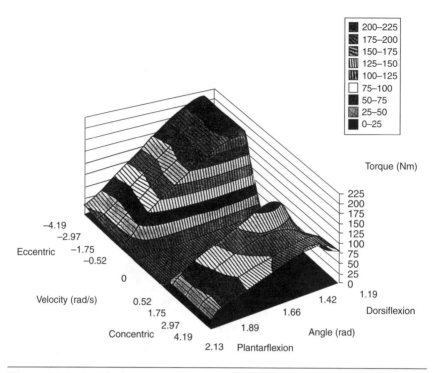

**Figure 21.4** Pre-bed rest topographical AE map (BR+EX group).

**Table 21.2 Significant Range of Motion Segments (in Radians) of KE Torque Loss for BR Subjects**

|            | 0.52 rad/s | 1.75 rad/s | 2.97 rad/s  | 4.19 rad/s  |
|------------|------------|------------|-------------|-------------|
| Concentric | 1.63–.44   | 1.63–.74   | 1.63–1.19   | 1.63–1.49   |
|            |            |            | .73–.44     |             |
| Eccentric  | 1.63–.44   | 1.63–.44   | 1.63–.44    | 1.63–.74    |

**Table 21.3 Significant Range of Motion Segments (in Radians) of KE Torque Loss for BR+EX Subjects**

|            | 0.52 rad/s | 1.75 rad/s | 2.97 rad/s | 4.19 rad/s |
|------------|------------|------------|------------|------------|
| Concentric | 1.48–.59   |            |            |            |
| Eccentric  | 1.48–.29   | 1.48–.29   | 1.48–.59   | 1.48–.43   |

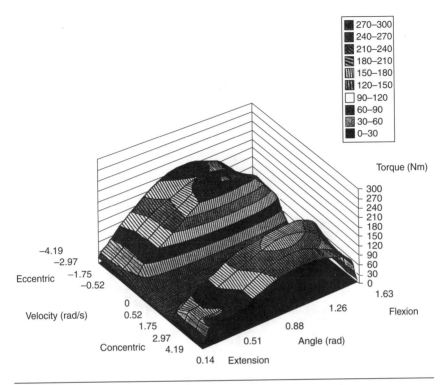

**Figure 21.5** Post-bed rest topographical KE map (BR group).

**Table 21.4 Significant Range of Motion Segments (in Radians) of AE Torque Loss for BR Subjects**

|            | 0.52 rad/s | 1.75 rad/s | 2.97 rad/s | 4.19 rad/s |
|------------|------------|------------|------------|------------|
| Concentric | 1.52–1.66  |            |            |            |
| Eccentric  | 1.19–1.66  |            | 1.19–1.50  | 1.19–1.50  |

**Table 21.5 Significant Range of Motion Segments (in Radians) of AE Torque Loss for BR+EX Subjects**

|            | 0.52 rad/s | 1.75 rad/s | 2.97 rad/s | 4.19 rad/s |
|------------|------------|------------|------------|------------|
| Concentric |            |            | 1.19–1.34  |            |
| Eccentric  |            |            |            |            |

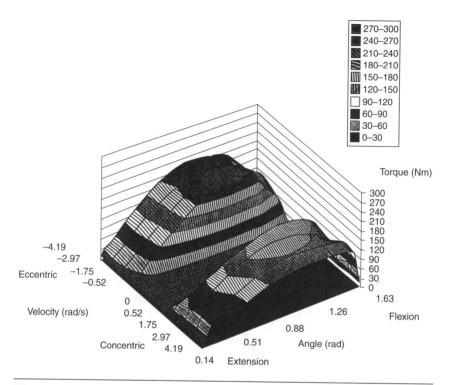

**Figure 21.6** Post-bed rest topographical KE map (BR+EX group).

constant load training as a countermeasure to strength loss. The KE and AE data show less strength loss to the BR+EX group at posttesting, helping to validate resistance training as a countermeasure to weightlessness. Three-dimensional topography illustrates isokinetic strength changes and graphically displays the efficacy of the countermeasure. Torque deficits in figures 21.9 to 21.12 were generally greater eccentrically than concentrically. However, when losses are expressed on a percentage basis, little difference is shown among contractile modes and velocities. A prior discussion emphasizes the importance of eccentric loading during unweighting (28). Also, the KE and AE exhibited significant losses while testing at extended muscle lengths regardless of group assignment.

All losses exhibited (see figures 21.9–21.12) may impair in-flight operational effectiveness, compromising astronaut health and safety (17). Angle-specific (0.78 rad) torque following 16 days of unloading showed a 12% loss to the KE (1). Present results obtained at a similar angle note slightly greater posttest losses (see figures 21.5 and 21.6). Longer unloading periods result in greater angle-specific torque (18–21%) losses (5, 12). Concentric AE losses, measured at a single velocity (1.04 rad/s), averaged 26% after a 5-week bed rest (15).

In the present study, in the BR group significant KE concentric and eccentric strength losses across all angles and velocities averaged 24% and 26%,

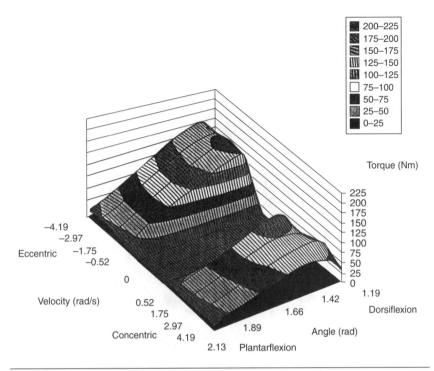

**Figure 21.7**   Post-bed rest topographical AE map (BR group).

respectively. Both contractile modes demonstrated losses exceeding 18 to 21% in the current study, particularly with the knee at flexed angles (> 0.78 rad). Concentric and eccentric AE losses (see figure 21.11) in the current study averaged 18% and 20%, respectively, across the examined angles and velocities, demonstrating significant strength loss. In the present study subjects kept their knees and ankles extended during bed rest, which shortened muscle lengths. Astronauts are in a similar posture during weightlessness. Greater rates of muscle atrophy occur at shortened muscle lengths (21, 26, 29). Strength loss, due to muscle shortening and atrophy, results from unloading (5). Shortened muscle lengths during bed rest may account for significant torque losses as the KE and AE are lengthened. Presumably, KE and AE would be unfamiliar exerting torque at stretched lengths following an extended period of muscle shortening and unloading. The greater strength loss at flexed knee and ankle angles may also be a function of a more optimal angle of pull. Thus angle-specific torque examinations may underestimate strength losses incurred throughout an entire range of motion (1, 5, 11, 12).

Percentage torque losses following four to five weeks of simulated weightlessness varied very little (5), if at all (11), by velocity or contractile mode. While absolute losses are greater eccentrically (see figures 21.9–21.12), present results expressed as a percentage agree with prior findings (5, 12). The present

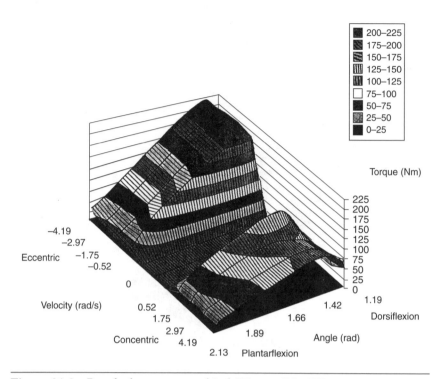

**Figure 21.8** Post-bed rest topographical AE map (BR+EX group).

study illustrates absolute concentric losses as treatment dependent, with group assignment impacting the range over which losses were observed (see figures 21.9–21.12). Figures 21.9 and 21.11, representing the angles and velocities of bed rest strength decrements and the magnitude (z axis) of torque loss, illustrate the impact of unloading on strength. Figure 21.9 shows an inverse relationship between concentric velocity and the area of significant strength loss. Comparing concentric portions among groups (see figures 21.9–21.12) illustrates constant load training's impact on KE and AE strength preservation. The BR+EX group (see figures 21.10 and 21.12) shows fewer areas of significant concentric strength loss per velocity, showing the countermeasure's effect. Unloading's impact on eccentric strength (see figures 21.9–21.12) does not appear treatment dependent, suggesting that constant load training had limited success at reducing eccentric strength loss.

Constant load training is regularly performed at a velocity approximating 1.04 rad/s (personal communication). Results for the BR+EX group (see figure 21.6) showing no significant concentric losses at moderate to high velocities (1.75–4.19 rad/s) suggest that training eliminated losses at higher speeds. Repetitive constant load concentric actions involve increasing motor unit recruitment per repetition to muscular failure (22). Maximal tension is greater as muscle lengthens. Conventional constant load resistance training involves

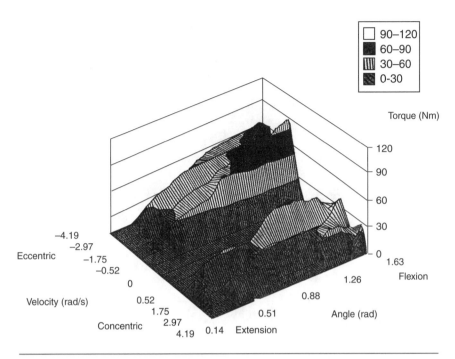

**Figure 21.9** Pre- to post-bed rest losses in KE torque (BR group).

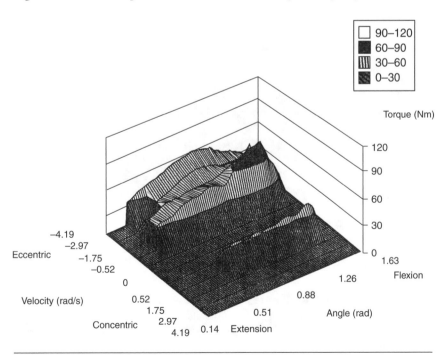

**Figure 21.10** Pre- to post-bed rest losses in KE torque (BR+EX group).

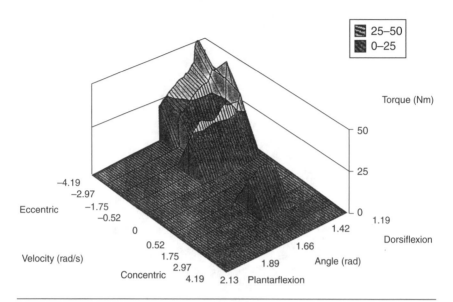

**Figure 21.11**    Pre- to post-bed rest losses in AE torque (BR group).

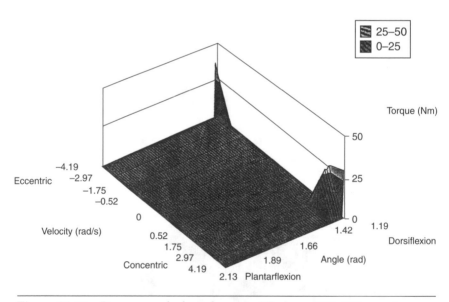

**Figure 21.12**    Pre- to post-bed rest losses in AE torque (BR+EX group).

submaximal eccentric loading (13, 18, 22). Greater tension is produced as muscles lengthen, stimulating neuromuscular adaptations for strength gain with eccentric actions (13, 22). The knee and ankle extensors perform eccentric actions to properly decelerate the body during locomotion, such as astronauts would require during emergency egress (29). Submaximal eccentrics have produced 1-g strength gains (19, 20, 27), however during bed rest such training appears insufficient at maintaining eccentric strength. Such effects may result from the unweighting-induced omission of lengthening actions for postural maintenance. Concentric and eccentric strength deficits (see figures 21.9–21.12) suggest requirements that need to be addressed through exercise countermeasures. Conventional constant load resistance exercise reduced concentric strength losses. However, eccentric losses still must be addressed through exercise countermeasures.

# Summary

Three-dimensional topography and isokinetic testing illustrate conventional constant load training's ability to reduce KE and AE strength losses incurred during simulated weightlessness. Thus it appears that free weight training eliminated some of the unloading-induced strength losses incurred during bed rest, particularly for the AE. Also, by combining isokinetic testing with three-dimensional topography, a broader understanding of strength performance resulting from unweighting in each treatment condition is established. Strength losses at flexed knee and ankle angles should be addressed through continued development of exercise countermeasures. Pre- to post-bed rest group differences (see figures 21.9–21.12) suggest that high-tension lengthening actions should be considered to minimize eccentric strength loss. Since conventional constant load devices do not offer sufficient eccentric loading, equipment with a high-tension eccentric component would be preferable. Isokinetic dynamometers offer high-tension eccentric loading and may operate in gravity-free environments. Thus isokinetic dynamometers may be preferable to conventional constant load equipment during space flight. To ensure successful in-flight performance and to hasten 1-g readaptation, pre- and postflight resistance training, involving concentric and eccentric contractions, may serve as an appropriate countermeasure to strength loss. The eccentric tension employed should be greater than that associated with conventional constant load training.

# References

1. Adams, G.R., B.M. Hather, and G.A. Dudley. 1994. Effect of short-term unweighting on human skeletal muscle strength and size. *Aviat. Space Environ. Med.* 65: 1116–21.

2. Atha, J. 1981. Strengthening muscle. *Exerc. Sport Sci. Rev.* 9: 1–78.

3. Bamman, M.M., M.S.F. Clarke, D.L. Feeback, R.J. Talmadge, B.R. Stevens, S.A. Lieberman, and M.C. Greenisen. 1998. Impact of resistance exercise during bed rest on skeletal muscle sarcopenia and myosin isoform distribution. *J. Appl. Physiol.* 84(1): 157–63.

4. Bamman, M.M., G.R. Hunter, B.R. Stevens, M.E. Guilliams, and M.C. Greenisen. 1997. Resistance exercise prevents plantar flexor deconditioning during bed rest. *Med. Sci. Sports Exerc.* 29(11): 1462–68.

5. Berg, H.E., G.A. Dudley, T. Haggmark, H. Ohlsen, and P.A. Tesch. 1991. Effects of lower limb unloading on skeletal muscle mass and function in humans. *J. Appl. Phys.* 70(4): 1882–85.

6. Berg, H.E., and P.A. Tesch. 1992. Designing methods for musculoskeletal conditioning in weightlessness. *The Physiologist* 35 (1Suppl.): S96-S98.

7. Buchanan, P., and V.A. Convertino. 1989. A study of the effects of prolonged simulated microgravity on the musculature of the lower extremities in man: An introduction. *Aviat. Space Environ. Med.* 60: 649–52.

8. Caruso, J.F., J.F. Signorile, A.C. Perry, B. LeBlanc, R. Williams, M. Clark, and M.M. Bamman. 1995. The effects of albuterol and isokinetic exercise on the quadriceps muscle group. *Med. Sci. Sports Exerc.* 27(11): 1471–76.

9. Colliander, E.B., and P.A. Tesch. 1990. Effects of eccentric and concentric muscle actions in resistance training. *Acta Physiol. Scand.* 140: 31–39.

10. Convertino, V.A. 1990. Physiological adaptation to weightlessness: Effects on exercise and work performance. *Exerc. Sports Sci. Rev.* 18: 119–66.

11. Dudley, G.A., M.R. Duvosin, G.R. Adams, R.A. Meyer, A.H. Belew, and P. Buchanan. 1992. Adaptations to unilateral lower limb suspension in humans. *Aviat. Space Environ. Med.* 63: 678–83.

12. Dudley, G.A., M.R. Duvosin, V.A. Convertino, and P. Buchanan. 1989. Alterations of the in vivo torque-velocity relationship of human skeletal muscle following 30 days exposure to simulated microgravity. *Aviat. Space Environ. Med.* 60: 659–63.

13. Dudley, G.A., P.A. Tesch, B.J. Miller, and P. Buchanan. 1991. Importance of eccentric actions in performance adaptations to resistance training. *Aviat. Space Environ. Med.* 62: 543–50.

14. Friman, G., and E. Hamrin. 1976. Changes of reactive hyperanemia after clinical bed rest for seven days. *Ups. J. Med. Sci.* 81(2): 79–83.

15. Gogia, P.P., V.S. Schneider, A.D. Le Blanc, J. Krebs, C. Kasson, and C. Pientok. 1988. Bed rest effect on extremity muscle torque in healthy men. *Arch. Phys. Med. Rehabil.* 69: 1030–32.

16. Greenleaf, J.E., R. Bulbulian, E.M. Bernauer, W.L. Haskell, and T. Moore. 1989. Exercise training protocols for astronauts in microgravity. *J. Appl. Physiol.* 67(6): 2191–204.

17. Hayes, J.C., M.L. Roper, A.D. Mazzocca, J.J. McBrine, L.H. Barrows, B.H. Harris, and S.F. Siconolfi. February 1992. Eccentric and concentric muscle performance following seven days of simulated weightlessness. *NASA Technical Paper 3182.*

18. Hortobayagi, T., and F.I. Katch. 1990. Role of concentric force in limiting improvement in muscular strength. *J. Appl. Phys.* 68(2): 650–58.

19. Johnson, B.L., J.W. Adamczyk, K.O. Tennoe, and S.B. Stromme. 1976. A comparison of concentric and eccentric muscle training. *Med. Sci. Sports Exerc.* 8: 35–38.

20. Jones, D.A., and O.M. Rutherford. 1987. Human muscle strength training: The nature of three different regimes and the nature of the resultant changes. *J. Physiol.* 391: 1–11.

21. Knowlton, G.C., and H.M. Hines. 1939. The effects of growth and atrophy upon the strength of skeletal muscle. *Am. J. Physiol.* 128: 521–25.

22. Komi, P.V., and J.T. Viitasalo. 1977. Changes in motor unit activity and metabolism in human skeletal muscle during and after repeated eccentric and concentric contractions. *Acta Physiol. Scand.* 100: 246–54.

23. Koryak, Y. 1995. Contractile properties of the human triceps surae muscle during simulated weightlessness. *Eur. J. Appl. Phys.* 70: 344–50.

24. LeBlanc, A., P. Gogia, V. Schneider, J. Krebs, E. Schonfeld, H. Evans. 1988. Calf muscle area and strength changes after five weeks of horizontal bed rest. *Am. J. Sports Med.* 16(6): 624–29.

25. LeBlanc, A.D., V.S. Schneider, H.J. Evans, C. Pientok, R. Rowe, and E. Spector. 1992. Regional changes in muscle mass following 17 weeks of bed rest. *J. Appl. Phys.* 73(5): 2172–78.

26. Lippmann, R.K., and S. Selig. 1928. An experimental study of muscle atrophy. *Surg. Gynecol. Obstet.* 47: 512–22.

27. Seliger, V., L. Dolejs, V. Karas, and I. Pachlopnikova. 1968. Adaptation of trained athletes' energy expenditure to repeated concentric and eccentric muscle contractions. *Int. Z. Angew Physiol. Einschl. Arbeitsphysiol.* 26: 227–34.

28. Stauber, W.T. 1986. A unique problem of muscle adaptation from weightlessness: The deceleration deficiency. Workshop on exercise prescription for long-duration space flight. *NASA Conference Publication 3051.*

29. Thomsen, P., and J.V. Luco. 1944. Changes in weight and neuromuscular transmission in muscles of immobilized joints. *J. Neurophysiol.* 7: 246–51.

30. Thornton, W.E., and J.A. Rummel. 1977. Muscular deconditioning and its prevention during space flight. *Biomedical results from Skylab* 191–97.

# Epilogue

Upon final analysis the reader is left to decide on the efficacy of many of the concepts and procedures laid out in this book. If there appears to be controversy between two chapters and authors then it should be explained that that is the nature of science. It is the essence of inferential investigation that a conclusion is sometimes drawn in one laboratory that does not exactly coincide with that drawn in another laboratory. That is how science and technology grow and evolve. It is the constant examination of data and the performance of validity studies based on the work of others that ultimately solves problems and answers questions. The critical reader of this text will not see obstacles to understanding but rather opportunities for future research.

Much of the material included in this book should be considered fundamental to research involving isokinetic dynamometry. The authors have made every attempt to include elements of relevant research that shed light on a constant search by practitioners to enhance the performance of their clients. The preceding chapters have presented, in technical nature, a model for test interpretation within the framework of specificity of testing and training while keeping focus on how one technology correlates with athletic performance. We have made no effort to hide the shortcomings of isokinetics or portray it as a panacea for the ills that plague the laboratory and field technician alike. Rather, we present an open view of how this technology device fits among the comprehensive tools utilized in the field of exercise science.

A framework has been built around grand protocols and far-reaching general subject matter in order to draw conclusions about specific populations. This work in no way strives to be the last word on isokinetic dynamometry or the use thereof. Instead, it strives to lay bare the heart of published research and point out ways in which the user may enhance both the validity and reliability of his or her exercise outcomes. In other words this book was written to encourage thought-provoking discussion, which hopefully will culminate in cutting edge research that contributes to the knowledge base of isokinetics.

# Index

The letters *f* and *t* after locators indicate figures and tables, respectively.

# About the Editor

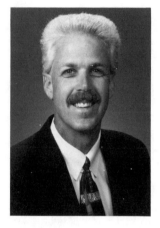

Prior to assuming his current position as Department of Health Sciences Laboratory coordinator at Florida Atlantic University, Lee E. Brown, MEd, CSCS, *D, began his career in teaching, coaching, consulting, and directing research and rehabilitation services in 1984. Since 1990, he has conducted isokinetic research.

Coauthor of numerous professional journal articles and abstracts and a frequent presenter at conferences in the United States, Germany, and the Netherlands Antilles, Brown has also coedited two other texts.

In addition, he is on the board of directors of the National Strength and Conditioning Association (NSCA) and a member of the American College of Sports Medicine (ACSM).

Currently a doctoral candidate in educational leadership at Florida Atlantic University, Brown attained his MEd in exercise science from Florida Atlantic University.

Brown resides in Coconut Creek, Florida with his wife Theresa. In his leisure time he enjoys trapshooting, running, and cycling.

# Other Books From Human Kinetics

## Periodization
## Theory and Methodology of Training
**(Fourth Edition)**

Tudor O. Bompa, PhD

1999 • Paperback • 424 pp

ISBN 0-88011-851-2 • $33.00 ($49.50 Canadian)

*Periodization: Theory and Methodology of Training* presents Tudor Bompa's latest refinements to the theory he developed. Formerly titled *Theory and Methodology of Training*, this long-standing classic has been translated into nine languages and has come to be regarded as the definitive reference on training theory. Now in its fourth edition, it's even better organized, easier to read, and more up-to-date than before.

## Designing Resistance Training Programs
**(Second Edition)**

Steven J. Fleck, PhD, and William J. Kraemer, PhD

1997 • Hardback • 288 pp

ISBN 0-87322-508-2 • $42.00 ($62.95 Canadian)

Written by two of the world's leading experts on strength training, this second edition of the most widely read professional text on the topic has been completely revised, updated, and expanded. The result is a state-of-the-art guide to developing individualized training programs for both athletes and fitness enthusiasts. This book is also an excellent undergraduate textbook for courses in resistance training prescription.

## Facilitated Stretching
**(Second Edition)**

Robert E. McAtee

1999 • Spiral • 152 pp

ISBN 0-7360-0066-6 • $16.95 ($24.95 Canadian)

When *Facilitated Stretching* was published in 1993, it was the first book to present "PNF" stretching in an easy, illustrated format for athletes, coaches, and fitness professionals. Now, the fully updated and expanded edition of *Facilitated Stretching* is even more user-friendly, with a greater emphasis on effective self-stretching that makes PNF techniques accessible for everyone.

To request more information or to order, U.S. customers call 1-800-747-4457, e-mail us at humank@hkusa.com, or visit our website at www.humankinetics.com. Persons outside the U.S. can contact us via our website or use the appropriate telephone number, postal address, or e-mail address shown in the front of this book.

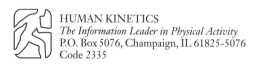

HUMAN KINETICS
*The Information Leader in Physical Activity*
P.O. Box 5076, Champaign, IL 61825-5076
Code 2335

## DATE DUE